Design, Development, and Deployment of Cutting-Edge Medical Devices

Ricardo Pateiro Marcão
ISLA Santarém, Portugal

Stéphanie Coelho Monteiro
Institute for Systems and Robotics, Portugal

IGI Global
Scientific Publishing
Publishing Tomorrow's Research Today

Vice President of Editorial Melissa Wagner
Managing Editor of Acquisitions Mikaela Felty
Managing Editor of Book Development Jocelynn Hessler
Production Manager Mike Brehm
Cover Design Phillip Shickler

Published in the United States of America by
IGI Global Scientific Publishing
701 East Chocolate Avenue
Hershey, PA, 17033, USA
Tel: 717-533-8845
Fax: 717-533-8661
Website: https://www.igi-global.com E-mail: cust@igi-global.com

Library of Congress Cataloging-in-Publication Data

Names: Marcao, Ricardo, 1987- editor
Title: Design, development, and deployment of cutting-edge medical devices / edited by Ricardo Marcao, Stéphanie Monteiro.
Description: Hershey, PA : IGI Global Scientific Publishing, [2025] | Includes bibliographical references and index. | Summary: "The primary objective of the book is to provide a thorough and multifaceted exploration of the entire lifecycle of advanced medical devices, from conceptual design to real-world deployment"-- Provided by publisher.
Identifiers: LCCN 2024055619 (print) | LCCN 2024055620 (ebook) | ISBN 9798369385982 h/c | ISBN 9798369385999 s/c | ISBN 9798369386002 eISBN
Subjects: LCSH: Medical instruments and apparatus--Design and construction | Medical instruments and apparatus--Technological innovations
Classification: LCC RA418.5.M4 D47 2025 (print) | LCC RA418.5.M4 (ebook) | DDC 610.28/4--dc23/eng/20250408
LC record available at https://lccn.loc.gov/2024055619
LC ebook record available at https://lccn.loc.gov/2024055620

British Cataloguing in Publication Data
A Cataloguing in Publication record for this book is available from the British Library.

Table of Contents

Detailed Table of Contents

As technology reshapes industries, gamification has emerged as a key strategy, using game design elements in non-game settings to boost motivation and collaboration, especially in healthcare. This study examines gamification's role in enhancing teamwork among healthcare professionals, addressing a gap in existing research. A quantitative survey of 164 employees from organizations using gamified systems was analyzed through multiple linear regression. Results show that game elements, such as dynamics and mechanics, positively impact collaboration, trust, and engagement. Dynamics foster a collaborative environment and positive social interactions, while mechanics involving collaborative challenges and rewards strengthen team cohesion. This study highlights gamification as an effective tool for improving internal collaboration in healthcare, offering practical insights for organizations implementing such systems. Findings reinforce the importance of gamification in creating trust-based cultures, boosting performance, and enhancing satisfaction for both professionals and patients.

The research was conducted with the aim of determining whether Green Marketing can be considered a competitive advantage in the cosmetics sector. Given the increase in environmental awareness and the growing demand for sustainable products, understanding the impact of Green Marketing is essential for companies seeking to differentiate themselves in the market and attract conscious consumers. The main objective of the research was to evaluate the effectiveness of Green Marketing in providing a competitive advantage, analyzing both the practices of companies and the perception of consumers. To this end, the research used a qualitative approach that included interviews with representatives of cosmetics companies and focus groups with consumers. The research underlines the importance of addressing challenges such as cost and lack of awareness to promote more sustainable consumption and broaden the acceptance of eco-friendly products.

Electroencephalography (EEG)-based Brain-Computer Interface (BCI) technology has appeared as a promising path for healthcare, contributing to novel solutions for detecting, treating, and dealing with neurological conditions. By capturing and construing the electrical activities of brain signals, EEG-based BCIs empower direct brain communication with external devices, circumventing traditional neural conduits. This chapter delves into the progress of EEG-based BCI devices, emphasizing their implication in healthcare, the technical challenges tangled, and their potential to transform patient care. The key objective is to deliver a detailed exploration of the development procedure of EEG-based BCI devices, emphasizing their applications in healthcare. The chapter includes the principles of EEG signal acquisition, the design and engineering of BCI systems, the employment of machine learning algorithms for signal decoding, and the clinical validation required for medical use. Moreover, it will discuss the prospective effect of these devices on healthcare and future research directions.

This chapter provides a detailed exploration of effective leadership practices and performance assessment strategies critical to managing remote healthcare teams in the digital health era. It begins by analyzing leadership styles, such as transformational, servant, and transactional leadership, and how these can address unique challenges in virtual environments, such as communication gaps, security, and system integration. Through a review of various assessment frameworks and methods, the chapter highlights tools and metrics suited to evaluate remote healthcare team performance effectively. Real-world case studies from renowned institutions, including Cleveland Clinic, Mayo Clinic, and UCSF, showcase the successful deployment of leadership

Foreword

In the rapidly evolving field of medical device innovation, the interplay between advanced technologies and healthcare outcomes defines the trajectory of modern medicine. This publication, "Design, Development, and Deployment of Cutting-Edge Medical Devices," offers a comprehensive exploration of this transformative domain, addressing key challenges and opportunities with exceptional depth and clarity.

The significance of this book lies in its ability to bridge the gap between technical innovation and its practical application in global healthcare systems. By examining topics such as advanced diagnostic tools, therapeutic devices, and the integration of artificial intelligence, robotics, and telemedicine, this book provides a roadmap for navigating the complexities of medical device design and deployment. Its focus on sustainability, user-centered design, and global challenges further underscores its relevance in today's healthcare landscape.

What sets this work apart is its interdisciplinary approach, bringing together insights from leading researchers, clinicians, and industry experts. Each chapter reflects a commitment to excellence, offering both theoretical frameworks and practical case studies that illustrate the real-world impact of these innovations. The editors, Ricardo Pateiro Marcão, PhD, MBA, PMP®, and Stéphanie Monteiro, have curated a remarkable collection of contributions that not only push the boundaries of medical technology but also address the ethical, regulatory, and human-centered dimensions that underpin its success.

Having reviewed the table of contents and abstracts, I am deeply impressed by the breadth and depth of the topics covered. This book goes beyond technical exploration, delving into critical aspects such as clinical validation, regulatory frameworks, and the challenges of global deployment. It serves as a vital resource for researchers, practitioners, and policymakers seeking to understand and shape the future of medical devices.

I am confident that this publication will inspire innovation and collaboration across disciplines, fostering new ideas and solutions that will ultimately improve patient care worldwide. It is an invaluable addition to the literature, providing a platform for meaningful dialogue and forward-thinking strategies in medical device development.

I strongly recommend this book to anyone interested in advancing the field of medical devices. It is a pioneering work that will leave a lasting impact on the industry and beyond.

Vasco Ribeiro Santos
Polytechnic Institute of Tomar, Portugal & ISLA Santarém, Portugal & GOVCOPP, Portugal & CITUR, Portugal

Preface

In an era defined by rapid technological advancements and an ever-increasing demand for innovative healthcare solutions, the development and deployment of cutting-edge medical devices stand at the forefront of global healthcare transformation. This book, "Design, Development, and Deployment of Cutting-Edge Medical Devices", represents a collaborative effort to explore the dynamic intersection of biomedical engineering, healthcare delivery, and patient-centered innovation.

The journey to this publication has been both inspiring and illuminating. This book is a testament to the remarkable contributions of researchers, engineers, clinicians, and industry experts from across the globe who responded to our call for chapters with unparalleled enthusiasm and expertise. Together, we have sought to create a resource that not only highlights the state-of-the-art in medical device innovation but also addresses the practical challenges of bringing these technologies from concept to clinical practice.

The chapters in this book delve into diverse topics, including principles of biomedical engineering, technological breakthroughs like AI and robotics, regulatory landscapes, and the critical importance of user-centered design. Each contribution reflects a commitment to excellence and a shared vision of improving healthcare outcomes through technological advancement. Beyond technical insights, the book also engages with broader themes such as sustainability, ethical considerations, and the collaborative efforts required for global deployment.

We extend our deepest gratitude to all the authors for their rigorous research and thoughtful perspectives. We also thank the reviewers and editorial team for their invaluable feedback and meticulous attention to detail. Finally, we acknowledge the patients, practitioners, and visionaries who inspire us to push the boundaries of innovation.

It is our hope that this book will serve as a catalyst for further exploration, fostering collaboration across disciplines and encouraging new ideas that will shape the future of healthcare. Whether you are a researcher, a medical professional, or an industry leader, we invite you to engage with these chapters and join us in this exciting journey of discovery and transformation.

Let us continue to innovate, collaborate, and improve lives.

Ricardo Pateiro Marcão
ISLA Santarém, Portugal

Stéphanie Coelho Monteiro
Institute for Systems and Robotics, Portugal

Acknowledgment

We would like to express our deepest gratitude to all those who contributed to the creation and success of this book, **"Design, Development, and Deployment of Cutting-Edge Medical Devices."**

First and foremost, we extend our heartfelt thanks to our families, whose unwavering support and encouragement have been our greatest source of strength throughout this journey. To our parents – namely Mrs. Maria do Rosário Pinto Coelho, Mr. Adão Monteiro Mendes, Dr. Maria de Fátima Caldeira Pateiro Marcão, and Dr. Guilherme Morais da Costa Marcão – thank you for your love, guidance, and unwavering belief in us. To our siblings, Dr. Cindy Coelho Monteiro and Dr. Eduardo Abel Pateiro Marcão, your encouragement and understanding allowed us to dedicate the time and energy required for this project.

We owe a profound debt of gratitude to Dr. Patrícia Correia David, whose unparalleled expertise in the pharma and medtech world has been instrumental in shaping our journey. From the very beginning, she provided invaluable guidance, inspiring us to navigate this intricate field with confidence and purpose. Her mentorship, unwavering support, and contributions, including co-authoring one of the chapters in this book, have been nothing short of transformative. This work would not have been possible without her insights, passion, and dedication.

We are also deeply grateful to the authors, reviewers, and collaborators who contributed their expertise and insights to this publication. Your dedication and commitment to advancing knowledge in the field of medical devices have made this book possible.

Finally, we acknowledge all the researchers, healthcare professionals, and industry experts whose work continues to inspire innovation and drive progress in the medical device field.

Thank you for being part of this endeavor.

Chapter 1
Financial Planning and Performance Evaluation:
A Comprehensive Study in Healthcare Organizations

Cláudia Trinca
ISLA Santarém, Portugal

Ricardo Marcão
https://orcid.org/0000-0003-3277-3078
ISLA Santarém, Portugal

ABSTRACT

This chapter explores the critical role of financial planning, highlighting core concepts, essential tools, challenges, and current trends. Effective financial planning serves as a decision-making framework, enabling management to prioritize goals and adapt strategies to internal and external dynamics. By creating budgets and consistently monitoring financial indicators, organizations can evaluate performance through metrics like profitability, liquidity, and operational efficiency. These tools identify areas requiring improvement and guide the implementation of corrective measures to achieve desired objectives. The chapter emphasizes that financial planning fosters transparency and accountability, vital for attracting investors and building trust among shareholders and stakeholders. It enables organizations to anticipate challenges, adapt to shifting market conditions, and reduce uncertainty, thereby enhancing resilience and strategic agility.

DOI: 10.4018/979-8-3693-8598-2.ch001

1. INTRODUCTION TO FINANCIAL PLANNING AND ORGANIZATIONAL PERFORMANCE ASSESSMENT

Financial management practices play a key role in the success and sustainability of companies in various sectors (Sugianto et al., 2024; Hadijah & Karmila, 2024; Ibrahim, 2024). Efficient financial management involves making the right investment choices, maximizing performance and implementing strategic approaches that fit the organizational environment. In recent years, researchers have shown a growing interest in exploring the complex aspects of financial management strategies to improve the performance and competitiveness of companies. This chapter develops an analysis of financial management strategies, focusing on performance, investment choices and strategic approaches, seeking to enrich existing knowledge in this field.

Financial management encompasses a broad set of activities designed to efficiently manage an organization's financial resources in order to achieve its goals. It involves planning, organizing, directing and controlling a company's financial operations.

Improving performance remains a central objective in financial management strategies and is constantly sought to strengthen operational effectiveness, increase productivity and improve profitability (Brigham & Ehrhardt, 2019).

Effective financial management is essential for boosting the performance of organizations in both the public and private sectors. This area involves various tasks, such as creating budgets, preparing financial reports and planning strategies, all with the aim of maximizing the use of available resources (Brigham & Ehrhardt, 2013). In the public context, financial management is often constrained by regulatory standards and budget limits that can reduce the flexibility and efficiency of the practices adopted (Modell, 2009). Public entities need to comply with strict requirements to ensure transparency and accountability, which can occasionally hinder the implementation of innovative financial solutions (Hood & Peters, 2004). On the other hand, private companies tend to have greater autonomy to adopt adjustable financial strategies that favor efficiency and increased profits (Jensen, 2001). These organizations are motivated by the quest to maximize shareholder returns, which often leads to the adoption of more agile and adaptable financial management practices (Fama & French, 2002).

The implementation of effective budgetary practices is essential to boosting the performance of organizations, ensuring an efficient use of resources and solid financial stability (Libby & Lindsay, 2010; Abernethy & Brownell, 1999; Horngren et al., 2013). In the context of the public sector, well-structured and flexible budgeting processes make it possible to optimize the use of scarce resources to achieve public service objectives. On the other hand, in the private sector, an adaptable budgeting approach facilitates agile responses to market changes (Libby & Lindsay, 2010). In this way, organizations that adopt robust budgetary practices have fewer financial variations and sounder financial health in general.

2. DEFINITION AND CONCEPTS OF FINANCIAL PLANNING

Financial management is a widely studied field Ortega (2008). According to Baca (2010), there are a variety of methods for evaluating investments in the business sector, which plays an essential role in any country's economy. The financial literature forms the fundamental basis for management, for drawing up formal planning and tackling complex problems, as well as making difficult decisions in companies, especially in volatile and segmented markets, it is essential to use analysis and evaluation tools based on proven and effective methodologies, such as the scientific method and to carry out these tasks efficiently, it is not enough to resort to simplistic approaches such as common sense, experience without critical reflection or prejudices, Baca (2010). The financial literature indicates that attention should be directed towards the management of company debt, with a view to optimizing its use and focusing on financial restructuring (Ortega, 2008). One of the management practices that has contributed to the increase in corporate financing is the use of debt, and good financial management reflects the company's operational efficiency, which sends a positive signal to investors and regulators (Ortega, 2008). According to Baca (2010), takeovers do not have a significant impact on the managers hired to make decisions in large listed companies, in terms of share valuation, contrary to some previous studies, which suggested that shareholders benefited financially from takeovers. According to Ortega (2008), when dealing with the planning and evaluation of investment projects, he stresses that one of the essential skills for a manager is knowledge of research methodology, i.e. the scientific method. So what is the relevance of this method in formal planning? Ortega (2008) argues that the rigorous application of the planning process is the starting point for all administrative activity. Planning involves making the right decisions about what actions to take in the future. According to Bak (2012), planning is crucial to the success of any economic activity. The author points out that uncertainty is present in all economic systems, so it is necessary to carefully analyze the impact of potential decisions on financial results. Bak (2012) also states that, in a free market system, planning means making rational decisions based on microeconomic criteria, representing a shift from material planning to a focus on financial planning.

Financial planning is considered an essential tool for companies to make informed decisions and achieve their financial goals. Without proper planning, it would be difficult, for example, to obtain credit from a bank, support the growth of a new company or improve the cash flows of an existing company. Mazzarol (2005) reviewed several studies on formal planning in small companies and points out that, although it is not possible to clearly prove the benefits of this type of planning for small companies, it is fundamental for large organizations and those with expansion objectives. In addition, he stresses that formal planning is indispensable for companies seeking state support or funding. Gansel (2005) points out that there is a positive link between planning and business success, citing various studies which show that financial planning is one of the most important tools in managing a company. According to Ortega (2008), financial strategy must be an integral part of the decision-making process of managers, and it is crucial that those involved in business administration know how to draw up good financial planning. With regard to formal planning in different dimensions, Mazzarol (2005) states that there is a relationship between the size of the company and the adoption of formal planning. The larger the company, the more likely it is to implement formal planning, as these organizations tend to employ qualified professionals with the necessary skills. In addition, he mentions the study by Unni (1984), which concludes that the majority of small companies do not adopt any type of formal business planning.

According to Nolan & Foran (1983), the main objective of strategic planning is to develop a support structure for decision-making, in order to optimize the distribution of capital resources and foresee possible contingencies. They argue that when the operating environment changes, management must face new options and make decisions that need to be evaluated taking into account the organization's objectives. On the other hand, Bak (2012) sees planning as a decision-making process in which a future vision for the company is defined and the methods for achieving it are established.

3. ORGANIZATIONAL PERFORMANCE AND ITS INDICATORS

In today's global competitive context, organizations need to be able to evaluate their objectives, such as cost per unit, profits, subjective performance (e.g. quality and satisfaction), and define appropriate strategies to achieve them. A business process consists of a set of activities carried out to achieve common goals, based on clearly defined business objectives (Hammer & Champy, 1994; Keung and Kawalek, 1997). These processes are fundamental to achieving organizational goals. Magretta and Stone (2002) pointed out that performance measurement and indicators are essential for turning an organization's mission or strategy into reality. Indicators and strategies are closely interlinked: without indicators, a strategy is useless, and without a strategy, indicators serve no purpose. Edwards and Thomas (2005) argued that Key Performance Indicators (KPIs) are sets of data used to measure and evaluate performance, representing a company's ultimate level of efficiency and effectiveness. According to Vucomanovic et al. (2010), KPIs are the basis for evaluating the success of businesses and projects.

KPIs (Key Performance Indicators) make it possible to measure performance in companies and industries, as well as facilitating benchmarking. They are also used as a means of communication between stakeholders, keeping them constantly informed about improvement efforts. Parmenter (2007) pointed out that KPIs must have certain characteristics, such as: being measurable, monitored frequently, relevant to the CEO (Chief Executive Officer) and the senior management team, understood by all employees, linking responsibility to individuals or teams, and having a significant and positive impact. McCrindell (1997), identified the best performance indicators in five dimensions: strategic objectives justifying the service's raison d'être and its objectives, costs/efficiency the resources allocated to the service and the efficiency in transforming the inputs, results of service provision the degree of success of the service in achieving the strategic objectives, quality reflecting the experience of users, fair access related to equity in access to the service.

Performance measurement in organizations is still heavily focused on financial data for control and coordination purposes (Atkinson & McCrindell, 1997; Atkinson et al., 1997). Several studies have investigated the effectiveness of balancing measures in performance evaluation systems (Bremser & Barsky, 2004; Sávioz & Blum, 2002). Establishing the link between performance, strategy and organizational purpose is a complex task. Given this complexity, many advocate the use of multiple perspectives and measures to assess organizational performance (Venkatraman & Ramanujam, 1986). The choice of relevant indicators influences the operation and direction of the organization. In addition, it is essential to define clear objectives, aligned with the strategy and accepted by those involved (Parmenter, 2007). Measuring and improving performance also depends on the appropriate selection of effective models and indicators (Meng & Minoque, 2011).

Sawang (2011) investigated the link between the perceived relevance and effective use of indicators, both financial and non-financial, that reflect innovation performance in small and medium-sized enterprises.

Organizations' financial indicators and their variability are relevant both to individuals who have a direct connection to the company (such as managers, owners and employees) and to those who are indirectly involved (such as cooperation partners, creditors and the press). The analysis and understanding of the role and importance of financial indicators, combined with the efficient resolution of management challenges, can be achieved by creating an integrated system for evaluating these indicators, within a broad context of analyzing organizational performance. Several researchers (Lau, Sholihin, 2005; Fernandes et al., 2006; Craig, Moores, 2005) have studied the holistic evaluation of corporate performance, which encompasses both financial and non-financial indicator systems. However, the practical implementation of these systems faces challenges, as there is no uniform methodology for identifying, classifying, measuring and evaluating financial and non-financial indicators.

Financial indicators are fundamental criteria in assessing business performance, Hopwood (1972) argues that financial metrics can encourage positive behavior on the part of subordinates, due to their objectivity and the low uncertainty associated with these measurements. Kaplan and Atkinson (1998) highlight two main reasons for the widespread use of financial performance indicators. Firstly, these metrics, such as profit, are directly linked to the long-term objectives of organizations, which are generally financial in nature. Secondly, financial indicators, when chosen correctly, offer a global view of a company's performance. An aggregate metric, such as the profitability of a company or a specific division, summarizes the success of the strategies and operations implemented.

Financial metrics are often seen as "retrospective" indicators, as they reflect the result of previous actions, with a predominantly quantitative focus (Cohen et al., 2008). Kaplan and Norton (2008) developed the balanced scorecard (BSC), which includes a set of financial indicators, and this method is widely used worldwide to assess the performance of organizations. For example, the application of the BSC to assess the performance of small and medium-sized enterprises has been analyzed in the UK context (Sousa et al., 2006), in the performance of manufacturing companies (Fernandes et al., 2006), in the tourism sector (Phipips and Louvieris, 2005) and in the strategic planning of family businesses (Craig and Moores, 2005).

Financial indicators are often expressed in the form of financial ratios. These ratios are a strategic management tool that offers key stakeholders a summarized and organized way of transforming the voluminous data in financial statements (such as balance sheets, income statements and cash flows) into useful information. Financial ratios represent a numerical or quantitative relationship between two elements or variables and can be presented as percentages or fractions (Suarez, et al., 2011). Although theoretically they are divided into 5 categories, in practice, especially in the case of small companies, 3 groups of ratios are used:

- Activity ratios measure the efficiency with which the company carries out its daily tasks, such as debt collection and stock management.
- Liquidity ratios assess the company's ability to meet its short-term obligations.
- Solvency ratios measure a company's ability to meet its long-term obligations.

In terms of non-financial indicators, Browne et al. (1997) observed that organizations adopt a variety of methods to analyse their performance, often segmenting the business into specific processes for this assessment. In general, each process receives its own performance indicators. Rolstadas (1998) pointed out that assessing organizational performance involves a complex interaction between factors such as effectiveness, efficiency, quality, productivity, work environment, innovation and profitability. To be successful, each organization needs to identify performance indicators and then establish measures and metrics that are strategically aligned with its particular reality (Leong et al., 1990; Mapes and Szwejczewski, 1997).

3.1 Quality

uality is fundamental to the success of any company. Today, customers expect high quality products, and companies that manage to offer such products at competitive costs gain prominence in the market. uality is assessed mainly on three fronts: the resources used, the end products and the production processes. Many companies prioritize quality, making a commitment to customer satisfaction with their products and services (Heckl and Moormann, 2010; Badri et al., 1994).

White (1996) identified eight dimensions for measuring quality: characteristics, reliability, conformity, durability, ease of maintenance, aesthetics and perceived quality. Among these, conformity is widely supported by empirical evidence related to quality. Gosselin (2005) discussed various ways of measuring quality, such as customer satisfaction, quality of resources and end products, costs associated with quality and the volume of complaints. De Toni and Tonchia (2001) addressed indicators such as machine reliability, rework, quality system costs, customer satisfaction, returns, quality of resources and end products, as well as the reliability of products and machines. Neely and Platts (2005) listed performance, characteristics, reliability, comfort, technical durability, ease of maintenance, aesthetics, perceived quality, human value and added value as elements for measuring quality.

3.2 Flexibility

Flexibility is understood as the ability of companies to perform multiple functions simultaneously, using various resources, such as labor and equipment, among others. Neely and Platts (2005) analyzed those factors such as the quality of materials, the quality of production, product innovation, modifications to existing products, delivery capacity, the adaptation of volumes and the variety of characteristics are effective indicators of flexibility. De Toni and Tonchia (2001), highlighted volume flexibility, product diversity, the ability to adapt to product changes, process modification and expansion as indicators of flexibility performance.

White (1996) addressed various aspects of flexibility, such as perceived flexibility compared to competitors, adaptability of processes compared to the market, perceived flexibility in products, speed of response to changes in the product mix, cycle and set-up times, time to replace tools and adaptation of accessories. Other indicators included the average increase in daily setups, perceived flexibility in volume, efficiency in carrying out multiple tasks, proportion of programmable equipment, equipment downtime, availability of manpower, use of pull systems, interruptions caused by failures and supplier lead times, all of which are essential for a flexibility strategy in production organizations.

3.3 Time

Time is a crucial element in the productive performance of organizations. Time-oriented production has become a central concern for companies in the sector, which are thus seeking to gain a competitive advantage over their competitors (Koufteros et al., 1998). De Toni and Tonchia (2001) identified manufacturing lead time, delivery time, compliance with deadlines, delivery frequency and the launch rate of new products as performance indicators associated with time.

Neely and Platts (2005) highlighted indicators such as time to introduce products to the market, distribution times, reliability of deliveries to customers, supply times, supplier reliability, production lead time, standard and actual lead times, waiting times, preparation, material handling, stock rotation, order fulfillment time and average flexibility time. White (1996) used metrics such as lead time, cycle time, the interval between receiving the customer's order and delivery, order processing time, response time, the percentage of punctuality for urgent orders, time for processing documentation and materials, distance traveled, decision-making time, percentage of entry into the market ahead of competitors, time to break even, time between design and arrival on the market, average time between innovations, number of changes to projects and engineering time as time metrics linked to strategy. White (1996) also defined speed as a measure of time in his research.

3.4 Security

In recent years, it has been noted that the reliability of complex work systems to achieve safety objectives in organizations depends on both the work structures and the arrangements put in place (Mearns et al., 2003). Parmenter (2009), in his book, pointed to the level of risk and perceived safety, the accident rate, the degree of collaboration between workers, the safety attitude of managers and employees, the level of exposure to physical risk in the workplace and the accessibility of safety information as the main safety indicators. In the UK, the main metrics for assessing safety performance include lost time due to accidents and the accident rate (Flin and O'Connor, 2000; Mearns et al., 2003).

3.5 Financial Performance

Historically, financial metrics have been the most effective for evaluating company performance, such as sales volume, profits or the rate of return on equity and assets. As external investors are very interested in this type of information, companies are encouraged to use financial indicators for their internal performance assessment (White, 1996). Various studies and organizations use different metrics to measure their financial performance. In this analysis, the financial measures suggested by Parmenter (2009), in his book The Main Performance Indicators (KPIs), were adopted. Among the measures used are the cost of goods sold in relation to sales, cost of waste as a percentage of total sales, accounts receivable turnover, cash flows, days in inventory, receipt period, net profit, sales volume, number of profitable customers, return on equity, sales per product, sales growth rate, return on assets and return on invested capital.

3.6 Cost

Cost-based performance metrics are of great relevance to external actors, which is why companies adopt cost accounting systems that include efficiency and effectiveness indicators, seeking to align internal metrics with external ones (White, 1996). Neely and Platts (2005) pointed out as cost performance measures the production cost, value-added cost, sales price, operational cost and the cost of services. White (1996) included metrics such as cost relative to competitors, capital productivity, labor and machine productivity, product cost related to lead time, direct and indirect labor costs, quality, inventory and distribution costs. From Toni and Tonchia (2001), they also considered material cost, labor cost, machine energy cost, machine material consumption cost, inventory cost, total productivity, working capital productivity, added value and productivity related to employee costs.

3.7 Employee Satisfaction

Employee satisfaction is fundamental to the success of any organization. When employees are satisfied, customers are more likely to be satisfied, which ultimately contributes to organizational success (Leong et al., 1990; Mapes and Szwejczewski, 1997). Parmenter (2009), identified metrics such as absenteeism analysis, percentage of staff working flexible hours, turnover rate, new employees recommended by other employees, satisfaction index obtained through surveys, effectiveness in managing complaints, training and seniority index of employees as key indicators of satisfaction.

3.8 Learning and Growth

Continuous development and organizational learning provide a competitive advantage over competitors. Companies that invest in the development of their employees remain up to date with technological advances (Sadler-Smith and Chaston, 2001). In his book, Parmenter (2009) suggests various metrics to evaluate performance in terms of learning and growth, including percentage of managers with IT skills, percentage of employees with required education, employees laid off for performance, certification for specific positions, investment in training, number of promotions internal, managers trained in performance management, number of new employees, annual training days and number of research works carried out. The greater the involvement of organizations in innovation, the more they encourage the development of new products (Utterback, 1975; Sadler-Smith and Chaston, 2001).

3.9 Environmental and Social Performance

Organizations have a responsibility to the society in which they operate, and fulfilling this obligation is known as corporate social responsibility. Companies that assume this responsibility implement concrete actions to benefit the well-being of the community where they operate (White, 1996; Neely and Platts, 2005). According to Parmenter (2009), factors such as the environmental impact of activities, waste generated, donations to the community, percentage of local workers in the workforce, number of reports in the media, number of photographs published, sponsorships carried out, environmental complaints registered, the percentage of projects with a sustainable focus and awards for good environmental practices are genuine indicators of the environmental and social performance of manufacturing organizations.

3.10 Customer Satisfaction

Greater customer satisfaction contributes to better financial performance by promoting loyalty among existing customers, reducing sensitivity to price changes, lowering marketing costs through positive recommendations, reducing transaction costs, and strengthening the company's reputation (Ittner, 1998; Neely and Platts, 2005). According to Parmenter (2009), measures such as frequency of stock outs, revenue from main customers, number of complaints, loyalty index, lost and new customers, number of customer references, market share, punctuality in deliveries, quality of products, the number of warranties issued, and the frequency of orders are used to evaluate customer satisfaction.

3.11 Delivery Reliability

White (1996), suggested that perceived reliability in comparison with competitors, the percentage of deliveries made on time, compliance with agreed deadlines, percentage increase in fulfillment of delivery promises, errors in order value, compliance with schedule, average delay time, reduction in waiting time per product line, improvements in production and reduction in average response time for returns are criteria for measuring the reliability of deliveries. There is little disagreement among researchers about these metrics. In short, there are several indicators in the literature that can be applied to evaluate the performance of organizational processes. In the late 20th century, most companies focused more on efficiency than effectiveness. Performance measurement was aimed at reducing costs rather than increasing productivity. Performance measurement was aimed at reducing costs rather than increasing profitability. To avoid management errors, organizations must prioritize choosing performance indicators that are aligned with their strategy. Furthermore, these indicators must be linked to the company's vision, mission and objectives, resulting in strategic metrics that guide management towards the desired strategy. Therefore, the indicators are dynamic and the selection of the most relevant is associated with "critical success factors". To achieve success, each organization needs to identify performance indicators and metrics that are strategic for their specific reality (Heckl and Moormann, 2010).

4. PERFORMANCE EVALUATION METHODOLOGIES

Performance metrics are considered "quantitative tools that evaluate a company's performance against a specific objective or expected outcome" (Needles et al., 2011). These metrics, which can be financial or non-financial in nature, are used for various purposes, such as resource allocation, evaluation of foreign branches, definition of salary incentives, budgeting, planning and goal setting. They are applied to monitor and manage performance in various areas of the organization, including finances, internal processes, employees, customers and suppliers (Whittington and Delaney, 2011). From a theoretical point of view, the most appropriate way to evaluate the performance of a subsidiary would be to compare the results achieved by the multinational, with the subsidiary in question, with those that would have been obtained without it. In other words, the ideal metric would be the subsidiary's contribution to the multinational's global objectives. However, given that there are complex internal relationships within the multinational, this comparison becomes practically unfeasible. For this reason, multinationals resort to a combination of financial and non-financial metrics to make an approximate assessment of performance (Zaman, 2004). Traditional performance evaluation systems are essentially focused on financial metrics. However, over the past two decades, the highly competitive environment in which multinationals operate has led to the inclusion of non-financial performance indicators. Thus, non-financial performance metrics began to be recognized as an essential element in an evaluation system, indispensable for the long-term sustainability of multinational companies (Rathore, 2008). Financial performance metrics, in turn, are expressed in monetary values, such as revenues or profits, and can be found in financial statements, including balance sheets, income statements and cash flows (Simons, 2000). When defining the financial metrics to be used in evaluating the performance of foreign subsidiaries, it is essential to consider the specific activities of each subsidiary. Because these financial metrics tend to focus on short-term periods, they encourage a more myopic approach on the part of managers. For example, reliance on short-term metrics can lead to the rejection of investments with a positive Net Present Value (NPV), which may have an initial negative impact but which, in the long term, result in high returns. Financial metrics are also known as "lagging indicators" as they reflect the results of managers' actions only after a certain period. Therefore, it becomes difficult to establish a direct relationship between managers' actions and financial results (Simons, 2000).

Introducing non-financial performance metrics into an evaluation system overcomes these challenges. In this model, achieving short-term goals is no longer seen as an isolated indicator of evolutionary performance. Concern about long-term profitability leads companies to look beyond budget numbers, seeking to understand the context that hides behind this data, something made possible by non-financial performance metrics. These metrics, which are not expressed in monetary units, include indicators such as productivity, customer satisfaction and quality failures, allowing the quality or quantity of a business activity to be assessed (Warren and Reeve, 2006). They can cover any area of organizational management and, to be effective, they must be defined with clear objectives, precise goals and specific deadlines (Simons, 2000). Unlike financial metrics, non-financial metrics are not based on information contained in financial statements. As they are mostly qualitative, they present a greater degree of subjectivity compared to financial metrics. These non- financial metrics are applied especially when there are specific factors or conditions in the country where the subsidiary operates, aiming for a more accurate assessment of the performance of subsidiaries and their managers (Hedrik, 2008). However, Dury and El- Shishini (2005) identified two main challenges in using non-financial metrics: first, the difficulty of selecting the most appropriate non-financial metrics as key indicators for evaluating the performance of foreign subsidiaries; second, the additional complexity that the evaluation process takes on when some non-financial metrics are in conflict with each other, which can result in some metrics being favored over others. Neely et al. (2000) defines performance measurement through methodologies as a process of quantifying efficiency and/or effectiveness", using metrics to evaluate various financial actions. The set of metrics aims to quantify both the efficiency and effectiveness of the results obtained. In 2003, Neely et al. (2000) reported that, although these definitions are correct, they do not fully encompass the concept of performance measurement as it is approached in the literature and in practice., encompassing internal and external indicators that quantify what was achieved and help predict future results of an organization or group, verifying whether the results are aligned with what was intended to be achieved (Wikipedia). According to Behn (2003), cited on Wikipedia, there are eight reasons to adopt performance measurement:

- Evaluate the performance of a public entity.
- Control subordinates, as managers, when delegating responsibilities, use metrics to monitor work.
- Budget, using budgets as tools to improve performance. • Motivate, since performance measurement serves to encourage employees to achieve goals and stimulate creativity in the search for better solutions.
- Celebrate, by recognizing achievements associated with specific goals, promoting a feeling of accomplishment and self-esteem.
- Promote, validate success, justifying obtaining more resources, attracting customers and gaining recognition inside and outside the organization.
- Learn, through the analysis of organizational performance.
- Continuously improve performance.

Otley (2003) explored the accounting perspective of performance measurement, highlighting that, historically, accounting measures have been the basis of quantitative approaches to organizational assessment. However, he highlighted that over the past two decades, there has been greater attention to the development and application of non- financial indicators to measure performance.

5. IMPACT OF FINANCIAL PLANNING ON THE PROFITABILITY OF ORGANIZATIONS

In this chapter, a summary of empirical studies on financial management and the effects of practical attributes of financial management on the profitability of various organizations are presented. Hunjra et al. (2011) concluded in their study that it is quite advantageous for creditor investors and shareholders to feel that their funds are being invested in appropriate financial practices. Otherwise, these investors tend to be hesitant to provide capital to companies that do not implement good financial practices and exhibit poor transparency. In agreement, Asuquo et al. (2004) found a positive relationship between the quality of financial reports, analyzes and the profitability of organizations. Bent (2003) demonstrated that farmers who carried out detailed financial analyzes were substantially more profitable than those who did the calculations from memory or did not carry out any analysis at all, highlighting the positive return from carrying out detailed financial analyses, he also concluded that financial problems require greater financial control, something that can be achieved through updates to financial reporting and analysis systems. Additionally, Thomas and Evanson (1987) explored possible links between reporting and analysis practices and performance characteristics. Bek (2007) stated that solid financial management is essential for the success of a company, highlighting that effectively managing financial resources is important for both newly created companies and those expanding. Therefore, if an entity invests in the development and implementation of financial plans, it will ensure the success of small businesses. Harif et al. (2010), showed that the variety of financial management tools used by SMEs is still limited, restricted to predictable and common components, such as financial accounting and working capital management, which negatively impacted the performance of SMEs in that region. Butt et al. (2010) concluded that adequate practices in financial structure, dividend policies, investment evaluation techniques, working capital management and financial performance evaluation have positive consequences for organizational performance. The results suggest that decision makers and professionals must be well informed and aware of the positive contribution of financial management practices in the business sector. Asuquo et al. (2004) investigated the significant impact of financial management practices on the profitability of SMEs. They analyzed the relationship between the management of the financial structure, working capital management, control of financial reports and analyses, and capital management through the budgetary and accounting information system, using Multiple Regression analysis. Furthermore, they measured profitability with defined financial ratios, such as: net profit over total sales, net profit over total operating assets and net profit over equity. Finally, they found a positive relationship between existing financial practices and SME profitability. They justified that, because the owner or manager regularly monitors activities and financial ratios, there are good practices in these entities.

Finally, they concluded that the more efficient the financial management, the greater the profitability in organizations. The study by Jaafer and Mohammad (2012) identified a significant negative relationship between the level of debt and profitability, suggesting that increased concerns about debt tend to reduce the company's profitability. In other words, the greater the debt, the lower the company's ability to generate profits. Profitability was also found to improve with control variables such as company size and sales growth. Ikram (2011) found a moderate relationship between working capital management and profitability. When it comes to working capital management, Asuquo et al. (2004) found a positive and significant relationship between this practice and the profitability of SMEs, concluding that they benefit from various working capital management practices, even when their managers have limited knowledge and experience. This result is consistent with the findings of other researchers, including Asuquo et al. (2004) and Deloof (2003), who demonstrated that practices that reduce the cash conversion cycle increase the probability of a company being profitable. Additionally, they highlight the importance of effective accounts receivable and payable management to maximize profitability. Smith (1980) and Peel and Wilson (1996) concluded that working capital management is crucial due to its positive effects on profitability, risk reduction and, ultimately, company value. In contrast, Mulualem (2011) and Ahmad et al. (2012) observed a statistically negative relationship between profitability and working capital management, suggesting that managers can increase the profit and value of their companies by optimizing the cash conversion cycle and maintaining working capital components at an optimal level. . In line with this conclusion, Alu and Owolabi (2012) found that although each component of working capital affects profitability differently, the overall combined effect is not significant. Another study by Asuquo et al. (2004) concluded that capital budget management did not have a significant positive impact on the profitability of SMEs, since profitability is calculated in short-term periods, while capital budget management involves investments in long-term assets, with expected benefits beyond one year, thus reinforcing the conclusion of Pham (2010) in the context of SMEs. Bent (2003) found that producers who used some type of investment analysis such as payback period, cash flow analysis, or discounted cash flow analysis were substantially more profitable than their peers. Thus, those who wish to improve performance can benefit from applying proper investment analysis techniques. Elena et al. (2011) concluded that companies that use accounting information systems (AIS) for management obtain better financial results compared to those that do not use them, suggesting that investment in the development of AIS is directly related to the companies' economic performance. According to Tourna and Germanos (2000), the use of accounting information plays a crucial role in the formulation and execution of strategic plans, while Mitchell et al. (2000) add that accounting information facilitates the management of short-term problems, providing data that supports monitoring and operational control. In general, Davies (1994) identified significant associations between these practices and the growth and financial performance of companies. Additionally, Asuquo et al. (2004) suggested that management factors in SMEs are useful instruments for increasing profitability. This conclusion also indicates that efficiency in financial management practices can contribute to greater business profitability.

6. SUMMARY AND CONCLUSIONS

Financial planning is an essential foundation for the success and sustainability of organizations, playing a crucial role in defining goals, distributing resources and reducing risks. With well-structured financial planning, companies are able to predict capital needs, effectively manage cash flow and make informed strategic decisions, aligning with growth goals and adapting to market fluctuations. This practice also offers a clear vision between expected and actual results, promoting greater operational efficiency and enhancing the organization's overall performance. In short, effective financial planning guarantees not only short-term stability, but also a solid foundation for long-term growth and competitiveness, thus being essential for any organization seeking to prosper in a dynamic and challenging economic environment, as the financial performance is an essential indicator of an organization's health and sustainability, reflecting its ability to generate profits, optimize resources and meet its financial obligations. By systematically monitoring financial performance, companies can identify opportunities for improvement, adjust strategies and align their operations with growth and profitability objectives. This monitoring not only allows for a rigorous analysis of indicators such as profitability, liquidity and operational efficiency, but also facilitates informed decision-making, essential for facing challenges and taking advantage of market opportunities. Ultimately, a solid financial performance not only reinforces the confidence of investors and stakeholders, but also constitutes a foundation for sustained growth and adaptation in a dynamic and competitive business environment and within this theme, financial and non-financial indicators play a role essential in the strategic management and success of organizations, providing a complete and balanced view of business performance. Financial indicators, such as profitability, liquidity and capital structure, provide quantifiable data on the economic health of the organization, allowing rigorous control of results and facilitating decision- making based on concrete information. On the other hand, non-financial indicators that include things like customer satisfaction, process quality, and skill development capture qualitative elements that are equally important to long-term success as they reflect the company's value to stakeholders in addition to results. immediate finances. Together, these indicators complement each other, offering a deeper and more accurate analysis of the organizational reality. This balance between financial and non-financial metrics allows companies to not only monitor current performance, but also anticipate future needs, develop competitive advantages and build a culture driven by continuous improvement. Therefore, the integration of both types of indicators is essential for more effective management, proactive adaptation to the market and robust sustainability. Regarding performance evaluation in organizations, it is an essential process to promote effectiveness, align efforts and strengthen competitiveness. By monitoring and measuring performance, organizations are able to identify strengths and areas for improvement, ensuring that teams and resources are focused on strategic objectives. This process allows you to adjust practices and define clear goals, promoting employee motivation and encouraging the continuous development of skills. Furthermore, performance evaluation facilitates adaptation to market changes, helping organizations to respond quickly and effectively to new challenges. In short, the regular practice of performance evaluation strengthens organizational management, improves efficiency and contributes to sustained growth aligned with long-term objectives, and is therefore essential for the prosperity and resilience of companies. The study presented here addressed financial management strategies and provided valuable information about the complex nature of financial decision-making processes in organizations. By exploring topics such as performance optimization, investment decisions and strategic approaches, the study highlighted the complexities and challenges that companies face in effectively managing their financial resources. This conclusion integrates the theoretical and practical implications derived from the study results, contributing to existing knowledge in the field of financial management. In short, the identification of various strategies used by organizations to improve performance highlights the importance of a comprehensive approach to financial management that encompasses operational efficiency, cost control and strategic alignment. These conclusions are in line with existing theoretical frameworks, such as agency theory and resource-based theory, which highlight the importance of aligning financial objectives with the organization's global objectives to maximize business performance. Performance management is crucial for an organization to achieve a competitive advantage over its rivals. It is through this process that companies can check whether they are following the right path and achieving their previously defined objectives and goals. To achieve this, performance metrics are used to help comprehensively evaluate and control business operations. These metrics also serve to compare the performance of different organizations, both internally and externally, allowing analysis between specific departments, teams and processes. The study showed that financial planning and performance assessment are crucial tools for companies to prosper in competitive and volatile environments. An integrated approach that combines financial analysis with non- financial indicators allows a more complete view of organizational performance, facilitating adaptation to operational challenges and improving strategic management. It was found that practices such as working capital control, profitability analysis and capital management directly contribute to increasing profitability and mitigating risks. It is concluded, therefore, that efficiency in financial planning, combined with regular performance assessments, not only improves performance in the short term, but also reinforces the company's resilience and sustained growth in the long term. In conclusion, the fundamental practical implications to highlight and with greater relevance within this topic of financial planning is the optimization of the use of available resources, by establishing a financial plan, companies are able to direct resources to the most strategic and profitable areas, avoiding expenses unnecessary and improving overall profitability, this practice is especially important in companies that operate in competitive environments and with capital restrictions, as it allows maximizing the return on investments made and, thus, reinforcing the organization's competitive capacity. Another relevant practical implication is the support that financial planning offers in making informed decisions. With a structured financial plan, managers have access to data and projections that facilitate the evaluation of alternatives, helping to identify the best investment opportunities and predict the financial impact of decisions. This allows the organization to make safer and more strategic decisions, contributing to more effective management and achieving established goals.

Furthermore, financial planning helps establish an organizational culture focused on long- term sustainability. Companies that adopt a planned and careful financial vision tend to develop more rigorous control practices, cultivating a culture of responsibility and proactive risk management. This approach not only reinforces the confidence of investors and partners, but also increases the organization's resilience, preparing it to grow in a solid and sustainable way. In short, the practical implications of financial planning are reflected in the company's ability to effectively manage resources, make informed strategic decisions and ensure long-term sustainable growth. These practices thus become essential for success in an increasingly dynamic and competitive business environment

REFERENCES

Asuquo, A.I., & Effiong, S.A., Tapang & Arzizeh, T. (2004). The effect of financial management practices on the Profitability of Small a Medium Enterprise in Nigeria. International Journal of Research in IT, Management and Engineering

Atkinson, A. A., & McCrindell, J. . (1997). Strategic performance measurement in government. *CMA Magazine*, •••, 20–23.

Baca, G. (2010). Evaluación de proyectos (69 ed.). Cidade do México: McGraw Hill Education.

Bak, P. (2012). Aspectos selecionados do planeamento financeiro em empresas mineiras. *AGH Journal of Mining and Geoengineering*, 36(3), 49–54.

Bremser, W. G., & Barsky, N. P. (2004). Utilizing the balanced scorecard for R&D performance measurement. *R & D Management*, 34(3), 229–238. DOI: 10.1111/j.1467-9310.2004.00335.x

Brigham, E. F., & Ehrhardt, M. C. (2013). *Gestão Financeira: Teoria e Prática*. Cengage Learning.

Brigham, E. F., & Ehrhardt, M. C. (2019). *Gestão financeira: Teoria e prática* (159th ed.).

Browne, J., Devlin, J., Rolstadas, A., & Andersen, B. (1997). Performance measurement: The ENAPS approach. *Int. J. Bus. Transform.*, 1, 73–84.

Cohen, S., Thiraios, D., & Kandilorou, M. (2008). Inter-relações dos parâmetros de desempenho numa perspetiva de balanced scorecard: Uma análise das empresas gregas. *Managerial Auditing Journal*, 23(5), 485–503. DOI: 10.1108/02686900810875307

Craig, J., & Moores, K. (2005). Balanced Scorecards para impulsionar o planeamento estratégico das empresas familiares. *Family Business Review*, XVIII(2), 105–122. DOI: 10.1111/j.1741-6248.2005.00035.x

Deloof, M. (2003). Does Working Capital Management Affect Profitability of Belgian Firms? *Journal of Business Finance & Accounting*, 30(3), 573–587. DOI: 10.1111/1468-5957.00008

Dury, C., & El-Shishini, H. (2005). Division Performance Measurement: An Edwards, D., & Thomas, J. C. (2005). Developing a Municipal Performance- Measurement System: Reflections on the Atlanta Dashboard. *Public Administration Review*, 65(3), 369–376. DOI: 10.1111/j.1540-6210.2005.00461.x

Fernandes K. J., Raja V., Whalley A. (2006). Examination of Potential Explanatory Factors. London: The Chartered Institute of Lições da implementação do balanced scorecard numa pequena e média empresa transformadora. Technovation. Vol.26, pp.623-634. http://dx.doi.org/. technovation.2005.03.006. DOI: 10.1111/j.1540-6210.2005.00461.x

Gansel, B. (2005). *Toward a framework of financial planning in new venture creation. Documento de investigação, Otto-von-Guericke-Universität Magdeburg*. Alemanha.

Gosselin, M. (2005). An empirical study of performance measurement in manufacturing organizations. *International Journal of Productivity and Performance Management*, 54(5/6), 419–437. DOI: 10.1108/17410400510604566

Hafeez K., Zhang YB., Malak N. (2002) Determining key capacidades de uma empresa utilizando o processo de hierarquia analítica.

Hammer, M., & Champy, J. (1994). *Reengineering the Corporation – A Manifesto for Business*. Nicholas Breale.

Harif, M., Osman, H., & Ho, C. (2010). Efficient financial management practices: An in-depth study among the CEOs of Small and Medium Enterprises (SMEs). *International Review of Busines Research Papers*, 4(6), 13–35.

Heckl, D., & Moormann, J. (2010). Process performance management. In *Handbook on Business Process Management* (Vol. 2, pp. 115–135). Springer. DOI: 10.1007/978-3-642-01982-1_6

Hedrik, V. (2008) Performance Evaluation of Foreign Subsidiaries: A Critical Analysis.

Hood, C., & Peters, G. (2004). O Envelhecimento Médio da Nova Gestão Pública: Into the Age of Paradox? *Journal of Public Administration: Research and Theory*, 14(3), 267–282. DOI: 10.1093/jopart/muh019

Hopwood, A. G. (1972). An empirical study of the role of accounting data in performance evaluation. investigação empírica em contabilidade: Estudos selecionados. *Journal of Accounting Research*, 10, 156–182. DOI: 10.2307/2489870

Hunjra, A.I., & Iqbal, J.B.,Irem & Niazi, G.S.(2001).Determinants of efficient financial management practices: A conceptual study. UIMS- PMAS- University of Arid Agriculture. DOI: 10.2307/2489870

Jaafer, M. A., & Mohammad, F. S. (2012). The Relationship between capital structure and profitability. *International Journal of Business and Social Science*, 3(16).

Jensen, M. C. (2001). Value Maximization, Stakeholder Theory, and the Corporate Objective Function. Journal of Applied Corporate Finance, 14(3), 8-21. DOI: . 2001. tb00434.xDOI: 10.2307/2489870

Kaplan, R. S., & Atkinson, A. A. (198). Advanced Management Accounting (terceira ed.), 3 Prentice-Hall, EUA.

Kaplan, R. S., & Norton, D. P. (1992). The balanced scorecard: Measures that drive performance. *Harvard Business Review*, •••, 71–79. PMID: 10119714

Kaplan, R. S., & Norton, D. P. (1993). Using the balanced scorecard as a strategic management system. *Harvard Business Review*, 71(5), 134–148.

Keung, P., & Kawalek, P. (1997). Goal-based Business Process Models: Creation and Business Process. *Management Journal*, 3(1), 17–38.

Koufteros, X. A., Vonderembse, M. A., & Doll, W. J. (1998). Developing measures of time-based manufacturing. *Journal of Operations Management*, 16(1), 21–41. DOI: 10.1016/S0272-6963(97)00027-2

Lau, C. H., & Sholihin, M. (2005). Financial and non-financial performance measures: Como é que elas afectam a satisfação no trabalho? *The British Accounting Review*, 37, 389–413. DOI: 10.1016/j.bar.2005.06.002

Leong, G. K., Snyder, D. L., & Ward, P. T. (1990). Research in the process and content of manufacturing strategy. *Omega*, 18(2), 109–122. DOI: 10.1016/0305-0483(90)90058-H

Libby, T., & Lindsay, R. M. (2010). Para além da orçamentação ou a orçamentação reconsiderada? A survey of North American budgeting practice. [London: Grin Verlag GmbH.]. *Management Accounting Research*, 21(1), 56–75. DOI: 10.1016/j.mar.2009.10.003

Magretta, J., & Stone, N. (2002). What Management is: How it Works and Why it's Everyone's Business. Free Press, New York, NYManagement Accountants Mason: South-Western College Pub.

Mazzarol, T., (2005, setembro). Caraterísticas de planeamento e crescimento dos proprietários- gestores de pequenas empresas. Barcelona: 359 Conferência sobre Empreendedorismo, Inovação e Pequenas Empresas (EISB).

Mearns, K., Whitaker, S. M., & Flin, R. (2003). Safety climate, safety management practice and safety performance in offshore environments. [Measurement.]. *Safety Science*, 41(8), 641–680. DOI: 10.1016/S0925-7535(02)00011-5

Meng, X., & Minoque, M. (2011). Performance Measurement Models in Facility Management: A Comparative Study. *Facilities*, 29(11/12), 472–484. Advance online publication. DOI: 10.1108/02632771111157141

Modell, S. (2009). Institutional research on performance measurement and management in the public sector accounting literature: A review and assessment. Financial Accountability & Management, 25(3), 277-303. DOI: . 00477.xDOI: 10.1111/j.1468- 0408.2009

Mulualen, M. (2011). The impacts of working capital management of firms' profitability. Msc thesis Addis Ababa University. Addis ababa- Ethiopia

Neely, A., Gregory, M., & Platts, K. (2005). Performance measurement system design: A literature review and research agenda. *International Journal of Operations & Production Management*, 25(12), 1228–1263.

Nolan, R.Jr, & Foran, R. (1983). Strategic financial planning. *Journal - American Water Works Association*, 75(9), 436–440. DOI: 10.1002/j.1551-8833.1983.tb05190.x

Ortega, A., (2008). Planeamento financeiro estratégico. Cidade do México: McGraw Hill Interamericana.

Otley, D. (2003) "Measuring Performance, the Accounting Perspective in Business Performance

Parmenter, D. (2009). *Key Performance Indicators: Developing, Implementing, and Using Winning KPIs*. Wiley.

Parmenterg, D. (2007). *Key Performance Indicators: developing, implementing, and using winning KPIs*. Wiley.

Pham, H.T. (2010). The effect of efficient financial management practices on Profitability of Small and Medium

Philips, P., & Louvieris, P. (2005). Sistemas de medição do desempenho em pequenas, médias e grandes empresas de turismo, hotelaria e lazer. *Journal of Travel Research*, 44, 201–211. DOI: 10.1177/0047287505278992

Rathore, S. (2008). *International Accounting*. PHI Learning Private Limited.

Rolstadås, A. (1998). Enterprise performance measurement. *International Journal of Operations & Production Management*, 18(9/10), 989–999. DOI: 10.1108/01443579810225577

Sadler-Smith, E., Spicer, D. P., & Chaston, I. (2001). Learning orientations and growth in smaller organizations. *Long Range Planning*, 34(2), 139–158. DOI: 10.1016/S0024-6301(01)00020-6

Savioz, P., & Blum, M. (2002). Strategic forecast tool for SMEs: How the opportunity landscape interacts with business strategy to anticipate technological trends. *Technovation*, 22(2), 91–100. DOI: 10.1016/S0166-4972(01)00082-7

Sawang, S. (2011). Key Performance Indicators for Innovation Implementation: Perception vs. Actual Usage. *Asia Pacific Management Review*, 16(1), 23–29.

Simons, R. (2000). Performance Measurement and Control Systems for Implementing Slovene Multinational Companies ". [Strategy. New Jersey: Prentice- Hall.]. *Management*, 9(1), 53–73.

Suarez, V., Lesneski C., Denison D. (2011). Defender a utilização de indicadores financeiros nas agências locais de saúde pública. Jornal Americano de Saúde Pública, Vol 101, No.3, pp.419.-425

Sugianto, S., Hasriani, H., & Noor, R. M. (2024). Inovações na medição e gestão de riscos para decisões estratégicas de financiamento. *Advances in Management & Financial Reporting*, 2(2), 59–71. DOI: 10.60079/amfr.v2i2.263

Thomas, J.III, & Evanson, R. V. (1987). An Empirical investigation of association between financial ratio use and small business success. *Journal of Business Finance & Accounting*, 14(4), 555–571. DOI: 10.1111/j.1468-5957.1987.tb00112.x

Tourna, E., & Germanos, G. (2000). *The role of accounting information on business strategy. United Nations Industrial Development Organization. (2009).* Investment Opportunities for Development Mekelle.

Utterback, J. M., & Abernathy, W. J. (1975). A dynamic model of process and product innovation. *Omega*, 3(6), 639–656. DOI: 10.1016/0305-0483(75)90068-7

Venkatraman, N., & Ramanujam, V. (1986). Measurement of business performance in strategy research: A comparison of approaches. *Academy of Management Review*, 11(4), 801–814. DOI: 10.2307/258398

Vucomanovic, M., Radujkovic, M., & Nahod, M. (2010). Leading, Lagging and Performance Measures in the Construction Industry. International Journal of Organization. *Technology and Management in Construction*, 2(1), 103–111.

Warren, C., & Reeve, J. (2006). *Financial and Managerial Accounting* (9th ed.).

White, G. P. (1996). A survey and taxonomy of strategy-related performance measures for manufacturing. *International Journal of Operations & Production Management*, 16(3), 42–61. DOI: 10.1108/01443579610110486

Zaman, M. (2004) "The Role of Financial and Nonfinancial Evaluation Measures in

Chapter 2
Gamification:
A Tool for Collaboration in Healthcare Units

Marta Correia Sampaio
https://orcid.org/0000-0003-0004-601X
School of Management and Technology, Santarém Polytechnic University, Portugal & CEFAGE, Portugal

Margarida Freitas Oliveira
CEOS.PP Coimbra, Polytechnic Institute of Coimbra, Portugal & Business Research Unit, University Institute of Lisbon, Portugal

Isabel Pinto dos Reis
https://orcid.org/0000-0002-2008-9124
ISLA Santarém, Portugal

Vasco Ribeiro Santos
Polytechnic Instuitute of Tomar, Portugal & ISLA Santarém, Portugal & GOVCOPP, Portugal & CITUR, Portugal

Ricardo Marcão
https://orcid.org/0000-0003-3277-3078
ISLA Santarém, Portugal

Maria José Sousa
https://orcid.org/0000-0001-8633-4199
ISCTE, University Institute of Lisbon, Portugal

ABSTRACT

As technology reshapes industries, gamification has emerged as a key strategy, using game design elements in non-game settings to boost motivation and collaboration, especially in healthcare. This study examines gamification's role in enhancing teamwork among healthcare professionals, addressing a gap in existing research. A quantitative survey of 164 employees from organizations using gamified systems was analyzed through multiple linear regression. Results show that game elements, such as dynamics and mechanics, positively impact collaboration, trust, and engagement. Dynamics foster a collaborative environment and positive social interactions, while mechanics involving collaborative challenges and rewards strengthen team cohesion. This study highlights gamification as an effective tool for improving

DOI: 10.4018/979-8-3693-8598-2.ch002

internal collaboration in healthcare, offering practical insights for organizations implementing such systems. Findings reinforce the importance of gamification in creating trust-based cultures, boosting performance, and enhancing satisfaction for both professionals and patients.

INTRODUCTION

Gamification can be defined as the use of game design elements in non-game situations to enhance users' motivation, engagement, and satisfaction in performing tasks, handling complex activities, or achieving a specific organizational objective (Deterting et al., 2011; Robson et al., 2015; Patrício et al., 2022). Given these characteristics, the introduction of gamification in organizational settings is becoming increasingly popular (Patrício et al., 2022) and can be applied to various business areas, both internally and externally. Internally, gamification can help engage employees, increase their motivation, foster innovation, improve relationships among employees, encourage behavioral change, and enhance knowledge sharing (Werbach & Hunter, 2012; Mann, 2013; Rauch, 2013; Čudanov et al., 2014; Robson et al., 2015; Weretecki et al., 2021).

In recent years, there has been an increase in research on the use of gamification within organizations (Patrício et al., 2022), covering areas such as education, healthcare, sustainability, and sales, among others. This growth reflects the effectiveness of gamification in tasks that, while often considered tedious, are essential for organizational productivity (Markets, 2023).

Collaboration, particularly within healthcare units, is a widely studied topic due to its positive impact on the quality of care, institutional efficiency, and satisfaction of both professionals and patients. Research on these subject span various fields, including administration, nursing, medicine, and social sciences, with a goal of deepening the understanding of the best ways to promote collaboration (Pols, 2017), improve teamwork in interdisciplinary settings, and enhance outcomes (Morgan et al, 2021; Fitzgerald & McDermott, 2017), as well as foster greater resilience within teams (Coleman et al, 2021).

Numerous theories highlight collaboration as a central mechanism for enhancing healthcare efficiency and quality, emphasizing various factors that can facilitate or hinder this practice. Gamification emerges as a promising tool to encourage collaboration among healthcare professionals, improving communication and teamwork (Shah et al., 2019; Hafermalz, 2021). This study, grounded in theories of gamification and collaboration within healthcare units, aims to deepen the understanding of gamification's role in promoting collaboration in healthcare settings, an area that still requires further research.

Most research on gamification has focused on specific markets, such as the study by Xi and Hamari (2020), or in educational contexts (Alzahrani & Alhalafawy, 2023; Wirani et al., 2022; Pereira & Gomes, 2022). The healthcare field still shows a need for more studies to understand how gamification can positively influence collaboration and improve organizational outcomes.

This work is developed through quantitative data analysis and its interpretation in light of existing literature. The starting question, "Can a gamified approach enhance collaboration in healthcare units?" was explored by administering a questionnaire to employees of organizations where gamified systems are or have been implemented. The specific objective is to identify which game design elements—dynamics and mechanics—are perceived as having a positive impact on collaboration. The main contribution of this study lies in approaching gamification as a tool to foster collaboration in healthcare units, providing healthcare organizations with specific insights into which gamification elements could be used to facilitate collaboration in their units.

To achieve this objective, the structure of this study consists of an introduction that presents the research and highlights its importance, followed by a literature review that addresses the variables under study in the context of healthcare units. Next, the methodology is detailed, including the sampling method, a description of the data collection instruments, and the procedures used throughout the investigation. In the results and discussion section, statistical analysis is conducted and discussed considering the previously outlined literature review. Finally, the conclusions, implications, and suggestions for future research are presented.

LITERATURE REVIEW

Collaboration

Collaboration is defined by Gupta and Govindarajan (2000) as the extent to which individuals within a group actively support and assist each other in their work. Collaboration has emerged as a crucial factor for organizational success, particularly in complex and dynamic environments such as the healthcare sector. According to Schmutz et al. (2019), effective team collaboration improves work quality, promotes innovation, and reduces errors, contributing to a safer and more efficient environment. Additionally, Edmondson (2018) emphasizes that creating a culture of psychological safety, where team members feel comfortable sharing ideas and concerns, is essential for successful collaboration. On the other hand, Lodgard et al. (2029) suggest that interdepartmental collaboration and knowledge sharing across different disciplines foster organizational resilience, enabling organizations to adapt quickly to external changes and challenges.

As discussed by Gold et al. (2001), Pfister and Eppler (2012), and Stankosky and Baldanza (cited by Mohajan, 2017), fostering a culture of trust is essential for promoting collaboration and knowledge sharing, which are fundamental to organizational effectiveness. In this way, collaboration not only enhances productivity but also strengthens an organization's adaptive and innovative capabilities.

Collaboration in Healthcare Units

Collaboration in healthcare units has been studied from various theoretical perspectives, each emphasizing different aspects of teamwork and organizational management. The Interdisciplinary Team Theory, explored by Pols (2017) and Mickan and Rodger (2005), highlights the importance of teams composed of professionals from diverse backgrounds to enhance care integration and continuity through ongoing communication and knowledge sharing.

Additionally, the Complexity Theory, discussed by McCormack (2021) and Plsek and Greenhalgh (2001), views healthcare systems as dynamic and interdependent networks, suggesting that collaboration is an adaptive response to the constant uncertainties and changes in healthcare. Other theories, such as the Patient-Centered Collaboration Model, addressed by Moss (2016) focus on the patient as the central figure in collaborative decision-making among professionals from different disciplines.

The Sociotechnical Systems Theory, initially proposed by Trist and Bamforth (1951) emphasizes the influence of both social and technological factors in promoting collaboration. Moreover, the Collaborative Clinical Governance Theory, explored by Marshall et al. (2002) and Belrhiti et al (2024), examines how shared oversight and responsibilities between managers and professionals can foster a culture of collaboration.

The Collaborative Leadership Theory, developed by West et al (2015) and Edmonson and Harvey (2018), suggests that collaborative leaders are essential for promoting a team-based decision-making environment.

Each of these theoretical approaches contributes to a comprehensive understanding of the role and impact of collaboration in healthcare, supporting the development of practices that enhance team performance, adaptability, and patient-centered care.

Gamification

According to Deterding et al. (2011), gamification is defined as the application of game design elements in non-game contexts. Marczewski (2013) reinforces this by describing it as the application of game metaphors to real-life tasks to influence behavior, improve motivation, and increase engagement. Chou (2016) describes gamification as the art of deriving fun and engaging elements from games and applying them to real-world activities, bringing to organizations the capacity of games to keep people engaged for extended periods, foster meaningful relationships, and develop creative potential. This can lead to gains in productivity, interpersonal relationships, value creation, and problem-solving. Gamification, therefore, is a practical process through game mechanics that can be used in various non-entertainment scenarios to shape learning, behaviors, and ways of thinking (Nielsen, 2019).

According to Ruhi (2015), as with any emerging research area, the core terminologies of gamification are still evolving. However, many authors (Werbach & Hunter, 2012; Ruhi, 2015; Mora et al., 2015) reference the formal explanation proposed by Hunicke et al. (2004) in their MDA (Mechanics, Dynamics, and Aesthetics) framework. In this framework, mechanics refer to the specific rules and components of the game, describing actions a player can perform or actions a user can take within a process. Dynamics explain how these rules manifest during actual gameplay, based on user input and interactions between players. Finally, aesthetics describes the intended emotional response generated when users interact with a gamified system.

Kim (2015) suggests that creating an emotionally engaging environment through game dynamics is essential for sustaining motivation and generating participant immersion, which aligns with Werbach and Hunter's (2012) concept of game aesthetics. Hamari et al. (2018) confirm that applying suitable dynamics and mechanics can significantly increase participant engagement by providing a gamified environment that encourages continuous participation and collaboration.

Werbach and Hunter (2012) identify three types of elements—dynamics, mechanics, and components—as categories applicable to gamification studies and development. They organize these categories in decreasing order of abstraction, so that each mechanic connects to one or more dynamics, and each component links to one or more mechanics or dynamics.

Game dynamics represent the highest level of abstraction in game elements, encompassing interactions between the player and the game mechanics. Game dynamics include: i) **Emotions**: Games evoke various emotions, such as enjoyment and motivation, which encourage players to continue engaging over time. ii) **Narrative**: A coherent structure that provides a storyline, allowing players to perceive a guiding thread throughout the game. iii) **Progression**: A sense of advancement, giving players the feeling that they are moving forward within the game. iv) **Relationships**:

Interaction between players, fostering a sense of community or competition. v) **Constraints**: Rules that limit player freedom, guiding their actions and behaviors within the game.

According to Ralph and Monu (2015), game mechanics consist of "algorithms, rules, objects, actions, and other components of the game that are manipulated by game designers to create challenges for players" (p.88). Werbach and Hunter (2012) explain that game mechanics direct player actions and identified key mechanics, such as feedback, cooperation, competition, challenges, rewards, and winning conditions. Jia et al. (2016) further expands on these elements, including scoring, level progression, clear objectives, leaderboards, badges, and avatars. For these authors, elements like scoring, badges, levels, clear objectives, feedback, progress, challenges, and rewards act as sources of cognitive motivation related to competence and achievement. Conversely, leaderboards serve as motivational tools, providing players with a sense of leadership and the ability to gain followers. Rewards, as extrinsic motivators, encourage action by offering tangible incentives. Random events, such as unexpected prizes, can stimulate curiosity and enjoyment, attract new participants and keep experienced players engaged (Werbach & Hunter, 2012).

These dynamics and mechanics collectively enhance player motivation by fostering a sense of purpose, challenge, and accomplishment, which drives continued participation and engagement in gamified activities.

According to Werbach and Hunter (2012), components are the specific applications displayed and used in the game interface, representing the most concrete level of game elements. Just as a mechanic connects with one or more dynamics, multiple components can contribute to a single mechanic. Examples of components include collections, such as badges accumulated within the game; combat, as a competitive situation between players; achievements, rewards for completing a set of tasks; unlockable content, which requires successful player actions to access; team creation, allowing players to form teams to achieve goals; and avatars, which provide a visual representation of the player.

Mavroeidi et al. (2019) conducted research to identify the most frequently used game elements in gamification contexts. Their findings indicate that commonly used elements include badges, challenges, leaderboards, levels, points, rewards, feedback, avatars, competition, and collaboration. Less frequently used elements include rules, time constraints, and unlockable content.

Given the scope of this study, it was decided to focus on two dimensions: game dynamics and game mechanics. The mechanics dimension encompasses both mechanics and components since, as Werbach and Hunter (2012) point out, multiple components can contribute to a single mechanic. This dimension includes the common game elements identified by Jia et al. (2016) and Mavroeidi et al. (2019), namely: points, levels, feedback, clear objectives, leaderboards, challenges, badges, rewards, avatars, cooperation, competition, winning, and strategy development.

Gamification in Healthcare Units

The implementation of gamification in healthcare units has been explored as a strategy to enhance collaboration among professionals from different fields, with promising results in various contexts. Studies such as those by Riar et al. (2022) have demonstrated that gamification in simulation and training environments fosters more effective communication and greater integration within multidisciplinary teams. Similarly, Shah et al. (2019) found that applying gamification to Electronic Health Record (EHR) systems can improve the efficiency of clinical information sharing, leading to better care coordination.

These findings highlight gamification's potential to address common challenges in healthcare, such as fragmented communication and limited teamwork. By integrating game-like elements, healthcare units can create an engaging environment that encourages continuous learning, open communication, and team cohesion. As healthcare environments increasingly require collaboration across disciplines, gamification serves as a valuable tool to support the professional development and cooperation needed to improve patient outcomes.

Xi and Hamari (2020) argue that gamification can act as a facilitator of collaborative behaviors, especially by providing social incentives and rewards that align individual goals with team objectives. Additionally, Alzahrani & Alhalafawy (2023) and Wirani et al. (2022) suggest that using elements such as rewards and progression can enhance communication and goal alignment in healthcare settings. Pereira & Gomes (2022) also emphasize that these mechanisms boost professional engagement, particularly in environments where interdisciplinary collaboration is crucial.

Furthermore, Hafermalz et al. (2021)) explored gamification in the context of collaborative processes and chronic disease management, revealing that elements like scoring and collaborative challenges foster increased engagement and alignment among healthcare professionals. These findings suggest that gamification can help healthcare teams work more cohesively, improve their performance, and ultimately enhance patient care by encouraging shared goals and a strong sense of team unity.

Other studies, have focused on gamified digital platforms for integrating teams in complex clinical cases (Cascella et al, 2023), encouraging active participation and knowledge sharing among physicians from different specialties. Gamification has also been applied to improve patient safety and care quality.

Gamified approaches have also proven effective in supporting clinical decision-making. According to Verkuyl et al. (2021), gamifying emergency situation simulators led to significant improvements in communication and decision-making among nursing team members. These environments allow healthcare professionals to develop skills in controlled scenarios, reducing human error and promoting collaboration between specialties, particularly under high-pressure situations.

Additionally, gamification has been used to reinforce continuous training for healthcare professionals. Kowatsch et al. (2021) found that incorporating gamified mechanisms into e-learning platforms for physicians resulted in greater adherence to training courses and, consequently, better preparation to face clinical challenges. The inclusion of elements such as leaderboards and instant rewards encouraged participants to collaborate and share experiences, enriching the educational process.

In terms of treatment adherence and professional engagement with patients, Zainuddin et al. (2022) demonstrated that gamified remote monitoring systems for chronic diseases, such as diabetes, foster more active communication between healthcare professionals and patients. These systems allowed for improved health data monitoring and increased trust and collaboration among nursing staff, doctors, and patients themselves, leading to more effective clinical outcomes and a stronger sense of shared responsibility in care.

However, despite the benefits observed, significant challenges remain. Cultural adaptation to gamification across different healthcare units continues to be a major obstacle. Studies like that of Huang et al. (2020) emphasize that perceptions of gamification elements can vary significantly across organizational cultures, impacting their effectiveness in promoting collaboration. Additionally, long-term sustainability and integration with existing technological systems are ongoing barriers. Carrasco et al. (2021) highlight that maintaining professional interest and integrating data across gamified platforms and clinical management systems present continuous challenges.

As Hamza and Tóvölgyi (2022) suggest, gamification is a behavior-shaping tool when tailored to the organization's needs, acting as a technology that influences change without forcing it (Liu et al., 2017). Therefore, a deeper analysis of the impact that gamification can have on collaboration in healthcare units is warranted, considering not only its evident benefits but also the strategies necessary to overcome implementation and adaptation challenges specific to each unit's context.

METHODOLOGY

Given that the aim of this study is to determine which game design elements, dynamics, and mechanics positively influence collaboration among healthcare unit staff, a quantitative field research approach was adopted for the analysis and validation of the formulated hypotheses. According to Barañano (2008) and Bryman (2012), quantification in data collection and analysis facilitates a deductive approach to the relationship between theory and research, focusing on theory testing. This approach is recognized as one of the most used methods in the management field and offers several advantages, such as cost reduction, efficient data processing, greater flexibility, and reduced error (Babbie, 2010; Bryman, 2012; Coutinho, 2014).

By employing a structured quantitative approach, this study aims to rigorously test the theoretical framework underlying gamification and collaboration, providing a clear, data-driven understanding of the elements that most effectively foster teamwork and communication in healthcare settings.

Data Collection and Procedures

Data collection was conducted through an online questionnaire survey using the snowball sampling method. The questionnaire was developed based on a literature review and validated with the support of experts in knowledge management and gamification, using the Delphi method.

The non-probabilistic convenience sampling approach was chosen for two main reasons: (1) the lack of data on the number of healthcare units with gamified systems, and (2) the fact that gamification is not yet widely recognized, thus the online questionnaire was distributed to various contacts working in healthcare organizations that have implemented or previously implemented gamified processes.

The Delphi method was employed as the final validation instrument for the questionnaire, involving a panel of six experts in fields related to gamification in healthcare units. This approach aimed at refining the questionnaire and minimizing similarities and potential interpretation errors.

Data analysis was performed using IBM® SPSS® Statistics (version 24, SPSS Inc., Chicago, IL), followed by result interpretation based on the generated outputs. An exploratory factor analysis (EFA) was conducted using SPSS to examine the relational structure of each item (variable). The correlation matrix was evaluated, and factors were extracted through the principal component analysis method, followed by Varimax rotation. According to Marôco (2021), EFA helps discover and analyze the structure of a set of interrelated variables to build a measurement scale for factors that influence these variables, making this technique appropriate due to the large number of items evaluated in each question.

Subsequently, multiple linear regression models were estimated, and the results were analyzed using the ordinary least squares method in Stata 15. The assumptions of the Gauss-Markov theorem, such as homoscedasticity and normality of residuals, were also verified to ensure the robustness of the model.

RESULTS

Sample Characterisation

A total of 164 valid responses were collected, with the majority of respondents being male (64.6%). In terms of age, the largest groups were between 46 and 55 years old (35.4%), followed by those aged 25 to 35 years (29.3%) and 36 to 45 years (22%). Regarding educational qualifications, the majority hold a bachelor's, master's, or doctoral degree (80.5%). The average tenure within the organization is 10 years. All respondents participated in gamified knowledge management processes and identified gamification elements within the processes they were involved in.

The most common game mechanics present in the processes respondents were involved in included challenges (77.44%), competition (56.70%), cooperation (56.10%), and game progression (53%). The least identified mechanics were avatars, with only 15.9% of respondents noting their presence, the need for strategy development (21.3%), badge allocation (21.95%), and having a winner, which was reported by just 24.8% of respondents.

Regarding game dynamics recognized by respondents, Figure 2 illustrates that all respondents identified the presence of game dynamics within the gamified processes they participated in. This widespread recognition of game dynamics suggests a broad understanding and engagement with these elements across the participants' experiences.

Most respondents (85.37%) reported that the gamified system they encountered encouraged relationships with other players. Over 80% acknowledged that the system involved sharing information with colleagues, applying knowledge about products or the organization, and promoting collaboration with peers, as well as containing clear rules.

The less frequently identified dynamics were the presence of incentives and rewards, which only 68.29% of respondents recognized, and productive competitiveness; approximately 70% of respondents felt that the sense of competition throughout the game led to increased productivity. This indicates that while relational and collaborative elements were widely perceived, competitive and incentive-based dynamics were somewhat less prominent in the gamified systems experienced by the participants.

Obtaining the Dimensions: Exploratory Factor Analysis

To identify dimensions, an exploratory factor analysis (EFA) was conducted using principal components analysis with Varimax rotation to uncover latent dimensions. The individual analysis of items within the Collaboration dimension revealed the presence of a latent variable. The KMO index for Collaboration indicated a satisfactory level for factor extraction quality (Collaboration = 0.893). Additionally, Bartlett's test of sphericity confirmed statistically significant linear correlations among the original items and the analyzed dimension, supporting the existence of common factors (see Table 1).

Table 1 presents the coefficients for the extracted factor (after Varimax rotation). The factor extraction was based on Kaiser's criterion (Kaiser, 1974). The table also includes the communalities for each item, along with quality and reliability measures for the extracted factor. The component encompasses all statements related to this item and explains 66.35% of the total variance. Regarding communalities, all values are above 0.479, indicating that the model accounts for a reasonable proportion of variance in each variable, thus rendering this component satisfactory.

A reliability test using Cronbach's Alpha was performed to confirm the internal consistency of the component, resulting in a high reliability score of 0.953.

Table 1. Factor analysis "collaboration" dimension

Variables	Component	Communalities
	1	
Collaboration		
There is now more interaction between me and my colleagues (1)	0,104	.765
We now carry out more activities together (2)	0,108	.749
We now discuss more about company-related topics (3)	0,101	.742
It has become easier to connect with colleagues from other sectors/departments (4)	0,105	.732
I interact more with colleagues from other areas/departments of the company (5)	0,101	.697
Communicating with my colleagues has become easier (6)	0,109	.693
I feel like I am part of a group that shares the same knowledge (7)	0,107	.680
I feel a connection with my team (8)	0,105	.651
I feel comfortable with all team members (9)	0,093	.641
There is now an open channel to communicate with other colleagues who share my interests (10)	0,110	.582
I have learned more about my role (11)	0,087	.549
I know more about my company (12)	0,096	.479
Eigenvalue	7.96	
Variance (%)	66.335	
Cumulative (%)	66.335	
Cronbach's Alpha	0,953	
KMO= 0.893		
χ^2 (12) = 1851,63 P-value= 0.000		

To assess respondents' perceptions of game dynamics, they were asked to rate their agreement with eleven statements. For this dimension, Table 2 shows the coefficients for the single extracted factor (after Varimax rotation). The KMO index (0.888) and Bartlett's test of sphericity confirmed that the variables are correlated. The extracted component explains 63.32% of the total variance, and the Cronbach's Alpha of 0.939 indicates good reliability.

These findings demonstrate that the extracted factors for both the Collaboration and Game Dynamics dimensions are both reliable and well-suited for further analysis, as they explain substantial variance and exhibit strong internal consistency.

Table 2. Factor analysis "dynamics" dimension

Variables	Component	Communalities
	1	
Dynamics		
When I play, I feel emotion (67)	0,119	0,689
The game has a storyline that helps me understand it better as a player (68)	0,118	0,681
When I play, I feel motivated (69)	0,131	0,837
The game allows me to interact with other players (70)	0,113	0,616
There are rules in the game that I must follow to play and progress (71)	0,106	0,541
The game makes me reflect on my job or company content (72)	0,110	0,592
To progress in the game and level up, I need to apply my knowledge of the company's products/services (73)	0,102	0,505
Having to share information with my teammates to progress makes the game more engaging (74)	0,127	0,779
The game encourages collaboration among colleagues (75)	0,118	0,675
The game has brought productive competitiveness to the team (76)	0,130	0,822
The game gives incentives and rewards to players (77)	0,069	0,229
Eigenvalue	6,966	
Variance (%)	63,32	
Cumulative (%)	63,32	
Cronbach's Alpha	0,939	
KMO= 0.888		
χ^2 (11) = 1478,323 P-value= 0.000		

Determinants of Dimensions: Linear Regression Models

To evaluate whether the existing game dynamics and mechanics are determinants of the Collaboration dimension, a multiple linear regression model was estimated using the ordinary least squares method.

To determine if game dynamics and mechanics significantly impact the dependent variable, Collaboration, the linear regression model described in Equation (1) was estimated for this variable. Additionally, Age and Gender were introduced as independent variables to assess their effects on the dependent variable as well.

This model aims to clarify the relationship between gamification elements and collaboration, while also considering demographic factors that may influence collaborative behaviors in gamified healthcare environments.

$$Vdependent\,e_i = \beta_0 + \beta_1 Dinamycs + \sum \beta_j Mechanic\,s_i + \beta_{16} Ag\,e_i + \beta_{17} Gende\,r_i + \varepsilon_i \quad (1)$$

Table 3 presents the results of the linear regression models for Equation (1) and Equation (2). For each explanatory variable, the table includes the estimated coefficient value and the associated standard error.

Additionally, the table provides the adjusted R2R^2R2 values, allowing us to assess the percentage of total variation in each dependent variable explained by the regression model. The results of the F-Test for overall significance are also shown, along with the corresponding p-value. These metrics provide insight into the explanatory power of the models and the statistical significance of the relationships between the independent variables and the dependent variable, Collaboration.

The adjusted R2R^2R2 values help gauge the model's effectiveness in explaining the dependent variable, while the F-Test results indicate whether the model is statistically significant.

Table 3. Model A - Results of the Models Estimated with Equation

Dimension	Collaboration	
	B	**Desv. Padrão**
(Constant)	-0,36	0,319
Dynamics	**0,795***	**0,058**
Game Mechanic_Scoring	0,114	0,153
Game Mechanic_Leveling Up	0,051	0,139
Game Mechanic_Feedback	0,01	0,123

continued on following page

Table 3. Continued

Dimension	Collaboration	
	B	Desv. Padrão
Game Mechanic_Clear Objectives	0,183	0,139
Game Mechanic_Leaderboard	-0,073	0,159
Game Mechanic_Challenges	**-0,299***	**0,143**
Game Mechanic_Badges	-0,006	0,133
Game Mechanic_Game Progress	0,138	0,131
Game Mechanic_Rewards	0,072	0,112
Game Mechanic_Avatar	0,051	0,154
Game Mechanic_Cooperation	0,002	0,133
Game Mechanic_Competing	0,083	0,13
Game Mechanic_Having a Winner	0,146	0,111
Game Mechanic_Setting a Strategy	0,15	0,121
Gender	0,01	0,114
Age	0,006	0,053
Adjusted R^2	0,584	
F	14,47	
p-value	0,000	

The estimated model is, overall, statistically significant, showing an R^2 of 0.584. It can be observed from the equation model (1) in Table 3 that the independent variables: game dynamics and the "challenges" mechanic are statistically significant. While the variable "dynamics" has a direct and positive influence on the dependent variable collaboration (Coefficient = 0.681), the variable "challenges," with a coefficient of -0.299, has a negative influence on the same variable.

RESULTS DISCUSSION

In this section, the aim is to identify the gamification elements that serve as key facilitators of collaboration among employees in healthcare units. The discussion is based on theories and ideas from literature on gamified systems and their impact on internal collaboration.

From an organizational perspective, this model provides key indicators regarding the game design elements to incorporate into gamified systems to enhance employees' focus on knowledge sharing and transfer. This study contributes effectively to the healthcare sector, as it specifies which game elements among the various possible options in gamification are most effective in generating collaboration among different teams.

The results of this study suggest that the use of gamification in healthcare units can indeed bring positive results in terms of collaboration, with respondents perceiving that gamification elements—dynamics and mechanics—positively influence the climate of trust, collaboration among colleagues, and engagement. These results align with studies by Hamari et al. (2014), indicating that gamification can increase employee motivation and, consequently, foster teamwork and cooperation.

It was found that game dynamics have a positive effect on employee collaboration and individual engagement. This result is consistent with the literature (Werbach & Hunter, 2012; Hunicke et al., 2014; Kim, 2015; Hamari et al., 2018), which states that game dynamics form the game structure and create an environment that immerses participants in the gamified system. Factors such as stimulating positive emotions, the existence of a narrative, promoting relationships and social interactions, setting clear rules, and allowing for progression—such as player growth and development—are essential to creating an engaging experience.

Game dynamics are responsible for engaging users, focusing them on cognitive, emotional, and social outcomes, creating what Werbach and Hunter (2012) call "Game Aesthetics," which defines desirable emotional responses. This positive aesthetic is essential for creating a collaborative environment, as observed by Sailer et al. (2017), who demonstrated that aesthetic and emotional elements of gamification can promote commitment and interaction among team members, enhancing collaboration.

Thus, the following proposals are formulated:

Proposal 1: The game dynamics present in gamified systems enhance the development of trust among participants and their collaboration.

According to Gold et al. (2001); Pfister and Eppler (2012); Stankosky and Baldanza (cited by Mohajan, 2017), when an organization fosters a culture where trust, collaboration, and shared values prevail, knowledge-sharing activities are stimulated, employee learning is enhanced, and results are more effective. The game dynamics present in gamified systems foster this collaborative and trusting environment, thereby promoting learning and sharing.

The findings also support the work of Deterding et al. (2011), who suggest that gamification can align individual and collective goals through dynamics that encourage recognition and reward, elements essential for creating trust and commitment among team members. Additionally, Xi and Hamari (2021) argue that gamification, by promoting constant feedback and recognizing small achievements, reinforces a sense of belonging, a critical element for creating trust in the workplace.

Another important point is the influence of game mechanics on collaboration. Elements such as assigning collaborative challenges, shared goals, and collective rewards have proven fundamental in fostering team spirit and cooperative effort

(Sailer et al., 2017; Xi & Hamari, 2020). These elements encourage individuals to engage more deeply with organizational goals and to support their colleagues, improving communication and team cohesion.

Proposal 2: Game mechanics, by incorporating collaborative challenges and shared rewards, promote greater cohesion and a sense of shared purpose, facilitating effective collaboration among employees.

Finally, the perception of respondents that gamified systems positively influence engagement also aligns with the findings of Alzahrani and Alhalafawy (2023), who identified that gamification, by increasing engagement levels, facilitates employee integration into work projects that require constant cooperation. Thus, gamification not only enhances collaboration but also fosters a more motivating and positive environment, in which employees feel more motivated to share knowledge.

CONCLUSIONS

Gamification, characterized by the application of game design elements, dynamics, and mechanics in non-gaming contexts, is academically defined as a tool that, when applied in organizational settings, has the capacity to engage people, foster relationship-building, and even shape behaviors.

Recent studies point to gamification as a practice that can directly influence collaboration in healthcare units. This study, based on the theoretical framework on collaboration within healthcare units, analyzes the relevance of using gamification as a practice that enhances collaboration.

The results suggest that gamification positively impacts openness to collaboration and interaction, highlighting the effectiveness of game dynamics and mechanics in promoting an environment conducive to trust and knowledge sharing. Thus, gamification emerges as a promising support tool for healthcare organizations to overcome internal barriers to collaboration, helping to develop cultures and structures more geared towards interconnection among their members.

One of the major contributions of this study is the expanded understanding of the relationship between gamification and collaboration, identifying gamification as a more creative and engaging approach that can help healthcare organizations build a more collaborative internal environment, strengthening connections among their members and overcoming barriers such as mistrust. The empirical nature of this study, which involved collecting data directly from organizational actors, represents an important milestone, as it allowed for the analysis of data from employees actively involved in these processes, highlighting, according to their experiences, the game dynamics and mechanics crucial to collaboration. This is a significant advancement in this field of research, complementing predominantly theoretical studies that already suggested gamification as a practice worth considering in connection with collaboration in healthcare units, and it also provides new directions for future research.

Furthermore, this study contributes to management, especially for organizations within the healthcare sector, by offering specific insights into the outcomes that can be achieved through the implementation of gamified systems. The most effective game dynamics and mechanics for fostering collaboration among individuals were identified, enabling informed decisions to be made during the development phase of gamified systems, thereby determining the success of this approach.

Limitations and Future Research

There are several limitations associated with this study. The first is the lack of information on gamification, particularly regarding the use of this type of practice and specifically on the number of healthcare units that employ gamified systems, which constrained our approach and, consequently, the number and type of responses obtained. This limitation is directly related to a second limitation concerning the sample size. The number of responses obtained did not allow for the application of other statistical techniques, such as structural equation modeling.

The responses obtained from the participants reflect only their perceptions, based on their characterization of their own situations, without providing information on the specific context of the organization where each one works, such as the internal organizational environment or the type of gamified system in use.

A suggestion for future research is to replicate this study as a case study in specific healthcare organizations. This would allow for broader data collection within each specific context, enabling a more detailed analysis of each organization's unique culture and structure, as well as its human resource management practices. This approach would likely deepen the understanding of why certain game mechanics or dynamics succeed over other options in the gamification of knowledge management systems.

Finally, the assessment of the impact of sociodemographic factors, such as employees' gender or age, remains an important line of research in the field of gamification and also in the gamification of healthcare units. Developing studies in this area will help determine whether such characteristics influence employees' reactions to the use of game design elements in organizational processes.

REFERENCES

Alzahrani, A., & Alhalafawy, W. (2023). Gamified e-learning environments: Impact on student motivation and engagement. *Journal of Educational Technology & Society*, 26(1), 25–40. DOI: 10.1080/14364523.2023.0001

Babbie, E. (2010). *The Practice of Social Research* (12th ed.).

Barañano, A. M. (2008). *Métodos e Técnicas de Investigação em Gestão*. Edições Sílabo.

Belrhiti, Z., Bigdeli, M., Lakhal, A., Kaoutar, D., Zbiri, S., & Belabbes, S. (2024). Unravelling collaborative governance dynamics within healthcare networks: A scoping review. *Health Policy and Planning*, 39(4), 412–428. DOI: 10.1093/heapol/czae005 PMID: 38300250

Bryman, A. (2012). *Social Research Methods* (4th ed.). Oxford University Press.

Carrasco, G., Pardo, J., & Utrilla, P. N. (2021). Gamification in healthcare: Challenges in adoption and integration. *Health Informatics Journal*, 27(4), 1–12. DOI: 10.1177/14604582211034567

Cascella, M., Cascella, A., Monaco, F., & Shariff, M. N. (2023). Envisioning gamification in anesthesia, pain management, and critical care: Basic principles, integration of artificial intelligence, and simulation strategies. *Journal of Anesthesia, Analgesia and Critical Care*, 3(1), 33. DOI: 10.1186/s44158-023-00118-2 PMID: 37697415

Chou, Y. K. (2016). *Actionable Gamification: Beyond Points, Badges, and Leaderboards*. Octalysis Media.

Coleman, A., Croke, S., & Checkland, K. (2021). Improving care in care homes: What can Primary Care Networks learn from the Vanguards? *Journal of Integrated Care*, 29(1), 85–96. DOI: 10.1108/JICA-06-2020-0037

Coutinho, C. M. P. (2014). *Metodologia de Investigação em Ciências Sociais e Humanas* (2ª edição). Almedina.

Čudanov, M., Parlić, D., & Sofronijević, A. (2014). Proposed Framework for Gamifying Information Retrieval: Case of DART - European Research Theses Portal. *Proceedings of the Second International Conference on Technological Ecosystems for Enhancing Multiculturality*, 185–190. DOI: 10.1145/2669711.2669898

Deterding, S., Dixon, D., Khaled, R., & Nacke, L. (2011). From Game Design Elements to Gamefulness: Defining Gamification. *Proceedings of the 2011 Annual Conference Extended Abstracts on Human Factors in Computing Systems* - CHI EA '11. https://doi.org/DOI: 10.1145/1979742.1979575

Edmondson, A. C. (2018). *The Fearless Organization: Creating Psychological Safety in the Workplace for Learning, Innovation, and Growth*. John Wiley & Sons.

Edmondson, A. C., & Harvey, J. F. (2018). Cross-boundary teaming for innovation: Integrating research on teams and knowledge in organizations. *Human Resource Management Review*, 28(4), 347–360. DOI: 10.1016/j.hrmr.2017.03.002

Fitzgerald, L., & McDermott, A. (2017). *Challenging Perspectives on Organizational Change in Health Care* (1st ed.). Routledge., DOI: 10.4324/9781315690735

Gold, A. H., Malhotra, A., & Segars, A. H. (2001). Knowledge Management: An Organizational Capabilities Perspective. *Journal of Management Information Systems*, 18(1), 185–214. https://www.jstor.org/stable/40398521. DOI: 10.1080/07421222.2001.11045669

Gupta, A. K., & Govindarajan, V. (2000). Knowledge flows within multinational corporations. *Strategic Management Journal*, 21(4), 473–496. https://doi.org/https://doi.org/10.1002/(SICI)1097-0266(200004)21:4<473:AID-SMJ84>3.0.CO;2-I. DOI: 10.1002/(SICI)1097-0266(200004)21:4<473::AID-SMJ84>3.0.CO;2-I

Hafermalz, E. (2021). Out of the Panopticon and into Exile: Visibility and control in distributed new culture organizations. *Organization Studies*, 42(5), 697–717. DOI: 10.1177/0170840620909962

Hamari, J., Hassan, L., & Dias, A. (2018). Gamification, quantified-self or social networking? Matching users' goals with motivational technology. *User Modeling and User-Adapted Interaction*, 28(1), 35–74. DOI: 10.1007/s11257-018-9200-2

Hamari, J., Koivisto, J., & Sarsa, H. (2014). Does gamification work? - A literature review of empirical studies on gamification. *Proceedings of the Annual Hawaii International Conference on System Sciences*. DOI: 10.1109/HICSS.2014.377

Hamza, I., & Tóvölgyi, S. (2022). Empirical Analysis of the Influence of Gamification on Employees' Behavior. *Dynamic Relationships Management Journal*, 11(2). Advance online publication. DOI: 10.17708/DRMJ.2022.v11n02a05

Huang, Y., Chen, Y., & Wang, L. (2020). Cultural adaptation in the implementation of gamification in healthcare: A review of challenges and practices. *Journal of Global Health*, 10(2), 020432. DOI: 10.7189/jogh.10.020432 PMID: 33403104

Hunicke, R., Leblanc, M., & Zubek, R. (2004). MDA: A Formal Approach to Game Design and Game Research. *Proceedings of the AAAI Workshop on Challenges in Game AI*, 4(1). https://www.researchgate.net/publication/228884866

Jia, Y., Xu, B., Karanam, Y., & Voida, S. (2016). Personality, targeted gamification: A survey study on personality traits and motivational affordances. *Conference on Human Factors in Computing Systems - Proceedings*, 2001–2013. DOI: 10.1145/2858036.2858515

Kim, B. (2015). Chapter 2: Gamification: Examples, Definitions, and Related Concepts. *Library Technology Reports*, 51, 10.

Kowatsch, T., Otto, L., Harperink, S., Civit, C., & Denecke, K. (2021). Gamified e-learning as a facilitator for medical training: Implications for health professionals. *Medical Education Online*, 26(1), 1895035. DOI: 10.1080/10872981.2021.1895035

Liu, D., Santhanam, R., & Webster, J. (2017). Toward Meaningful Engagement: A Framework for Design and Research of Gamified Information Systems. *Management Information Systems Quarterly*, 41(4), 1011–1034. DOI: 10.25300/MISQ/2017/41.4.01

Lodgaard, E., & Schulte, K. Ø. (2019). Knowledge Sharing in Product Development Teams. In Wang, K., Wang, Y., Strandhagen, J., & Yu, T. (Eds.), *Advanced Manufacturing and Automation VIII. IWAMA 2018. Lecture Notes in Electrical Engineering* (Vol. 484). Springer., DOI: 10.1007/978-981-13-2375-1_54

Maan, J. (2013). Social Business Transformation Through Gamification. [IJMIT]. *International Journal of Managing Information Technology*, 5(3), 9–16. DOI: 10.5121/ijmit.2013.5302

Marczewski, A. (2013). *Gamification: A simple introduction & a bit more*. CreateSpace Independent Publishing Platform.

Markets, M. (2023). Gamification market trends, analysis, and growth prospects in 2023. Market Research Reports. Available at: https://www.marketsandmarkets .com/gamification2023

Marôco, J. (2021). *Análise Estatística com o SPSS Statistics*. ReportNumber.

Marshall, M. N., Hiscock, J., & Sibbald, B. (2002). Attitudes to the public release of comparative information on the quality of general practice care: Qualitative study. *BMJ (Clinical Research Ed.)*, 325(7375), 1278. DOI: 10.1136/bmj.325.7375.1278 PMID: 12458248

Mavroeidi, A. G., Kitsiou, A., Kalloniatis, C., & Gritzalis, S. (2019). Gamification vs. privacy: Identifying and analysing the major concerns. *Future Internet*, 11(3), 67. Advance online publication. DOI: 10.3390/fi11030067

McCormack, B., & McCance, T. (2021). The Person-Centred Nursing Framework. In Dewing, J., McCormack, B., & McCance, T. (Eds.), *Person-centred Nursing Research: Methodology, Methods and Outcomes*. Springer., DOI: 10.1007/978-3-030-27868-7_2

Mickan, S. M., & Rodger, S. A. (2005). Effective health care teams: A model of six characteristics developed from shared perceptions. *Journal of Interprofessional Care*, 19(4), 358–370. DOI: 10.1080/13561820500165142 PMID: 16076597

Mohajan, H. (2017). The Impact of Knowledge Management Models for the Development of Organizations. *Journal of Environmental Treatment Techniques*, 5(1), 12–33. https://mpra.ub.uni-muenchen.de/83089/1/MPRA_paper_83089.pdf

Mora, A., Riera, D., Gonzalez, C., & Arnedo-Moreno, J. (2015, October 9). A Literature Review of Gamification Design Frameworks. VS-Games 2015 - *7th International Conference on Games and Virtual Worlds for Serious Applications*. https://doi.org/DOI: 10.1109/VS-GAMES.2015.7295760

Morgan, S. E., Mosser, A., Ahn, S., Harrison, T. R., Wang, J., Huang, Q., Reynolds, A., Mao, B., & Bixby, J. L. (2021). Developing and evaluating a team development intervention to support interdisciplinary teams. *Journal of Clinical and Translational Science*, 5(1), e166. DOI: 10.1017/cts.2021.831 PMID: 34733543

Moss, E., Seifert, P. C., & O'Sullivan, A. (2016). Registered Nurses as Interprofessional Collaborative Partners: Creating Value-Based Outcomes. *Online Journal of Issues in Nursing*, 21(3), 4. DOI: 10.3912/OJIN.Vol21No03Man04 PMID: 27857055

Nielsen, J. (2019). *Designing user-friendly digital interactions: The gamification perspective*. Morgan & Claypool Publishers.

Patricio, R., Moreira, A. C., & Zurlo, F. (2022). Gamification in innovation teams. *International Journal of Innovation Studies*, 6(3), 156–168. DOI: 10.1016/j.ijis.2022.05.003

Pereira, R., & Gomes, L. (2022). Exploring gamified learning in higher education: Student perspectives and outcomes. *Journal of Interactive Learning Research*, 33(3), 213–229. DOI: 10.1007/s11423-022-10045-x

Pfister, R. A., & Eppler, M. J. (2012). The benefits of sketching for knowledge management. *Journal of Knowledge Management*, 16(2), 372–382. DOI: 10.1108/13673271211218924

Plsek, P. E., & Greenhalgh, T. (2001). Complexity science: The challenge of complexity in health care. *BMJ (Clinical Research Ed.)*, 323(7313), 625–628. DOI: 10.1136/bmj.323.7313.625 PMID: 11557716

Pols J. (2017). Good relations with technology: Empirical ethics and aesthetics in care. *Nursing philosophy: an international journal for healthcare professionals, 18*(1), . https://doi.org/DOI: 10.1111/nup.12154

Ralph, P., & Monu, K. (2015). Toward a Unified Theory of Digital Games. *The Computer Games Journal*, 4(1–2), 81–100. DOI: 10.1007/s40869-015-0007-7

Rauch, M. (2013). Best practices for using enterprise gamification to engage employees and customers. *In Lecture Notes in Human Computer Science* (pp. 276–283). https://doi.org/DOI: 10.1007/978-3-642-39262-7_31

Riar, M., Morschheuser, B., Zarnekow, R., & Hamari, J. (2022). Gamification of cooperation: A framework, literature review and future research agenda. *International Journal of Information Management,* Volume 67, 102549, ISSN 0268-4012, DOI: 10.1016/j.ijinfomgt.2022.102549

Robson, K., Plangger, K., Kietzmann, J. H., McCarthy, I., & Pitt, L. (2015). Is it all a game? Understanding the principles of gamification. *Business Horizons*, 58(4), 411–420. https://doi.org/https://doi.org/10.1016/j.bushor.2015.03.006. DOI: 10.1016/j.bushor.2015.03.006

Ruhi, U. (2015). Level Up Your Strategy: Towards a Descriptive Framework for Meaningful Enterprise Gamification. *Technology Innovation Management Review*, 5(8), 5–16. DOI: 10.22215/timreview/918

Sailer, M., Hense, J. U., Mayr, S. K., & Mandl, H. (2017). How gamification motivates: An experimental study of the effects of specific game design elements on psychological need satisfaction. *Computers in Human Behavior*, 69, 371–380. DOI: 10.1016/j.chb.2016.12.033

Schmutz, J. B., Meier, L. L., & Manser, T. (2019). How effective is teamwork really? The relationship between teamwork and performance in healthcare teams: A systematic review and meta-analysis. *BMJ Open*, 9(9), e028280. DOI: 10.1136/bmjopen-2018-028280 PMID: 31515415

Shah, M. K., Gandrakota, N., Cimiotti, J. P., Ghose, N., Moore, M., & Ali, M. K. (2021). Prevalence of and Factors Associated With Nurse Burnout in the US. *JAMA Network Open*, 4(2), e2036469. DOI: 10.1001/jamanetworkopen.2020.36469 PMID: 33538823

Trist, E. L., & Bamforth, K. W. (1951). Some Social and Psychological Consequences of the Longwall Method of Coal-Getting: An Examination of the Psychological Situation and Defences of a Work Group in Relation to the Social Structure and Technological Content of the Work System. *Human Relations*, 4(1), 3–38. DOI: 10.1177/001872675100400101

Verkuyl, M., Lapum, J. L., Hughes, M., Romaniuk, D., & Garcia, S. (2021). Emergency response training using gamification: Impact on collaboration among nurses. *Nurse Education Today*, 100, 104835. DOI: 10.1016/j.nedt.2021.104835

Werbach, K., & Hunter, D. (2012). For the Win: How Game Thinking Can Revolutionize Your Business. *In Wharton Digital Press*. Wharton Digital Press. DOI: 10.1017/CBO9781107415324.004

Weretecki, P., Greve, G., Bates, K., & Henseler, J. (2021). Information management can't be all fun and games, can it? How gamified experiences foster information exchange in multi-actor service ecosystems. *International Journal of Information Management*, 61, 102391. DOI: 10.1016/j.ijinfomgt.2021.102391

West, M., Armit, K., Loewenthal, L., Eckert, R., West, T., & Lee, A. (2015). *Leadership and leadership development in health care: The evidence base.*

Wirani, R., Sutanto, R., & Nugroho, D. (2022). The role of gamification in enhancing student engagement in online learning: A systematic review. *Education and Information Technologies*, 27(4), 567–589. DOI: 10.1007/s10639-021-10756-3

Xi, N., & Hamari, J. (2020). Does gamification affect brand engagement and equity? A study in the context of branded apps. *Journal of Business Research*, 109, 449–460. DOI: 10.1016/j.jbusres.2019.11.058

Zainuddin, N., Jaafar, M., & Harris, J. (2022). Gamified remote monitoring for chronic illness: Engaging patients and healthcare teams. *International Journal of Medical Informatics*, 162, 104749. DOI: 10.1016/j.ijmedinf.2022.104749

Chapter 3
Green Marketing and the Competitive Edge in the Cosmetics and Wellness Products Sector:
An Exploratory Research

Priscila Junkes
Polytechnic University of Cávado and Ave (IPCA), Portugal

Bruno Barbosa Sousa
https://orcid.org/0000-0002-8588-2422
Polytechnic University of Cávado and Ave (IPCA), Portugal & Applied Management Research Unit (UNIAG), Portugal

ABSTRACT

The research was conducted with the aim of determining whether Green Marketing can be considered a competitive advantage in the cosmetics sector. Given the increase in environmental awareness and the growing demand for sustainable products, understanding the impact of Green Marketing is essential for companies seeking to differentiate themselves in the market and attract conscious consumers. The main objective of the research was to evaluate the effectiveness of Green Marketing in providing a competitive advantage, analyzing both the practices of companies and the perception of consumers. To this end, the research used a qualitative approach that included interviews with representatives of cosmetics companies and focus groups with consumers. The research underlines the importance of addressing challenges such as cost and lack of awareness to promote more sustainable consumption and broaden the acceptance of eco-friendly products.

DOI: 10.4018/979-8-3693-8598-2.ch003

1. INTRODUCTION

Green Marketing emerged as a response to growing environmental concerns and increased consumer awareness of sustainability. Environmental issues are currently a priority worldwide, leading companies to adopt environmentally responsible practices in their marketing strategies. Green Marketing encompasses both the promotion of products with a lower environmental impact and the communication of sustainable practices, seeking to engage consumers in a more conscious way.

The demand for sustainable products reflects a significant shift in consumption patterns. Consumers are not only looking for products that meet their functional needs, but also those that are aligned with their environmental values. In the cosmetics sector, this trend is evident in factors such as the sustainability of packaging, the origin of ingredients and production processes, which are increasingly influencing purchasing decisions.

For companies, adopting Green Marketing not only meets consumer demands, but also represents a strategic opportunity to differentiate themselves in the market. Sustainable practices strengthen brand image, increase customer loyalty and provide a competitive advantage in an increasingly competitive environment. However, it is crucial that these practices are authentic, avoiding the phenomenon known as greenwashing, which can undermine consumer trust.

This study investigates how Green Marketing can provide a competitive advantage in the cosmetics sector, analyzing sustainable practices and their influence on consumer perceptions in Brazil and Portugal. The research adopts a qualitative approach, allowing a deeper understanding of consumer motivations and preferences regarding Green Marketing.

2. LITERATURE REVIEW

2.1. Green Marketing and Its Evolution

Constant changes in the market, technological innovations and regulatory requirements represent significant challenges for organizations, which need to find sustainable ways to position themselves (Moreira, 2015). In this scenario, green marketing emerges as a response to the demands for more responsible practices. This new approach, also known as environmental or ecological marketing, aims to reconcile environmental concerns with the essence of marketing, which is to encourage consumption (Brandão et al., 2011). Thus, companies are challenged to adopt strategies that not only promote sustainable products, but also align with the expectations of an increasingly conscious public.

Green marketing promotes awareness about the preservation of natural resources and collective responsibility (Monteiro et al., 2014). In recent years, sustainable development and social responsibility practices have become central to companies, given the pressure for viable and environmentally appropriate solutions (Dalmoro et al., 2009). Although often associated with ecological products, the concept of green marketing goes beyond this, encompassing broader sustainable management strategies. This evolution reflects the need for companies to adapt to a changing environment, where sustainability is a critical success factor.

With the growing relevance of conscious consumption and anti-consumption movements, green marketing has become a strategic tool for companies, giving them a competitive advantage by aligning their practices with environmental and social expectations (Monteiro et al., 2014; Moreira, 2015). In this context, this study seeks to understand how Green Marketing impacts the competitiveness of companies in a scenario of global changes, highlighting its importance not only for environmental preservation, but also for customer loyalty.

The evolution of green marketing can be divided into three phases, according to Purwanti et al. (2019). The first phase, called "environmental marketing", focuses on solving specific environmental problems, such as pollution and resource depletion, through reactive marketing practices. The second phase, "Environmental Green Marketing", expands the focus to technological innovations and sustainable products, recognizing that ecological practices bring competitive advantage and address global issues such as climate change. The third phase, "Sustainable Green Marketing", integrates sustainability as an essential strategy for companies, incorporating environmental costs into planning and production, aiming for a truly sustainable economy. These phases illustrate the transition from a reactive to a proactive approach, where sustainability is seen as an opportunity for innovation.

This progress reflects a shift in vision, where sustainability is not just a regulatory requirement, but a source of innovation and competitiveness. Green marketing requires a holistic approach, different from traditional marketing, focusing on the long term and integrating sustainable practices at all levels of the organization. This paradigm shift is essential for companies to stand out in an increasingly competitive and demanding market.

Silva et al. (2022) complement this view, highlighting that green marketing connects companies, consumers, and the environment through the "4 Ss ": Satisfaction, Safety, Social Acceptance, and Sustainability. Throughout the product life cycle, green marketing educates consumers and promotes environmental preservation, becoming key to attracting and retaining customers in a market increasingly oriented towards sustainability. In this way, green marketing becomes a strategy not only for communication, but also for relationships with consumers, who seek brands that reflect their values.

Sustainability, according to Hu et al. (2022), refers to the ability to meet current needs without compromising future generations, supported by economic, social and environmental pillars. Introduced by the Brundtland Commission in 1987, this concept gained traction in the 1980s and 1990s, integrating economic growth with environmental preservation. Global awareness has driven public policies and business practices focused on sustainability. This movement has not only shaped the way companies operate, but has also influenced consumer behavior, which now prioritizes sustainable practices.

Oliveira (2019) highlights that growing environmental awareness has led to the adoption of practices such as organic farming, biodiesel, and recycling, with companies and institutions promoting conscious consumption and sustainability through the principles of reducing, recycling, and reusing. This meets the growing consumer demand for environmentally friendly products and drives innovation. Thus, the integration of sustainable practices has become not only a response to market demands, but an opportunity for competitive differentiation.

Padilla and Collazzo (2022) emphasize that adopting everyday sustainable practices, such as recycling and reuse, is essential to preserve quality of life and ensure resources for future generations. Companies are rethinking their business models, recognizing that sustainability is not just a response to external pressures, but a strategic opportunity for innovation and long-term value. This perception is fundamental, as sustainability becomes a central pillar in contemporary business strategies.

Furthermore, the social aspects of sustainability have gained relevance, with corporate social responsibility becoming crucial for the survival of organizations. Companies that contribute positively to society differentiate themselves in conscious markets, making sustainability central to their strategies for a balanced future (Hu et al., 2022). In this context, integrated social responsibility, according to Steiner and Calgaro (2023), must be part of the company's daily operations, going beyond philanthropy.

Social responsibility goes beyond philanthropy and should be part of a company's daily operations. Companies that neglect environmental aspects, such as the preservation of fauna and flora, lose credibility and face social and environmental criticism (Santos & Luz, 2024). This understanding is vital, as corporate reputation is increasingly influenced by transparency and environmental responsibility.

On the other hand, Motta and Oliveira (2007) note that the focus on unbridled consumption aggravates environmental and social problems. Societal marketing emerges as a response, integrating social and environmental concerns into business strategies, promoting long-term well-being. Thus, reflection on the impacts of business actions becomes an essential component of the marketing strategy.

Eco-marketing, as an extension of societal marketing, aims to achieve a beneficial exchange for society and the environment, encouraging sustainable development. Companies that adopt green practices are able to differentiate themselves in the market, taking advantage of competitive opportunities linked to environmental responsibility (Motta & Oliveira, 2007). This differentiation is crucial in an environment where consumers are increasingly demanding regarding sustainability.

The long-term survival of companies depends on sustainable practices, and the growing pressure for environmental responsibility creates opportunities to stand out, contributing to a more balanced future (Motta & Oliveira, 2007). Thus, sustainability is seen not only as an obligation, but as a differentiation strategy that can generate significant economic benefits.

Green marketing emerges as a response to the increase in unbridled consumption and the consequent environmental degradation, problems that have intensified since the Industrial Revolution (Sá et al., 2017). This approach seeks to incorporate sustainability into business strategies, promoting environmentally friendly products that are aligned with the expectations of conscious consumers (Sá et al., 2017). However, according to Oliveira and Sousa (2019), the acceptance of these products is not always guaranteed, since many consumers are still reluctant to pay more for environmentally superior products, requiring specific marketing strategies to overcome this barrier. Therefore, effective communication and consumer education are essential for the success of green marketing.

Monteiro et al. (2014) emphasize that green marketing is not limited to the promotion of sustainable products, but involves a cultural transformation in companies, committing to environmental responsibility in all their operations. This effort is essential to attract consumers who seek environmental quality and wish to minimize the impact of their consumption choices. Thus, companies that adopt green marketing not only improve their image, but also contribute to the formation of a more responsible market.

Xavier and Chiconatto (2014) add that green marketing encompasses both consumer goods and services, with the aim of satisfying human needs and minimizing environmental damage. At the same time, Bashar et al. (2023) highlight the importance of integrating green marketing strategies internally, involving employees and consumers in the commitment to sustainability. This engagement is essential to create an organizational culture that values sustainability.

In addition to creating commercial value, green marketing also promotes a positive image of companies, which can generate a competitive advantage in the market (Dalmoro et al., 2009). However, as Brandão et al. (2011) point out, the implementation of this concept presents significant management challenges, requiring a comprehensive strategic approach that includes everything from the product life cycle to the " greening " of the marketing mix. These challenges require a serious commitment on the part of companies for green marketing initiatives to be effective and bring lasting results.

Therefore, implementing green marketing is not just a matter of compliance, but a strategic step towards sustainability. Companies that recognize the importance of this concept not only ensure their survival in a competitive market, but also position themselves as leaders in a sustainable future.

3. METHODOLOGY

The methodology adopted for this research aims to investigate whether Green Marketing can offer a competitive advantage to brands, using a qualitative approach. According to Denzin and Lincoln (2006), qualitative research is naturalistic, investigating phenomena in their natural contexts through interpretative practices that seek to understand the world in a holistic way. This approach allows for an in-depth and contextualized analysis, which is essential to understanding the dynamics of Green Marketing. Fonseca (2007) adds that qualitative researchers use phenomenological techniques, analyzing phenomena based on their own perceptions to extract meanings.

Serrano (2004) highlights that this approach is hermeneutic, phenomenological, and interpretative, and theory is constructed throughout the process of data collection and analysis, an approach known as "grounded theory" (Bogdan & Biklen, 1994). This continuous process of knowledge construction reflects the complexity of the phenomena studied, allowing for richer and more relevant insights. Costa et al. (2021) reinforce that knowledge is generated continuously as data are interpreted.

Carmo and Ferreira (2008) describe qualitative methods as humanistic, focused on the in-depth understanding of individuals' everyday experiences. The researcher is the main instrument of data collection, and it is crucial that the data accurately reflect the participants' expressions and behaviors. This relationship between researcher and participants is essential for the validity of the results obtained. Qualitative research does not aim at generalization, but rather at the applicability of the results to similar contexts.

To achieve the objectives of this study — to understand the role of Green Marketing in companies, identify whether it offers a competitive advantage, and assess its impact on image and customer loyalty — semi-structured interviews were conducted with representatives of companies in the cosmetics sector and a focus group with Brazilian and Portuguese consumers. Lanka et al. (2020) emphasize the value of qualitative research in obtaining multiple perspectives on a topic, analyzed in a subjective and interpretative manner. This approach allows for a more comprehensive understanding of Green Marketing practices and their implications for brand competitiveness.

This methodology will allow a detailed analysis of Green Marketing practices and their relevance as a competitive advantage in the cosmetics sector, considering both the companies' vision and the consumers' perceptions. Furthermore, the wealth of qualitative data generated can provide valuable information for the formulation of more effective strategies in this field. Qualitative research adopts several theoretical paradigms and methods, such as case studies, oral histories, interviews and ethnography, which allow a holistic understanding of social and human problems. According to Lanka et al. (2020), this approach aims to capture the experiences of participants in their natural contexts, integrating them into the organizational analysis.

Semi-structured interviews are a popular method for collecting qualitative data. Wahyuni (2012) highlights that this hybrid technique combines the structure of a pre-determined script with the flexibility to explore the themes in greater depth, promoting a richer understanding of the phenomenon studied. Sobh and Perry (2006) reinforce that interviews are essential to obtain relevant contributions to the case study. This flexibility is especially important in complex topics, such as Green Marketing, where nuances can reveal crucial information.

Another widely used method is the focus group, described by Malhotra (2002) as an effective technique for discussing issues of interest in a collaborative environment. Kitzinger (2000) points out that interaction between participants generates valuable insights, making this technique ideal for exploring perceptions and behaviors, especially in exploratory research. Morgan (1997) and Merton et al. (1990) indicate that the focus group is also useful for evaluating programs and generating new ideas. In this study, this method will be essential to capture the diversity of consumers' opinions and experiences regarding Green Marketing.

Data triangulation, according to Sobh and Perry (2006), is essential to ensure the reliability of the research, allowing the phenomenon to be observed from different perspectives. Wahyuni (2012) suggests that collecting data from multiple sources increases the relevance and consistency of the information, while Drucker-Godard et al. (2001) state that the integrity and competence of the researcher are crucial to the validity of the research. These aspects are particularly important when studying a dynamic and complex phenomenon such as Green Marketing.

In this study, these methods were used to investigate Green Marketing in the cosmetics sector. Interviews with companies and a focus group with Brazilian and Portuguese consumers allowed us to explore whether these practices offer a competitive advantage. In addition, analyzing consumer perceptions of sustainable brands can contribute to understanding how Green Marketing is perceived in the market. Data analysis involved triangulating information from the interviews and the focus group, seeking to identify patterns and trends relevant to the investigation.

4. ANALYSIS AND DISCUSSION OF RESULTS

The main objective of this study is to evaluate whether Green Marketing provides a competitive advantage for companies in the cosmetics sector. To this end, representatives of two companies were interviewed: Biocosméticos.ind (E1) and Bio Extratus (E2). Both work with natural and sustainable products, reinforcing practices such as the use of organic and vegan ingredients, in addition to demonstrating concern for sustainability and animal welfare.

The interviews, based on semi-structured questions, focused on three main objectives:

1. Understand the role of Green Marketing in organizations.
2. Assess whether these practices offer a competitive advantage.
3. Analyze the impact of Green Marketing on brand image and customer loyalty.

To achieve these objectives, the exploratory questions sought to identify the Green Marketing practices implemented by companies and how they influence consumer loyalty and purchasing decisions. Additionally, the contribution of these practices to the strategic positioning and sustainability of organizations was also assessed.

The qualitative methodology allowed the responses to be reflected and detailed, enriching the analysis of the role of Green Marketing as a strategy for differentiation and reputation strengthening in the cosmetics sector. This qualitative approach is essential to capture the nuances and complexities of the participants' perceptions.

In the analysis of data from the focus group, composed of 8 female participants, residing in Brazil and Portugal, aged between 24 and 41 and with varied academic backgrounds, six main themes were explored:

1. Perceptions about Green Marketing: Participants demonstrated a basic understanding of the concept, associating it with sustainable practices and ecological products.
2. Influence on Purchasing Decisions: The majority indicated that Green Marketing practices influence their purchasing choices, especially when they perceive transparency in companies' actions.
3. Communication and Transparency: Clear and honest communication about sustainable initiatives was highlighted as crucial to building trust in brands.
4. Personal Experiences: Participants shared experiences with green marketing products, pointing out both benefits and disappointments, especially regarding the quality and authenticity of the practices.
5. Barriers and Challenges: The main difficulties mentioned include high prices and distrust about the veracity of sustainable claims made by companies.

6. Future Expectations: Participants expect Green Marketing to evolve, with more transparency and greater accessibility to sustainable products.

These themes were analyzed to extract insights into the impact of Green Marketing on consumer perceptions and behaviors. The analyses carried out can contribute significantly to understanding the effect that sustainable practices have on the market and on the relationship between brands and customers.

5. DISCUSSION AND CONCLUSION OF THE DATA OBTAINED

The interviews conducted show that Green Marketing is understood and implemented in a detailed and conscious manner by the companies interviewed. The interviewees demonstrated a deep understanding of the concept, revealing that their green marketing practices are an authentic extension of the companies' environmental commitment, and not merely loyalty strategies. Both highlighted that their initiatives aim to positively impact the environment, reflecting a genuine focus on sustainability.

An essential aspect of Green Marketing is the **green marketing mix**, which encompasses sustainable practices across four main pillars: **Product, Price, Place and Promotion** .

Product: Companies that adopt green marketing must ensure that their products are designed in a sustainable manner, using natural ingredients, recyclable or biodegradable materials, and production methods that minimize environmental impact. Participants interviewed highlighted that companies aim to offer products that demonstrate environmental benefits, which is directly related to the adoption of environmentally friendly practices in product design and manufacturing.

Price: While sustainable practices may result in higher costs, companies must balance pricing with the value perceived by consumers. In Brazil, as identified in the responses of focus group participants, cost is a limiting factor for the adoption of sustainable products. Thus, companies need to educate consumers about the long-term value of green products and explore pricing strategies that make these items more accessible to different segments.

Place: Distribution of sustainable products should also consider reducing the carbon footprint by adopting more environmentally friendly transportation methods and distribution partners committed to green practices. In addition, promoting points of sale that highlight these products as part of a sustainability strategy can help increase awareness and availability to more conscious consumers, especially in markets with a more critical perception of Green Marketing, such as Portugal.

Promotion: Transparent communication and the promotion of sustainable certifications are crucial to avoid greenwashing and build consumer trust. The companies interviewed have demonstrated that they use multiple communication channels, such as labeling and digital media, to promote their green initiatives. In this context, educational campaigns that highlight the benefits of products and the authenticity of sustainable practices can help mitigate public distrust and increase consumers' emotional engagement with the brand.

Credibility remains a significant challenge for Green Marketing, with both interviewees highlighting the need to overcome public distrust. Post-consumer packaging recycling campaigns were identified as high-impact initiatives, as they directly engage consumers and foster a stronger bond with the brand. This active engagement demonstrates that sustainable actions can create a meaningful emotional connection with the public.

A brand's reputation, positively impacted by green marketing, contributes to consumer trust and loyalty. Even when there is no immediate purchase, associating a brand with sustainable practices reinforces its positive and responsible image. Transparency, clear communication about sustainable practices and the effectiveness of initiatives are essential elements for building and maintaining consumer trust.

Companies are clearly focused on communicating their sustainable practices through a variety of channels, including labeling, digital media, and in-person events. They are using certifications, audits, and direct engagement to ensure transparency and build trust. This effort is crucial to avoid greenwashing and meet the growing demand for environmentally responsible and natural products.

In short, Green Marketing not only helps companies differentiate themselves in the competitive cosmetics market, but also builds a solid base of loyal customers by aligning brand values with those of a growing audience that values sustainability. Effective Green Marketing strategies, therefore, are those that integrate authentic practices with clear and transparent communication, solidifying brands' position in the industry and meeting the expectations of increasingly conscious consumers.

The responses from focus group participants reveal a complex web of factors that influence the understanding and perception of Green Marketing in the cosmetics sector. The analysis shows that academic background and place of residence are significant determinants of how consumers understand and value sustainable practices. Participants with higher education and living in Portugal tend to have a more detailed and critical view of Green Marketing, which is reflected in a greater awareness and practical application of these concepts in their purchasing decisions. They expect high transparency, with detailed and verifiable information about products, as well as clear communication about the effectiveness and sustainability commitment of brands.

On the other hand, participants with less education or exposure to the topic, particularly in Brazil, reveal a more limited understanding and less consideration for sustainable practices. For these consumers, cost and lack of awareness about the benefits of sustainable products emerge as significant barriers to adopting conscious consumption practices. Lack of experience with sustainable products and the perception that product quality and performance may not meet their expectations are critical issues that brands need to address.

Brand loyalty is strongly influenced by personal values and the perceived authenticity of sustainable practices, especially among consumers with higher levels of education and living in Portugal. Although many participants see Green Marketing as a growing trend and essential for the future of the sector, the relevance of Green Marketing may vary based on cultural and educational factors.

In short, to gain and maintain consumer trust and loyalty, cosmetics brands must implement sustainable practices in a genuine and transparent manner, communicating clearly and in detail about the efficacy and benefits of their products. Education and awareness play a crucial role in promoting sustainable consumption, and brands must consider these variables when developing marketing and communication strategies to meet consumers' diverse expectations.

6. CONCLUSIONS

Analysis of the interviews and focus group reveals that Green Marketing, when applied in an authentic and transparent way, can offer a significant competitive advantage to brands in the cosmetics sector. The research shows that both companies and consumers genuinely value a commitment to sustainability, which can strengthen a brand's image and position in the market.

The interviewees emphasize that Green Marketing is not just a strategy to build customer loyalty, but rather an authentic expression of companies' environmental commitment. This is reflected in the way these brands integrate sustainable practices into their operations and in their communication with their consumers. Green Marketing helps to improve brand reputation, increase consumer confidence and, consequently, promote loyalty. The positive impact on brand image is evidenced by the association with sustainable practices, even when it does not result in an immediate purchase.

However, the interviews and focus group also indicate that the effectiveness of Green Marketing may vary based on factors such as educational attainment and place of residence. Consumers with higher educational attainment and who reside in more advanced environmentally conscious regions, such as Portugal, tend to demonstrate a more detailed and critical understanding of green marketing practices. These consumers expect full transparency and thoughtful information about products, which may increase their loyalty to brands.

On the other hand, consumers with less education or less exposure to the topic, such as those in Brazil, may have a more limited understanding and are more sensitive to factors such as the cost and performance of products, which may represent a barrier to the adoption of sustainable products. This scenario points to the need for adjustments in green marketing mix strategies.

Green marketing practices that focus on engaging consumers and concretely demonstrating the positive impact of sustainable actions tend to be most effective. Recycling campaigns and clear communication about sustainability practices are seen as key to building an emotional connection with the public and overcoming distrust. Transparency and authenticity are crucial to avoiding greenwashing and meeting the expectations of increasingly demanding consumers.

Therefore, Green Marketing offers a competitive advantage when it is implemented in a genuine, transparent way and aligned with consumer expectations. Brands that adopt and communicate sustainable practices effectively are able to not only differentiate themselves in the market, but also build a solid base of loyal and committed customers. The key to this competitive advantage lies in the ability to align authentic practices with clear communication, meet diverse consumer expectations and promote sustainability education.

7. RESEARCH LIMITATIONS

Research on the impact of Green Marketing on the competitive advantage of cosmetic brands faces several limitations that should be considered when interpreting the results. Firstly, the sample used is relatively small and specific, consisting of a limited number of interviews and a focus group. This may not capture the full diversity of perceptions and practices within the global cosmetics market, making it difficult to generalize the results to a wider audience.

Furthermore, the research focuses on participants from specific regions, such as Portugal and Brazil, which may limit the applicability of the findings to other markets with different cultural and economic dynamics. The lack of representation from other regions may affect the comprehensiveness of the conclusions.

Educational attainment and sustainability awareness also influence perceptions of Green Marketing, but the research may not have fully considered other socioeconomic and cultural factors that affect these perceptions. This may lead to a limited view of the impact of Green Marketing, without covering all relevant variables.

The research identified barriers such as lack of experience with sustainable products and cost as challenges to conscious consumption, but did not explore in depth other potential barriers, such as product availability in the market or the effectiveness of brands' communication strategies. This may result in an incomplete understanding of the challenges faced by consumers and companies.

Another important point is the potential response bias of interviewees and focus group participants. Their personal beliefs and experiences may influence their responses, which may introduce bias into reported perceptions. Furthermore, the cosmetics market and Green Marketing practices are constantly evolving, and current perceptions and practices can change rapidly with new trends, regulations and innovations, which may render research results obsolete over time.

Finally, the research focused mainly on aspects of awareness and perception, without addressing in depth the real effectiveness of Green Marketing practices in terms of brands' financial performance or effective environmental impact.

These limitations should be taken into account when analyzing the research results and considering possible future investigations that could provide a more comprehensive and detailed view of the impact of Green Marketing on cosmetic brands.

8. RESEARCH CONTRIBUTIONS

Research into Green Marketing and its influence on the competitive advantage of cosmetic brands offers several significant contributions to understanding the topic and developing effective strategies in the sector.

Firstly, the research provides a detailed insight into how Green Marketing is understood and implemented by companies in the cosmetics sector. The analysis reveals that green marketing practices are often an authentic extension of companies' commitment to sustainability, rather than merely strategies aimed at building customer loyalty. This understanding is crucial for brands that want to align their marketing practices with their true environmental initiatives, helping to avoid superficiality and greenwashing .

Furthermore, the research highlights the importance of transparency and clear communication about sustainable practices. Companies that take a genuine and detailed approach to sustainability tend to build a positive reputation and strengthen consumer trust. The evidence that recycling campaigns and other initiatives that directly engage consumers have a significant impact underscores the effectiveness of strategies that promote active engagement.

The research also links Green Marketing and consumer loyalty, showing that brands that demonstrate a genuine commitment to sustainable practices tend to attract and retain a loyal customer base. Understanding how factors such as educational background and geographic location influence the perception of Green Marketing is an important contribution to developing marketing strategies that consider cultural and educational variations among different target audiences.

Another important contribution is the identification of barriers to adopting sustainable practices, such as cost and lack of awareness. This insight is valuable for companies looking to overcome these barriers and improve the accessibility and attractiveness of their sustainable products. Understanding these challenges can help brands develop more effective strategies to promote conscious consumption and expand their customer base.

Furthermore, the research provides a basis for future research, suggesting areas that need further exploration, such as the actual effectiveness of Green Marketing practices in terms of financial performance and environmental impact. By addressing these gaps, future studies can provide a more comprehensive and detailed view of the impact of Green Marketing on the cosmetics sector.

In summary, the research contributes to the understanding of how Green Marketing can provide a competitive advantage for cosmetics brands, highlighting the importance of authentic practices, clear communication and consumer engagement. The findings offer valuable guidance for companies that want to align their marketing strategies with their sustainability initiatives and meet the expectations of an increasingly conscious and demanding audience.

REFERENCES

Alves da Silva, A., de São Pedro Filho, F., Vasconcelos de Melo, J., Veludo Watanabe, C. Y., dos Santos, M. C., & Imam, A. (2015). Innovating the Organization through the Green Marketing Strategy. *International Journal of Research en Social Sciences*, 11(2), 165–178.

Bashar, S., Wang, D., & Rafiq, M. (2023). Adoption of green supply chain management in developing countries: Role of consumer cooperation, eco-design and green marketing. *Environmental Science and Pollution Research International*, 30(40), 92594–92610. DOI: 10.1007/s11356-023-28881-3 PMID: 37495804

Bauer, M. W., & Gaskell, G. (2017). *Qualitative research with text, image and sound: a practical manual*. Editora Vozes Limitada.

Bento, K. D. (2020). Sustainability in shopping malls: The fusion between a green marketing tool and a competitive advantage strategy. *Revista Produção Online*, 20(3), 993–1016. DOI: 10.14488/1676-1901.v20i3.4049

Bogdan, R., & Biklen, S. (1994). Qualitative research in education: an introduction to theory and methods. Porto editora.

Brandão, M. R. M., de Oliveira Alexandre, M. L., Anez, M. E. M., & Costa, B. K. (2011). Stakeholder influence on the adoption of green marketing strategies. *Pretexto Journal*, 12(4), 2.

Carmo, H., & Ferreira, M. (2008). Research Methodology–Guide for Self-Learning (2nd edition). *Lisbon: Universidade Aberta, 15*, 16.

Costa, A. P., Moreira, A., & Sá, P. (2021). Reflections on Research methodologies: data analysis (Vol. 3). *Aveiro: University of Aveiro.doi:* DOI: 10.34624/dws9-6j98

Costa, C., Rocha, G., & Acúrcio, M. (2004). *Research methodology*. Faculty of Sciences of the University of Lisbon.

Coutinho, C. P. (2014). *Research methodology in social and human sciences*. Leya.

Dalmoro, M., Venturini, J. C., & Pereira, B. A. D. (2009). Green marketing: Social and environmental responsibility integrated into the marketing environment. *RBGN: Brazilian Journal of Business Management*, 11(30), 38–52. DOI: 10.7819/rbgn.v11i30.232

de Oliveira, C. P., & Sousa, B. M. (2020). Green consumer behavior and its implications for brand marketing strategy. In *Green Marketing as a positive driver for corporate sustainability* (pp. 69-95). IGI Global. Sustainable Management Practices: Green Marketing as A Source for Organizational Competitive Advantage. *Journal of Social and Environmental Management*, 18(4).

Denzin, N. K., & Lincoln, Y. S. (2006). Qualitative research design: Theories and approaches. *The Art of Medication.*

dos Santos, N. M., & da Luz, E. R. (2024). Social responsibility and sustainability under the influence of social marketing: A case study of a hospital. *Brazilian Journal of Business*, 6(3), e72215. DOI: 10.34140/bjbv6n3-017

Fonseca, J. R. S. (2008, July). Quantitative methods in sociology: difficulties of a research methodology. In *VI Portuguese Congress of Sociology–Social Worlds: Knowledge and Practices. Universidade Nova de Lisboa: Faculty of Social Sciences and Humanities* (p. 8).

Hu, H., Cohen, G., Sharma, B., Yin, H., & McConnell, R. (2022). Sustainability in health care. *Annual Review of Environment and Resources*, 47(1), 173–196. DOI: 10.1146/annurev-environ-112320-095157

Lanka, E., Lanka, S., Rostron, A., & Singh, P. (2020). Why we need qualitative research in management studies. *Journal of Contemporary Administration*, 25(2), e200297.

Monteiro, T. A., Giuliani, A. C., Pizzinatto, A. K., & de Toledo Pitombo, T. C. D. (2014). Consumer ecological awareness and green marketing: a case study on sustainable marketing practices in Brazil/ ecological awareness of the consumer and green marketing: a case study of sustainable marketing practices in brazil. [Santo Agostinho University Center]. *FSA Journal*, 11(2), 84–97.

Moreira, C. V. (2015). Green marketing as a sustainable competitive advantage for an organization. *Revista Foco*, 8(2), 133–144. DOI: 10.28950/1981-223x_revistafocoadm/2015.v8i2.183

Motta, S. L. S., & Oliveira, B. (2007). Ecological marketing as a competitive advantage. *REGE Management Journal*, 14(2), 49–59.

Nuryakin, N., & Maryati, T. (2022). Do green innovation and green competitive advantage mediate the effect of green marketing orientation on SMEs' green marketing performance? *Cogent Business & Management*, 9(1), 2065948. Advance online publication. DOI: 10.1080/23311975.2022.2065948

Oliveira, MLD (2019). Sustainable consumption behavior in thrift stores: an analysis of the influence of sociocultural factors on the purchase decision process.

Pacevičiūtė, A., & Razbadauskaitė-Venskė, I. (2023). The role of green marketing in creating a sustainable competitive advantage. *Regional training and development studies: journal of social sciences* ., (2), 89-98.

Padilla-Lozano, C. P., & Collazzo, P. (2022). Corporate social responsibility, green innovation, and competitiveness–causality in manufacturing. *Competitiveness Review*, 32(7), 21–39. DOI: 10.1108/CR-12-2020-0160

Purwanti, I., Abadi, M. D., Suyanto, U. Y., & Ahmad, S. T. I. E. K. (2019). Green marketing: Strategy for achieving sustainable competitive advantage in industry 4.0. *Management Bisnis*, 9(2), 176–193.

Radons, D. L., Battistella, L. F., & Grohmann, M. Z. (2012). Competitive advantage of companies: What is the influence of green innovation? *Brazilian Journal of Scientific Administration*, 3(3), 97–111.

Sá, J., Lins, N., Fonseca, R., & Santos, R. (2017). Green marketing-an analysis of Shell 's "make the future" campaign . *Veredas FAVIP: Electronic Journal of Science and Culture, 10* (1).

Serrano, G. P. (1994). *Investigation qualitative: straight and questioning* . Madrid: The wall .

Shaukat, F., & Ming, J. (2022). Impact of green marketing orientation on business performance: Case of Pakistani pharmaceutical industry. *Frontiers in Psychology*, 13, 940278. DOI: 10.3389/fpsyg.2022.940278 PMID: 36237687

Silva, P. C. D., Teixeira, R. L. P., & de Araújo Brito, M. L. (2022). The role of green marketing in advertising campaigns of cosmetics companies: an analytical and linguistic approach to the metaphorization of green: green marketing in cosmetics companies advertising campaigns: an analytical and linguistic approach to the metaphorization of Green. *Journal of Social and Environmental Management*, 16(2), e02996–e02996.

Sobh, R., & Perry, C. (2006). Research design and data analysis in realism research. *European Journal of Marketing*, 40(11/12), 1194–1209. DOI: 10.1108/03090560610702777

Sousa, T., Lopes, L., & Esteves, S. (2023). Sustainability and marketing: marketing strategies applied to green marketing and consumer perceptions. *IV International Meeting on Portuguese Language and Lusophone Relations*, 246-254. Steiner[1], VL, & Calgaro, C. Sustainability indicators and corporate social responsibility: a tool for assessing organizational sustainability indicators and corporate social responsibility: a tool for organizational assessment.

Veiga Neto, AR, de Paula Costa, F., Pereira da Silva, AW, Abbas El- Aouar, W., & de Lima Dantas, BL (2019). Environmental Marketing as a Business Strategy: Determining Factors According to Brazilian Advertisers. *Electronic Journal of Strategy & Business, 12* (1).

Wahyuni, D. (2012). The research design maze: Understanding paradigms, cases, methods, and methodologies. *Journal of applied management accounting research, 10* (1), 69-80.

Xavier, R. N., & Chiconatto, P. (2014). The Direction of Green Marketing in Organizations: Concept, Opportunities and Limitations. *Scientific-Electronic Capital Journal (RCC)- ISSN 2177-4153, 12* (1), 133-147.

Zhu, Q., & Sarkis, J. (2016). Green marketing and consumerism as social change in China: Reviewing the literature. *International Journal of Production Economics*, 181, 289–302. DOI: 10.1016/j.ijpe.2016.06.006

Chapter 4
Harnessing Brainwaves: Advancing EEG-Based Interfaces for Next-Generation Healthcare

Piyali Datta
https://orcid.org/0000-0001-9966-6619
Institute of Engineering and Management, Kolkata, India

Mousumi Laha
Institute of Engineering and Management, Kolkata, India

ABSTRACT

Electroencephalography (EEG)-based Brain-Computer Interface (BCI) technology has appeared as a promising path for healthcare, contributing to novel solutions for detecting, treating, and dealing with neurological conditions. By capturing and construing the electrical activities of brain signals, EEG-based BCIs empower direct brain communication with external devices, circumventing traditional neural conduits. This chapter delves into the progress of EEG-based BCI devices, emphasizing their implication in healthcare, the technical challenges tangled, and their potential to transform patient care. The key objective is to deliver a detailed exploration of the development procedure of EEG-based BCI devices, emphasizing their applications in healthcare. The chapter includes the principles of EEG signal acquisition, the design and engineering of BCI systems, the employment of machine learning algorithms for signal decoding, and the clinical validation required for medical use. Moreover, it will discuss the prospective effect of these devices on healthcare and future research directions.

DOI: 10.4018/979-8-3693-8598-2.ch004

1. INTRODUCTION

The human brain produces electrical signals which replicate a broad range of cognitive and motor activities. Electroencephalography (EEG) is a non-invasive process of recording electrical signals and it has been extensively used in clinical situations to identify and monitor neurological situations such as sleep disorders, epilepsy, and brain injuries to name only a few (Wolpaw et al., 2000; Blankertz et al., 2004). With BCI technology, EEG has extended new implications as a tool for rendering brain activity into actionable instructions to control external devices (Millan et al., 2004; Pfurtscheller et al., 2000). The importance of EEG-based BCIs in healthcare is in their capability to reinstate lost functions, improve cognitive abilities, and offer new forms of communication for people with severe infirmities. To exemplify, people with Amyotrophic Lateral Sclerosis (ALS) or locked-in syndrome can practice EEG-based BCIs to converse by picking letters or words deploying their brain activity (Blankertz et al., 2004). Likewise, these devices have been engaged in neuro-rehabilitation, permitting patients to recover motor regulators after a stroke by training neural paths through BCI-driven trainings (Pfurtscheller et al., 2000; Birbaumer et al., 2006).

1.1. Categories of BCI Systems

1.1.1 Invasive / Non-Invasive BCI System

In invasive type BCI system, microelectrodes are embedded inside the skull of the subject (e.g. Electrocorticography (ECoG)). On the contrary, the non-invasive BCI devices require observing electrical brain action by retaining the electrodes on the scalp (e.g. Electroencephalography (EEG)).

1.1.2 Synchronous / Asynchronous BCI System

The BCI system of synchronous type is cue-based, referring to the user yields particular mental states by undertaking certain mental tasks in a prescheduled period with a system-initiated control. The asynchronous type BCI system is not cue-based, rather the user has freedom to initiate any specific mental task that is deliberated as control signal. Therefore, the control is initiated by the user instead of the system.

1.1.3 Universal / Individual BCI System

Universal BCI systems allows the EEG data to be acquired from various subjects for feature extraction and classification which is appropriate for any person, whereas an individual BCI system only allows to collect the EEG data from individual subject assuming that no two individuals are identical.

Figure 1. (a) Different human lobes and their associated functionalities; (b) General steps of BCI system development.

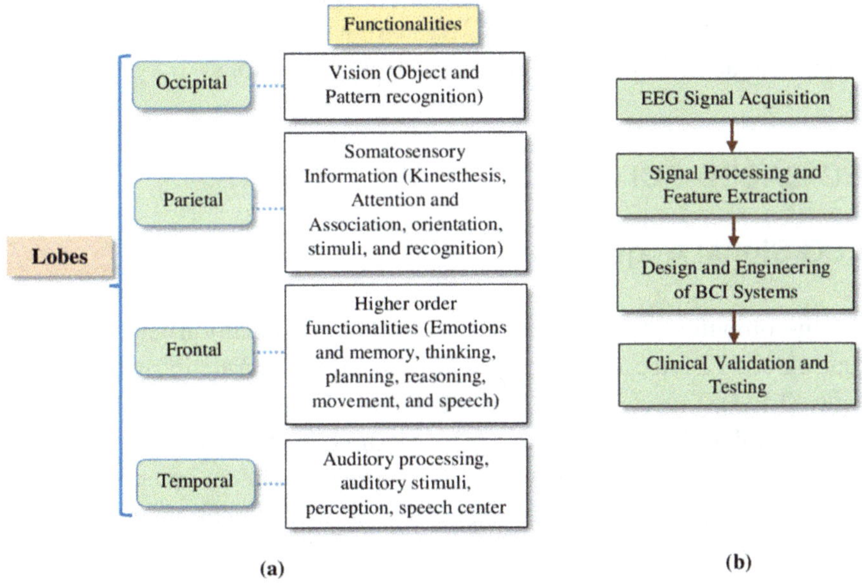

1.1.4 Offline / Online BCI System

In an offline BCI system, the EEG data are logged and captured deploying more electrodes. These records are archived and analyzed later to develop the BCI systems or for BCI research. The online BCI systems, on the flipside, are the real-time working systems providing feedbacks to the users.

1.1.5 Imagery / Mental Task BCI System

The imagery BCI systems belong to the user's point of view i.e. depend on the type of imaging function which the users are essential to accomplish such as motor imagery. BCI system for mental tasks comprises arithmetic tasks like visual tasks (e.g geometric figure rotation), visual counting tasks, and so on.

1.1.6 Exogenous / Endogenous BCI System

The Exogenous BCI systems are induced depending on stimulus that needs minimal training. The Endogenous BCI Systems are habitually self-generated being independent of any stimulus like cursor control applications.

2. EEG-BASED BCI DEVICES DEVELOPMENT

2.1 EEG Signal Acquisition

A brain-computer interface is a kind of direct communication between the human brain and external devices through brain activity signals, particularly electroencephalography (EEG) (Lee et al., 2023; Medina et al., 2024). EEG signal acquisition is the fundamental basis for BCI systems since it directly affects the interface's quality, accuracy, and efficacy. Thus, the article discusses various techniques that can be used for EEG signal acquisition in BCI systems based on principles, methodologies, and applications. This method of recording electrical activity generated by oscillations in the brain is known as EEG. The firings of neurons bring about these oscillations and produce voltage fluctuations that can be measured on the scalp and other parts of the head. The process of acquiring the signal includes electrodes that detect these electrical patterns, amplifiers for boosting weak signals, and analog-to-digital converters for preparing data for processing. For the majority of BCI systems, EEG is the preferred modality because it is non-invasive and economical while offering valuable information concerning real-time brain activity. However, the success in acquiring EEG depends highly on techniques that can capture accurate brain electrical activity while trying to minimize artifacts and noise. Figure 1(a) depicts various portions of human brain and their associated functionalities.

A. Electrode-Based EEG Signal Acquisition

Electrodes form a very crucial part in EEG acquisition. The configuration and type of electrodes used significantly affect the signal fidelity. Some of the most common types of electrode configurations include;

(i) Wet Electrodes:

Wet electrodes are highly considered as the highest quality for recording very clean and accurate brain activity. Using conductive gel or paste, these electrodes have low impedance hence resulting in minimizing noise and allowing proper neural oscillations measurements over a very wide frequency range. This is particularly useful for long-duration studies such as sleep monitoring and diagnostics of epilepsy where signal stability is very important. However, wet electrodes have disadvantages for instance the tremendous time in setting them up, which begins with preparation of the scalp and application of the gel.

(ii) Dry Electrodes:

Dry electrodes have found their convenient replacement for wet electrodes in bioelectrical signal recording, especially in such portable and wearable BCI applications. Made from materials like silver or gold, they can be avoid conductive gels and can set up quickly to offer greater user convenience.

(iii) Hybrids Electrodes

Hybrid electrodes combine features from wet and dry electrodes, for example, trace amount of gel in semi-dry setup. It retains the dual objective of practicality and quality of the signal. Hybrid electrodes are coming to be a potential solution for wearable BCIs especially in rehabilitation and gaming.

B. Scalp-Based EEG Acquisition Techniques

Acquiring EEG signals is done in standard systems like the 10-20 or the 10-10 international system that guarantees identical placements of scalp electrodes and standard coverage of brain regions. To increase spatial resolution to localize the brain activity appropriately, HD-EEG systems use between 64 to 256 electrodes. Preparation time, and computational demands for HD-EEG systems might be increased, and it can cause discomfort to the participants. In contrast, low-density EEG systems (8-32 electrodes) focus on easy setup, cost-effectiveness, and ease of use aspects that make them available for clinical and real-world applications. On the other hand, the systems offer reduced spatial resolution and decreased classification accuracy; hence there is a trade-off between practicality and detailed neural signal analysis.

a. Invasive and Non-Invasive Techniques

EEG involves placing electrodes on the scalp. Due to this safety, ease of use, and adaptability, this method has been popularly used in various domains, including healthcare, education, and assistive technologies, towards the development of a brain-computer interface. However, despite its popularity, the non-invasive technique always limits the spatial resolutions relative to invasive techniques and is susceptible to artifacts affecting data quality and precision. Conversely, invasive EEG is also termed as ElectroCorticoGraphy (ECoG), where the placement of electrodes are implanted under the skull directly on the cortical surface. This gives the following significant advantages: higher signal-to-noise ratio, better spatial localization, and high-frequency brain activity recording, thereby using it for more advanced applications, such as epilepsy research and BCIs for locked-in syndrome patients. Therefore, the invasiveness of ECoG poses surgical risks, affects ethics, and considerably limits adoption outside the clinic while making explicit trade-offs between precision and accessibility.

b. Advanced EEG Acquisition Techniques

The new approaches work well in improving the acquisition of EEG in BCIs and in enhancing traditional approaches to gain new avenues in applications. The portability of such a system is guaranteed, as wireless EEG systems using Bluetooth or Wi-Fi to send signals to processing units can enhance the ability to use it in the real world for applications in rehabilitation and gaming, for example. However, latency and electromagnetic interference might affect the functionality of these systems. Consumer-grade applications include relaxation, focus tracking, and entertainment applications, which the user-friendly wearable EEG system with integrated electrodes into a compact headband, cap, or helmet achieves. Another significant advancement is the integration of EEG systems with fNIRS for the real-time monitoring of electrical and hemodynamic brain activity. This dual-modality approach further enhances the character of brain activity, mainly for motor and cognitive tasks, with promising applications in neurorehabilitation and brain-behavior research. These advancements bring together improvements in the practicality, accessibility, and functionality of EEG-based BCI.

2.1.1 Artifact Management in EEG Acquisition

Artifacts are undesired signals interfering with EEG recordings, obscuring the actual brain activity patterns and thus interfering with the functionality of brain-computer interfaces (BCIs). Superior artifact management is essential to ensure reliable and accurate EEG data. Artifacts can be broadly classified into physiological and external types. Physiological artifacts originate from the physiologic activities of the human body, such as eye movement (electrooculography, EOG), muscle activity (electromyography, EMG), and cardiac signals (electrocardiography, ECG). These internal signals may overlap with neural activity, making data interpretation difficult. External artifacts arise from sources such as electromagnetic interference, or electrode motion and poor contact between the electrode and skin. Such artifacts are typically problematic in any mobile or real-world applications of EEG.

To overcome such issues researchers have taken recourse to hardware and software strategies. Hardware-based strategies are to design better electrode designs with improved stability and to take shielding action to minimize interference from external sources. This enhances the quality of source signal acquisition. Software approaches form the core of the post-processing EEG data as it involve sophisticated processing techniques like Independent Component Analysis and adaptive filtering. This has effectively separated and removed artifacts while leaving meaningful brain activity patterns. With both hardware and software approaches combined, artifact reduction supports significant improvements in the accuracy and reliability of BCIs for varied applications.

2.1.2 Signal Quality Metrics

Robust EEG performance is ensured only when signal quality is properly evaluated in real-time during acquisition. The SNR, or signal-to-noise ratio, is a measure of the clarity of the EEG signal relative to background noise. It provides the most basic indicator of data reliability. Another important parameter is impedance levels: high electrode-skin impedance means poor electrical contact, and higher recording fidelity with less noise that would otherwise have been picked up from loose or non-compatible electrode/skin interfaces. There are also spectral characteristics that need to be assessed; these are power distribution within various frequency bands, such as delta, theta, alpha, beta, and gamma, and also meaningful brain activity patterns. Monitoring during the data collection process ensures achievement both in terms of accuracy as well as usability in the acquired signals, hence enhancing effectiveness and reliability with regard to the applications of brain-computer interfaces.

2.1.3 Applications of EEG Signal Acquisition in BCIs

The techniques of EEG signal acquisition shape the applications of brain-computer interface systems, which have multiple uses and impacts in various disciplines. Medical diagnostics use EEG signals in following neurological conditions such as epilepsy, sleep disorders, and injuries to the brain providing insight into the patterns of activity related to the brain diagnosis and consequent treatment planning (Lee et al., 2023; Medina et al., 2024). Motor imagery BCIs help stroke victims regain their motor functions by exercising mental exercises on the restoration of motor functions. BCIs ensure the exploration of neuroplasticity in the brain and, therefore, help patients regain motor control and achieve a better quality of life. Communication is the other significant application for those with severe paralysis since BCI permits control of text, speech, or a cursor on a screen through brain signals, greatly enhancing their independence (Birbaumer et al., 2006). As far as gaming and entertainment, the interaction provided in EEG-based systems is based on the cognitive or emotional states of the player and, thus, allows for more immersive environments. These can measure the focus or levels of relaxation to change game dynamics. In addition to this, neurofeedback techniques in education and training are used to enhance learning and concentration by providing real-time feedback of brain activity so that the user can better optimize focus for better performance.

2.2 Signal Processing and Feature Extraction

In the context of BCIs, signal processing and feature extraction are some of the important phases to which raw EEG data is subjected before it is transformed into usable information that will ultimately be used for controlling devices or systems. This begins at the acquisition of EEG signals where rigorous techniques in signal processing can be considered-the intent being to clean up the data, extract relevant features, and prepare it for further analysis, classification, and interpretation by machine learning algorithms. These steps directly affect the accuracy, speed, and reliability of BCI systems, which makes signal processing and feature extraction a necessity for their performance.

2.2.1 Preprocessing of EEG Signals

Such signals, although very informative and useful for the assessment of brain activity, are noisy and affected by various artifacts. Physiological artifacts include eye movements (electrooculography, EOG), muscle activity (electromyography, EMG), or cardiac signals (electrocardiography, ECG). External artifacts may be from electromagnetic interference or electrode motion. Before the actual feature extraction process starts, it is essential that signal processing techniques be applied to clean the data and remove or reduce unwanted components. Filtering is the first step in this process. Filtering aims at removing unwanted frequencies not relevant to the pertinent brain activity. The signal of the EEG typically spans an extended frequency range, although relevant ones differ with type of cognitive or motor task. For instance, it is often described to be associated with a relaxed state in alpha waves (8–13 Hz), active concentration or even motor activity in beta waves (13–30 Hz), and drowsiness or light sleep in theta waves (4–8 Hz). Applying band-pass filters eliminates the frequency of signals outside the range of interest, cleaning up the data to be more relevant for feature extraction. Artifact removal techniques are applied beyond the basic filtering to reduce the influence of nonneural signals. For instance, artifacts such as Independent Component Analysis can separate the mixed signals into independent components, making it easier for one to identify and remove artifacts. The other most commonly used method is adaptive filtering, which adjusts dynamically based on varying noise levels and conditions, thereby offering robust real-time removal of artifacts.

Figure 2. General flow of raw EEG signal processing and classification.

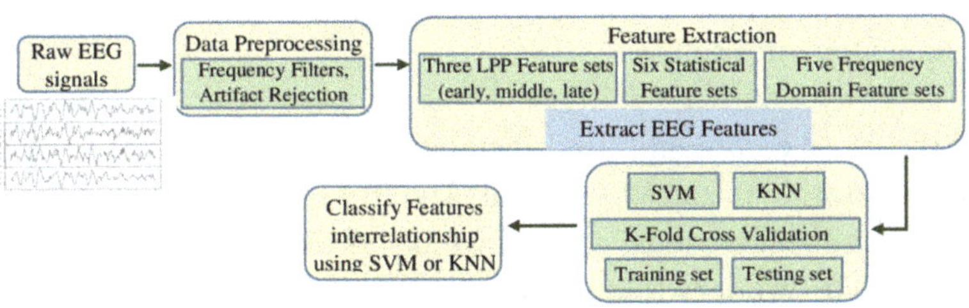

2.2.2 Segmentation of EEG Signals

Once the raw EEG data has been filtered, the next step is the segmentation of the signal into smaller epochs. Segmentation involves the division of the continuum of the EEG data into discrete time windows of 1 to 5 seconds, depending on an application. Each segment, or epoch, is examined in turn, ensuring a better capturing of the time resolution of brain activity associated with any specific event. For ERP-based BCIs, segmentation is typically based on stimuli or tasks. For a P300 speller system, for example, EEG data is segmented around the time when stimuli appear-on every screen flash, which may be a flashing letter or object associated with brain responses involving attention or recognition. Similarly, epochs are created during motor imagery tasks based on certain mental commands to detect brain activity patterns related to movement intentions. Segmenting the EEG signal is very important as that reduces the data to a time-specific window that could be analyzed for specific features that may have occurred in response to stimulus or even a cognitive task. This step aims to focus analysis on regions of the signal where it is most likely to be from significant brain activity while reducing computational complexity at the same time as maintaining the temporal integrity of data.

2.2.3 Feature Extraction from EEG Signals

The third primary operation in EEG signal processing, following preprocessing and segmentation, is feature extraction. Feature extraction can be defined as extracting and quantifying the specific features of the EEG signal representative of the underlying brain activity. The trained machine learning algorithms based on the data inferred, make interpretations about the intent of the user. Selection of appropriate features happens to play a major role in the performance of the BCI system because different features are sensitive to different kinds of brain activity. Many commonly practiced approaches extract features from EEG signals, which suit different kinds of brain activities or tasks.

A. Frequency Domain Features

One of the most commonly used methods for feature extraction is analyzing the **frequency domain** of the EEG signal. The EEG signal consists of oscillations across various frequency bands, each of which corresponds to different cognitive or motor states. The primary frequency bands of interest are:

- **Delta (1-4 Hz):** Associated with deep sleep or unconscious states.
- **Theta (4-8 Hz):** Linked to drowsiness, light sleep, and relaxation.
- **Alpha (8-13 Hz):** Typically observed during relaxed but alert states, such as when the eyes are closed.
- **Beta (13-30 Hz):** Associated with active thinking, problem-solving, or motor activity.
- **Gamma (30-100 Hz):** Linked to high-level cognitive functions, such as attention and sensory processing.

Feature extraction in the frequency domain usually operates by computing PSD (Power Spectral Density), which is a measure of the distribution of power across different frequency bands. In many BCI designs, perhaps one of the dominant features that pop up is this notion of relative power over certain frequency bands and its association with cognitive states or intentions. For example, increased alpha power is associated with relaxation, whereas increased beta power is often observed during motor imagery tasks. A commonly used feature in BCI systems is the power ratio between bands, such as an alpha/beta ratio.

B. Spatial Domain Features

Other than the frequency-based features, spatial features are crucial in spatially discriminating activity originating from different cortical regions. One of the most popular methods for extracting spatial features is CSP (Common Spatial Patterns). CSP is a technique of spatial filtering that aims to maximize variance for an EEG signal for a particular task such as motor imagery. The purpose of CSP is to find the spatial filters that maximize task-related activity, and minimize noise or unrelated brain signals. Then these spatial filters are used to extract features for classification from EEG data. Use of the CSP is best suited for applications such as motor imagery and movement-related BCIs, where the detection of brain activity associated with specific motor intentions is undertaken. This system can utilize spatial features to discover which parts of the brain are involved in processing the task and extract relevant signals for further analysis.

C. Time Domain Features

Spatial and frequency-domain features are quite common, although many applications of BCIs employ also time-domain features. They are based on raw EEG signals as well as on their statistical properties-mean, variance, or skewness of the signal within an epoch. Time-domain features are also easy to calculate but can be more useful where frequency or spatial domain features fail. The most common time-domain approach is Event-Related Potentials (ERPs). ERPs are a type of brain response that is time-locked to specific events or stimulation, such as a flashing letter in a P300 speller system or an effective cue for a motor imagery task. For example, the P300 is that positive deflection, appearing about 300 milliseconds after the presentation of a target stimulus, and its presence can be detected and used for BCI control.

D. Wavelet Transform

Another strong technique for feature extraction from EEG signals is the use of wavelets. While Fourier transforms provide only frequency information, wavelets allow a form of multi-resolution analysis that captures both the frequency and temporal characteristics of an EEG signal. The wavelet transform gives a time-frequency representation of the signal, which is well suited for non-stationary signals such as those typically arising in EEG. The features represented by wavelet coefficients become extracted in this de-composition of a signal, capturing how changes in brain activity occur over time, thus giving a more dynamic view of cognitive processes.

2.2.4 Classification and Interpretation of Features

The data then gets its features, relevant to EEG, which are applied to training the machine learning algorithms for classification. The goal of interpreting these features is in line with the intent or state of cognition of the user. Support Vector Machines (SVMs), LDA, and deep learning techniques are among some common algorithms that have been used here, with growing usage of BCI systems. Here, the features are mapped to specific commands or outcomes like moving a cursor on a screen, selecting a letter in a speller system, or controlling a robotic arm. The quality of the features extracted, the design of the classifier, and the number of training data used mainly determine the effectiveness of the classifier. Proper validation and testing must be performed to ensure that the system is capable of interpreting the user's intent accurately in real time.

2.3 Machine Learning and Classification

The BCI is an exciting frontier of neurotechnological possibility, one that allows people to communicate directly from the brain out to an external device. Yet it also points to the critical challenge in BCI systems: the interpretation of activity in the brain, captured by EEG signals, and translation into commands for prosthetic limbs, communication systems (Birbaumer et al., 2006), or other devices. One such aspect is the use of machine learning (ML), which provides a framework for identifying and decoding the intricate patterns contained in EEG data. This chapter delves into the application of ML in BCI by discussing classification, the issues of variability inherent in the EEG signal, and how these have been overcome in BCI designs to enhance their performance and adaptability.

2.3.1 The Role of Machine Learning in BCI

Machine learning, in the context of EEG-based BCIs, will mean training algorithms that recognize EEG patterns that could relate to such mental states or intentions (Lee et al., 2023; Medina et al., 2024). These states may include specific actions, such as motor imagery (moving an imaginary limb), selective attention, or even relaxation or concentration as types of emotions. The goal is to develop systems that translate mental states in real time into useful outputs, such as to operate a robotic arm, highlight letters in a speller system, or adjust the settings of some device, such as a wheelchair. EEG based BCI systems operate on recording electrical activity from the brain through sensors attached to the scalp, which, after processing, transforms into features to feed into learning algorithms. These are trained with some patterns within the data on specific mental states and would be able to classify a bit of new data as well as predict what a user wants. In that case, machine learning algorithms are crucial for the effectiveness of EEG-based BCIs because they provide a framework to decode and represent the electrical activity of the brain into commands for external devices.

A. Supervised Learning for Classification

One of the most commonly used machine learning paradigms in EEG-based BCIs is **supervised learning**, where the algorithm is trained on labeled data. In supervised learning, the training dataset consists of pairs of input features (EEG data) and the corresponding output labels (the intended mental states or actions). The machine learning model learns to map the EEG features to these predefined labels, allowing it to classify new, unseen EEG data into one of the known categories.

a. **Common Supervised Learning Algorithms**

Many supervised learning algorithms are applied to the classification of EEG signals for BCI systems, and each of them has its pros and cons. The most commonly used algorithm is:

- k-Nearest Neighbors (k-NN): It classifies a new data point depending on the majority class of its nearest neighbors in feature space. k-NN is simple, intuitive, and works well for most of the BCI applications, where the dataset is either small or moderately sized. However, it faces tremendous challenges with a large dataset due to high computation and sensitivity to noise in the data.
- Support Vector Machines (SVM): SVM is a classification algorithm in which data, in the majority, are classified using a hyperplane that best separates classes in high dimensional space. SVMs can be more efficient as they serve better for binary classifications and of late have been applied considerably to motor imagery BCIs to differentiate imagined hand movements from rest periods. SVMs are known to perform well on noisy data and well in high-dimensional feature spaces, though careful tuning of parameters such as the kernel and regularization term is needed.
- Deep Learning Algorithms: Latest of these promising algorithms are deep learning techniques, especially CNNs and RNNs developed for classifica-

tion purposes from EEG. These models can automatically learn the hierarchical representations from raw data without feature extraction by human beings. These models are very well-suited for spatial pattern recognition using CNNs and temporal processing capabilities in a sequential nature using RNNs. While deep learning models require as much labeled data as possible for effective training, they are also potentially more accurate than traditional machine learning models.

B. Training and Validation

The quality of the data used to train the machine learning algorithms determines their performance. For BCIs based on EEG, the training data are typically recorded in controlled experiments by directing participants to perform specific tasks, like imagining moving a limb or focusing attention on an object. Such tasks are labeled against the mental state they create and utilize the related EEG signals as input features in training the algorithm.

Testing the generalization capability of a learned model is typically carried out by splitting the dataset into two subsets, namely, the training subset and the testing subset. Here, the training data is used for training the model, and its generalization ability is tested against the testing data. Cross-validation techniques go even further; these aid in testing how robust the model is while preventing overfitting.

2.3.2 Challenges in Machine Learning for BCIs

While machine learning holds immense potential in BCI systems, several challenges must be addressed to ensure their successful implementation, particularly in the context of EEG signals (Lee et al., 2023; Medina et al., 2024).

A. EEG Signal Variability

One of the biggest challenges of making machine learning work with EEG-based BCIs is a large variance of EEG signals across different users and even across different sessions for the same user. In other words, the anatomy of people's brains and neural patterns are quite variable, and so a significant amount of differences will appear in EEG signals, even on the same task. This heterogeneity does make generalization of the models learned to users or sessions challenging as a model learned on data from one may not generalize well to data from another.

To these challenges, specific techniques were then developed to personalize the BCI system for each user. These techniques could be related to the adaptation of the machine learning model towards neural patterns of an individual or incorporating transfer learning.

Transfer learning involves the retraining of a predefined model by using a minimal amount of data belonging to a new user. Another such approach used is multi-session learning, wherein the model is actually trained on data from multiple sessions, so it could generalize better across time.

B. Feature Selection and Regularization

Feature selection is also one of the most significant aspects in the BCI system since there exist vast amounts of raw EEG data, all of which cannot be useful for classification. One feature could be some band of frequency or spatial pattern, and proper selection can drastically improve the model accuracy. The high-dimensionality of this dataset and overfitting make feature selection particularly difficult with respect to EEG data. The model learns to do well on the training data but fails to generalize to new data, which is known as overfitting. To counter overfitting, regularization techniques are utilized. Regularization methods like L1/L2 regularization penalize large weights in the model, preventing models from becoming overly complex and causing overfitting to the data.

Dimensionality is reduced with techniques like PCA or CSP for feature selection in order to extract relevant features.

C. Real-time Performance

Another requirement of machine learning for BCIs is real-time performance. In order to be practically useful, BCIs must extract EEG signals and make decisions in real time; such applications often need to offer low-latency outputs. Real-time classification is also computationally intensive in particular when deep learning models are applied. Thus, optimizing machine learning models towards real-time inference is an important step towards ensuring that BCIs can operate effectively in real-world application contexts, where fast user feedback is often required.

D. Data Imbalance

In most applications of BCI, data used to train the classifiers may be imbalanced; certain mental states or classes are underrepresented. For instance, a user may spend much more time resting or performing one type of action (e.g., imagining hand movements) than another. Such an imbalance can lead to biased classifiers that perform poorly on under-represented classes. Methods such as data augmentation, re-sampling, and class weighting can be highly helpful here as these techniques ensure the classifier is better trained on a more balanced representation of the data.

3. DESIGN AND ENGINEERING OF BCI SYSTEMS

The development of EEG-based BCI systems involves the integration of various hardware and software components of high importance ensuring the system works appropriately not only in terms of accuracy, reliability, and speed but also provide an intuitive and user-friendly interface for the end user. Not just the physiological requirements of EEG signal acquisition but also the computational complexities of signal processing and machine learning are considered by this design process, maintaining user comfort and system scalability.

This section briefly discusses the core parts of EEG-based BCI systems, especially how hardware and software can be integrated and some engineering challenges emerging in designing. It will look into some of the latest breakthroughs in BCI technology regarding wireless and wearable solutions with EEG that are revolutionizing the interaction patterns used with BCI technologies (Värbu et al., 2022; Wang et al., 2021).

3.1 Hardware Components in EEG-Based BCI Systems

These hardware components are made to capture electrical signals that come from the brain and then transmit them to an analysis device called a signal processing unit. The main components of this BCI are composed of EEG electrodes, a signal acquisition system, and amplifiers, with some setups containing additional accessories that include wireless transmission modules.

a. ***EEG Electrodes:*** The key source of recording electrical activity from the brain is EEG electrode. These sit on the scalp, following standardized international systems usually in 10-20 or 10-10 systems as discussed earlier; hence, uniformity is ensured in the placement of the electrode and coverage of different areas of the brain for better recording. EEG signal is largely a function of the quality and accuracy of electrodes selected.
b. ***Signal Acquisition Systems:*** Once the EEG electrodes capture the electrical activity from the brain, the raw signal must be transmitted to a processing unit for analysis. The signal-acquisition system is required to amplify the tiny electrical signals (on the order of microvolts) and transmit them to a central processing

unit. In BCIs, low-noise high-quality acquisition becomes critical as it goes into the interpretation of the signal.

These acquisition systems are typically composed of amplifiers that amplify the signals for an increase in strength and also analog-to-digital converters (ADCs), which are used to digitalize the analog signals for further processing. The type of amplifiers and ADCs employed in the acquisition system will significantly affect the performance of the BCI. These need also to be optimized with minimal noise and signal distortion while keeping latency as low as possible.

c. ***Wireless and Wearable EEG Systems:*** Connected electrodes to the signal processing unit through wires, which would limit the user's mobility and comfort, are required in traditional EEG systems. As BCI moves into more extensive real-world applications, more and more users are adopting the use of wire-free EEG systems. These systems use technology such as Bluetooth or Wi-Fi that can transfer EEG data wirelessly, thus giving increased freedom of movement to users and putting the system in a more desirable setting for daily use.

Wearable EEG systems integrate electrodes into compact, user-friendly headbands, caps, or helmets. These are lightweight and designed to be comfortable, making them ideal for long-term use in clinical, rehabilitation, or even home settings. All in all, wearable EEG systems are revolutionizing accessibility and usability in BCIs, letting users plug into neurorehabilitation equipment, communication aids (Birbaumer et al., 2006), or even gaming consoles with a more natural and seamless behavior.

The challenges for the wireless and wearable systems are to ensure reliable data transmission, minimum interference of signal, and power consumption management. With advancements in wireless communication protocols and energy-efficient designs, BCI applications will only open up more portable and accessible EEG-based BCI systems.

3.2 Software Components in EEG-Based BCI Systems

The software component of an EEG-based BCI is important to ensure that raw EEG data is processed, interpreted, and translated into meaningful actions. It involves several key stages, such as signal processing, feature extraction, classification, and user interface design (Lee et al., 2023; Medina et al., 2024).

a. ***Signal Processing:*** Signal processing is believed to be a very crucial stage in an EEG-based BCI system. Raw EEG signals contain a lot of noise and artifacts, which may result in failure in the correct interpretation of brain activity. Hence, signal processing algorithms clean up these unwanted components that would later reduce the quality of the signal before it is fed into feature extraction and classification. Common techniques applied include band-pass filtering where particular frequency bands of interest such as alpha, beta, or theta waves can be separated from the data stream, or artifact rejection techniques such as ICA or adaptive filtering for eye movement-related artifacts (EOG), muscle-related artifacts (EMG) or heartbeats-related artifacts (ECG). These initial stages allow the cleaning of data for better suitability to further analysis (Värbu et al., 2022; Wang et al., 2021).

b. ***Feature Extraction and Classification:*** Another major stage along the processing pipeline is feature extraction, from which relevant information is extracted from filtered EEG signals. The most widely applied features are frequency domain features including power spectral density, time-domain features such as waveforms or event-related potentials, and spatial features, like common spatial patterns or independent components. Those features are meant to represent different aspects of brain activity; with feature representation, specific mental states can be identified this case, motor imagery, attention, or relaxation. Once features are extracted, machine learning algorithms classify data to interpret the intent of the user as discussed earlier.
c. ***User Interface and Feedback***: Another integral part of BCI design is designing a user interface, which has to be an easy-to-use interface through which the individual can interact with the system. The user interface would have to provide appropriate real-time feedback to the user, meaning that the brain signals are being interpreted accurately, and the user could make adjustments if needed. In a clinical application, it might include controlling the arm of a robot or selecting text on a communication device. In a consumer application, it may include games or virtual environments. The interface needs to be as user-friendly as possible and accommodate the user's cognitive and physical abilities. Real-time feedback is particularly very crucial to train the user to control the BCI, for example, in motor imagery BCIs. Here, a subject can imagine that they are moving their limb to control a robotic prosthesis. Feedback is provided with visual or auditory cues within the interface and guides the user about how their mental state is being interpreted so that better performance is elicited.

3.3 Engineering Challenges in BCI Design

The design and engineering of EEG-based BCI systems pose numerous challenges that must be considered to enable the reliable, comfortable, and efficient operation of the system.

- User comfort and safety are of primary concern within the design of EEG-based BCIs, specifically with respect to electrode placement. Wet electrodes provide high-quality signals but are uncomfortable, especially when used for extended periods because gels or pastes have to be used. Dry electrodes are more comfortable but do not provide high-quality signals. Electrodes also need to sit securely on the head without slipping, allowing for irritation of the scalp or slipping of the electrodes. Safety considerations become issues for long-term or invasive systems, particularly in medical or rehabilitation use. Electrodes and ancillary hardware must be developed such that they cannot cause any injury to the skin or scalp, and the entire system must be considered for suitability for extended wear and use.
- ***Signal latency and real-time processing*:** For BCI systems to be effective, they need to be low-latency systems because they have to process user commands and execute them in real time (Birbaumer et al., 2006). This is particularly critical in applications like motor control or communication systems where the slightest delay can severely degrade the experience of the user. Hence, the phases of signal processing and classification should be optimized toward speed also, not at the cost of accuracy. Data transmission must be efficient with the proper hardware used, and software designed to actually process in real time must give feedback. Optimization of system performance also remains in terms of latency versus accuracy as a core engineering challenge.
- ***Scalability and User Adaptation*:** Another serious challenge in the engineering of these systems may be adapting the system to individual users. The brain activity of each person is unique, and therefore, the BCI must adapt to different users' neural patterns, cognitive states, and physical conditions. In some cases, one requires personal calibration and training protocols to optimize the system for each user, which may lead to complications during the design process.

4. CLINICAL VALIDATION AND TESTING

One of the most important steps would therefore be to determine and validate the clinical safety, efficacy, and usability of EEG-based BCI systems. Large-scale adoption of these systems in important areas of neurorehabilitation, assistive technologies for people with disabilities, and mental health treatments depends heavily on thorough and well-designed clinical trials. These studies evaluate the therapeutic values of BCI devices, understand the potential risks and side effects, and assist clinicians in better understanding the broader impact these technologies have on patients' lives. Clinical validation would include a wide variety of evaluations, ranging from physiological and psychological responses caused by BCI use to long-term studies designed to examine patient adaptation and the ability to personalize these devices. The following sections will detail the reason for clinical trials in the validation of EEG-based BCI, the methods involved, the challenges encountered during testing, and how this impacts the development and refinement of BCI technologies.

Clinical validation is important for EEG-based BCIs integration in mainstream health applications. In comparison, health-related BCIs can be different as they may require clinical validation and should be subject to strict medical standards due to the nature of application. It means that health-related BCIs must be tested with respect to their safety and effectiveness for specific patients with certain medical conditions. These devices aim at targeting users who have neurological disorders such as stroke, spinal cord injury, locked-in syndrome, epilepsy, or cerebral palsy, with therapies that were available previously being minimal or even of little effect.

The ultimate objective of clinical validation is to verify that the BCI system functions as expected in real clinical settings in providing measurable benefits to patients' conditions with no harm or discomfort incurred. Testing under these circumstances would involve testing not only the hardware and software components of the BCI but also its interplay with human physiology and psychology.

4.1 Types of Clinical Trials for EEG-Based BCIs

Clinical studies for EEG-based BCIs vary by the disease or condition being targeted, device functionality, and the developmental phase of the BCI system. Typically, these studies are phased and start with small pilot studies, followed by larger-scale, multicenter studies necessary to demonstrate short-term and long-term benefits of BCI systems.

4.1.1 Feasibility and Pilot Studies

First clinical trials often begin with feasibility and pilot studies. While the pilot studies are small-scale investigations intended to test the fundamental functionality as well as usability of the BCI system in actual clinical settings, feasibility studies assess the capability of integrating the BCI device effectively into the clinical workflow and its safe use by the patients with specific neurological conditions.

4.1.2 Randomized Controlled Trials (RCTs)

In the development of the BCI devices, their effectiveness is tested based on rigorous RCTs, where participants are assigned either to a treatment group that receives the actual BCI device or to a control group that receives an inert placebo or even standard treatment. RCTs provide maximum evidence relating to the therapeutic benefits of the BCI because they reduce bias and allow for the comparison of outcomes between groups.

4.1.3 Long-Term Studies and Adaptation

Long-term clinical studies should establish patients' adaptation to BCI systems over time. These studies evaluate the sustainability of improvement in cognitive or motor functions and the psychological and physiological effects of long-term BCI use. Patients that improve over the initial stages can start to show a decrease in returns followed by plateauing or even regression; these have to be investigated in finer detail so that adjustments can be made to the BCI device and the therapeutic approach.

4.2 Interdisciplinary Teamwork for Clinical Studies

Interdisciplinary teamwork may be required for clinical studies on EEG-based BCIs in such varied disciplines as engineering, neuroscience, medicine, psychology, and rehabilitation science. In all of these, the issue of system design, implementation, and patient care will be taken into account in close coordination.

- ***Collaboration with Clinicians*:** The development process for BCI systems for healthcare is centred on the clinician. Their input is crucial to determine appropriate populations for BCI intervention, clinically relevant outcome measures and how trials are designed to answer key questions about device safety and efficacy. Clinicians also provide crucial insight into how BCIs will be integrated into clinical practice and used either as a complement or enhancement of existing treatments.
- ***Participation by Neuroscientists and Engineers*:** Neuroscientists and engineers also feature prominently in validation. Neuroscientists provide in-depth knowledge of the electrical activity taking place in the brain so that they could accurately interpret EEG signals and identify which pattern of brain activity is most relevant to a specific clinical application. These systems are also designed and optimized by engineers, who ensure that the hardware and software of the BCI system are able to handle the complexity of processing

EEG signals and real-time feedback, as well as ensuring the device's safety and usability.

4.3 Clinical Validation and Testing Challenges

There are several challenges posed during the clinical validation and testing of EEG-based BCIs that restrain its development and diffusion.

a. Patient Variability

Among the big issues in BCI trials, some of them include tremendous variability between patients. EEG signals are extremely individualistic and highly susceptible to variations that vary in brain anatomy, cognitive abilities, and indeed motor functions. Such variations often make it difficult to make a system uniformly perform for all patients. Also, with time, the adaptability of a patient to a device varies greatly in terms of the specific conditions of the patient, the patient's preferences, and respective cognitive abilities. This variability requires personalized calibration of the BCI system, which is very expensive and time-consuming. Machine learning models and adaptive algorithms are used to individualize the system's performance to the specific patterns in neural inputs, but it remains an area where more research will be required for determining their usefulness.

b. Ethical and Privacy Issues

The employment of EEG-based BCIs in health care raises ethical issues on privacy concerns, especially in regard to the fact that a significant amount of sensitive neural information is collected and analyzed. With the fact that BCIs may potentially gain access into a person's mental state, therefore the storage, usage, and sharing of such information raise ethical management issues. Issues such as these need to come on the table to ensure patient privacy in the course of BCI use without predictable consequences and exploitation.

c. Cost and Accessibility

Another significant limitation of EEG-based BCIs to be widely used in healthcare is cost. Overall, the development and setup of the technology required for BCI devices are usually costly, both in terms of equipment and clinical infrastructure for testing and use. Progressing BCI technologies will require that these costs be toned down and accessibility improved to make this device available to a greater population of patients, especially in low-resource settings.

4.4 Incorporating Clinical Validation in Development of BCI

Outcomes of clinical studies and validation studies are important determinants for the foreseeable future of EEG-based BCI systems. Such studies are excellent sources of information on potential further optimizations of the said technologies that can be rendered more specific and tailored to meet patients' needs. In addition, the results from these trials contribute toward clinical guidelines that will serve as a basis for best practice in the use of BCI devices in healthcare. With further successful clinical trials, this technology is bound to gain more acceptance and be assimilated into the delivery of health care. Clinical validation, although tough, is necessary for ensuring that EEG-based BCIs are safe and effective for improved patient outcomes.

5. APPLICATIONS IN HEALTHCARE

5.1. Neurorehabilitation

It has been demonstrated that EEG-based BCIs have significant potential in neurorehabilitation, particularly for patients who are improving from stroke or traumatic brain injury. BCIs provide real-time feedback on their brain activity during motor tasks, making them useful in neural pathway reorganization and possible improvement of motor function (Värbu et al., 2022; Wang et al., 2021).

Case Study: EEG-Based BCIs in Neurorehabilitation for Stroke Recovery

- ***Background***

Stroke is considered one of the leading causes of long-term disability across the globe, as survivors suffer from impaired motor function. Recovery is often slow and incomplete, with many patients failing to regain full motor control, especially in the upper limb. Such traditional rehabilitation tools used are physiotherapy and occupational therapy, improving physical skills through exercises the number of repetitions could be limited based on the lesion degree and brain plasticity. In recent years, EEG-based Brain-Computer Interfaces (BCIs) have emerged as a promising technology for augmenting rehabilitation efforts, especially in patients recovering from stroke.

- ***Role of EEG-based BCIs in Stroke Rehabilitation***

The EEG-based BCIs should make neuroplasticity-the brain's ability to reorganize itself by forming new neural connections-effectively possible in the recovering stroke patient. BCIs provide an entirely new opportunity for engaging the brain at a finer grain of real-time feedback on its activity during motor tasks, which may help in "training" the patient by compensatory utilization of spared neural circuits for functional recovery. It aims not only at an increase in motor activity but also at better motor learning and adaptive behavior. While interacting with it in real time, during the course of interactions, patients' brains continuously provide feedback to the device, thus strengthening the neural pathways related to motor recovery.

Case Study: Using EEG-Based BCIs to Recover the Upper Limb Patient Background:

Mr. A is a 56-year-old male who had an ischemic stroke on the left side of the body that resulted in partial paralysis on the right. Even after six months of standardized rehabilitation, he regained little to no motor functions in his right arm and hand. The primary goals of Mr. A were to regain the ability to perform the activities of daily living, such as dressing and feeding himself, and to maximize the ability to grasp and manipulate objects.

- ***BCI Intervention*****:** Mr. A was recruited in a feasibility clinical study on EEG-based BCIs in neurorehabilitation. The study system was an EEG headset that picked up brainwave patterns responsible for motor imagery such as imagining to move his right arm. The BCI was fused with the robotic exoskeleton designed to facilitate arm movement. As he fantasized his right arm's movement, the BCI picked those waves and, based on the brain activity, converted them into robotics arm movements. The system allowed the user to receive direct visual feedback-by visualizing the virtual representation of his arm as he moved it or by showing the real movements of the robotic arm.
- ***Process*****:** During the rehabilitation sessions, Mr. A was encouraged to think through his right arm as if he were reaching out to grab something, lifting up a cup, or pressing a button. The BCI system, based on EEG, detected these brain signals and automatically gave feedback in the form of the movements of the robotic arm or virtual avatar that would indicate the correct movement. This feedback loop, over time, basically led his brain to strengthen the motor pathways and regain control over his right arm. BCI training sessions were performed for eight weeks; Mr. A attended five days in a week. These 30-minute sessions were meant to challenge him increasingly more complex movements as the brain had to adapt to increasingly difficult tasks.

- ***Results*:** At the end of the trial, Mr. A demonstrated significant improvements in both his physical and social/adaptive functioning. Objective measurements on Fugl-Meyer Assessment of Motor Recovery showed significant gains both in range of motion and strength in his right arm; he also showed greater dexterity and grasping capability which enabled him to hold and manipulate objects he could not previously manage. Subjectively, Mr. A reported a greater sense of independence and an improved quality of life, as he was able to perform basic tasks such as feeding himself and dressing with more ease. The voluntary movements pertaining to reaching and grasping improved significantly, and the patient gained more confidence in using his right arm for such activities. Additionally, EEG data showed that activity over regions of the brain controlling movement increased, and the BCI intervention had indeed enhanced neuroplastic changes in his brain.

Discussion

This case study demonstrates the possibility of EEG-based BCI in enhancing neurorehabilitation for stroke patients. Real-time feedback about brain activity, with support from a robotic assistant, mediated motor learning and facilitated functional recovery in Mr. A. BCI, used as a tool for motor imagery in association with the physical act of controlling a robotic exoskeleton, effectively activated neuroplastic mechanisms within the brain to favor functional reorganization and the recovery of motor control. The success of this intervention is consistent with others demonstrating that EEG-based BCIs can significantly contribute to stroke rehabilitation. Providing real-time feedback facilitates a patient's performance of specific motor tasks as well as induces the brain to change and adapt to newly established neural patterns. Furthermore, BCIs can be designed and built with each patient's individual needs in mind: the difficulty level as well as the feedback mechanisms can be tailored to enhance recovery.

5.2 Communication for Severely Disabled Patients

For patients with extremely severe disabilities, like ALS or locked-in syndrome, there is only one remaining lifeline communication channel provided by EEG BCIs: patients can now express their thoughts and needs by clicking on letters or phrases on a computer screen using mental imagery or attention-related tasks. Such communications can significantly improve quality of life and reduce caregiver burden (Birbaumer et al., 2006).

Case Study: EEG-Based BCI for Communication in a Patient with Locked-In Syndrome

- ***Background***

Locked-In Syndrome (LIS) is that state where patients are wholly conscious and aware but powerless to move or speak since all the muscles that may be considered under voluntary control have been rendered useless by complete paralysis, except for eye movements. This devastating condition is often caused by brainstem strokes, traumatic brain injuries, or neurodegenerative diseases like ALS (Amyotrophic Lateral Sclerosis). For these patients, communication is extremely challenging because they can neither speak nor communicate through other mechanisms of expression. Communication is indispensable to maintain dignity, reduce isolation, and improve quality of life. In the last few years, there has been a new wave of EEG-based Brain-Computer Interfaces (BCIs), which, for patients with severe disabilities, has become an essential tool to express their thoughts, needs, and emotions, purely on the basis of activity in their brain.

- ***Role of EEG-Based BCIs in Communication***

EEG-based BCIs determine the electrical activities taking place in the brain and translate them into commands that can operate external devices. In Locked-In Syndrome, BCIs typically rely on communication using mental imagery or attention-based tasks. Patients can focus on specific mental states - for example, a body part is envisioned moving - or concentrate on a particular object or letter that appears on the screen. The brainwaves are detected and interpreted by the BCI system to allow a person to select letters, words, or phrases on the screen and thus communicate his thoughts to caregivers and loved ones.

Case Study: Using EEG-Based BCI for Communication in a Patient with Locked-In Syndrome

- ***Patient Background*:** Ms. B is a 42-year-old female patient who, after having a severe brainstem stroke, developed Locked-In Syndrome. Previous to the stroke, she was completely independent and held a managerial job with a very active lifestyle. After the stroke, Ms. B lost speech and any motor movement in her body except for her eyes. At times, she could not effectively communicate with her family and caregivers as she could only use eye movements, which, though valuable, could not be used for complex communication or expressing her thoughts in real-time.

- ***BCI Intervention*****:** A BCI was therefore introduced to a communication-focused EEG-based BCI system. It utilized a non-invasive EEG headset with 32 electrodes to capture activity in the brain related to motor imagery tasks. In the training phase, Ms. B was required to focus her mental attention on one of two tasks: imagine moving her left hand or imagine moving her right hand. Both these mental states produced different patterns of brainwaves that the BCI system detected. A letter grid appeared in front of her, and with the concentration on the mental imagery tasks, Ms. B was selecting letters for words and sentences from the grid.
- ***Process*****:** In her initial few training sessions, Ms. B was using her left or right hand movements for some seconds as the system was recording the patterns of the brainwave. She soon mastered the selection of letters from the grid by using this system and calibrated the system so as to interpret her brain waves with a high degree of accuracy, allowing her to spell out words and phrases at a rate of about one letter per minute, though slow compared to other methods, it was much faster than with eye-tracking techniques. Secondly, the BCI used visual feedback and showed Ms. B the letters as she focused them. Those visual feedbacks served to complement her mental focus when using the system.
- ***Results*****:** After a period of weeks of training, the BCI, based on EEG, demonstrated for Ms. B a clear augmentation in her application of it to communicate. She could spell out short sentences indicating her basic needs, such as wanting something to eat or drink or being restless in bed. Much more importantly, it gave her the means of expressing much more complex thoughts and feelings that enhanced the quality of what little life was left for her. Ms. B could talk of wants for entertainment, engage in meaningful interactions with her family members, and become part of decisions related to her own care. Thirdly, the caregivers also indicated that BCI system minimized frustration and sense of isolation. She started experiencing considerable improvements in her emotional status due to enhanced possibility of communication. By getting such essential knowledge, the caregiver could meet up the needs and demands of the patient that reduced the stress psychologically and physically.

Discussion

This case clearly demonstrates that EEG-based BCIs have enormous potential to act as a communicator for Locked-In Syndrome patients. The system offered a non-invasive, real-time means of communication for Ms. B to express herself and convey her feelings and needs, thereby dramatically enhancing her independence and quality of life. Although the communication process was much slower than in a conventional sense, having meaningful conversations with loved ones was worth it. The BCI system enhanced the interaction between Ms. B and her caregivers, which, in turn led to improved care and emotional support for her. Challenges still exist, such as a practically slow rate of communication and the demand for training and adaptation by a patient. However, as BCI technology improves the accuracy, speed, and usability of the device, it promises to give people with severe disabilities the gift of having their voice back.

5.3 Mental Health Monitoring and Intervention

EEG-based Prospects for EEG-based BCIs can also be seen in the use of monitoring and modulating brain activity in depressed or anxietous patients, or those with other psychiatric disorders (Värbu et al., 2022; Wang et al., 2021). Neurofeedback training will help patients learn how to regulate their emotions or cognitive functions in BCIs that give them real-time feedback on states of the brain. This will present a non-pharmacological treatment alternative that can be molded to fit individual brain activity patterns.

Case Report: EEG-Based BCI for Monitoring and Intervention of a Patient with Depression

Background

Millions of people around the world have been afflicted with mental disorders, such as depression and anxiety disorders, which impair quality of life, compromise functioning, and are linked to high risks of chronicity. Patients are responsive to conventional treatments with pharmaceutical drugs and CBT. But studies show that this is not universally true. Besides this, the side effects of pharmacological interventions and the need for the time commitment of therapy can present a hindrance to the best possible care. Therefore, there has been a growing interest in non-invasive, imaginative ways to manage mental health. In this regard, EEG-based BCIs have shown promising use through real-time feedbacks of brain activity that can benefit from neurofeedback training; therefore, patients are taught how to regulate brain activity related to mood, cognition, and emotional states.

Case Study: EEG-Based BCI for Depression in a Patient

- ***Patient Background*:** Mr. C is a 35-year-old male patient who has been suffering from chronic depression for many years. Although Mr. C received standard treatment, including antidepressant medication and weekly sessions of CBT, he continued to experience such persistent major depressive symptoms as low energy, irritability, and even hopelessness. Thus, his depression proved resistant to multiple drug regimens, and he was referred for alternative treatment. Discussion with his psychiatrist led to his enrollment in a clinical study on the use of EEG-based BCI for monitoring and intervention in mental health conditions.

- ***BCI Intervention*:** The intervention was comprised of an EEG-based BCI system that monitored and modulated the activity of Mr. C in real time. This system had a cap containing multiple electrodes that detected brainwave patterns, especially in the frontal lobe, which is recognized to play a key role in mood regulation and cognitive function. Mr. C received neurofeedback training during an 8-week time span. The treatment aimed to stimulate in Mr. C brain waves usually associated with depressive states, such as low alpha activity and high theta activity, by stimulating alpha and beta waves.

    At every session, Mr. C was provided with tasks that required him to activate his mental capacity-for example, being asked to concentrate on calming imagery or listen to a calming sound. In this system, the visual feedback of his brainwave activity was clearly presented with a separate target range for each type of brainwave activity. Through real-time feedback, he learned to self-regulate his brain activity.
- ***Process*:** The neurofeedback training began with baseline assessments of Mr. C's brainwave activity, which showed decreased alpha waves and increased theta waves in the prefrontal cortex—both of which are typically indicative of states of depression. During the neurofeedback training, Mr. C learned to intentionally increase his production of alpha waves. Gradually, the training began to add complexity, forcing him to maintain the positive brain activity for increasingly longer periods of time. Based on the patterns of brain waves of Mr. C, the training session was individualized. Every training session was an accumulation of the previous one. Apart from BCI sessions, Mr. C was instructed on some relaxation techniques such as mindfulness and breathing exercises to help neurofeedback in combination.
- ***Results*:** At the end of the 8-week study, Mr. C showed improvement over his depressive episodes. Objective measures, such as the BDI, revealed that his depressive symptoms had abated in intensity by 40%. In contrast, subjectively Mr. C affirmed that he now had more energy, no irritability, nor was hopeless about his future. He further noted he was able to better control his emotions and stress and that that improved his personal and professional life. EEG data gathered in the sessions revealed enhanced patterns for brain activity, which included significantly increased alpha activity and decreased theta activity. These changes in EEG patterns were observed to parallel sub-

jective improvements reported by Mr. C regarding mood and cognition, thus showing that the neurofeedback treatment was indeed a resounding success in enhancing brain activity patterns associated with a more positive emotional state.

Discussion

This case study demonstrates the feasibility of the EEG-based BCIs for the treatment of mental disorders like depression. The real-time feedback from the BCI system enabled Mr C. to manage his brain waves. Prominent improvements in the depressed condition could be noticed in this patient. Targeting the dysregulated brainwave patterns typical of the depressive disorder, the BCI intervention offered an individualized, non-invasive approach compatible with regular treatments. Such EEG-based BCIs will not produce any side effects and can easily be made tailor-made for each patient's unique activity. Therefore, it would act as a very effective pharmacological therapy in those who do not respond well to drugs.

6. FUTURE DIRECTIONS

The future of EEG-based BCIs is really promising and good progress will be seen in technological domains pertaining to accuracy, usability, and accessibility. Advanced, user-friendly systems in healthcare towards a wide range of patients shall be an outcome of further research on signal processing, machine learning, and wearable technology (Värbu et al., 2022; Wang et al., 2021).

- The area of signal interpretation development is markedly improved. As machine learning algorithms, particularly deep learning models, continue to develop, BCIs will provide better decoding of brain signals in real-time, leading to better device control. This will, therefore make BCIs more adaptable to individual users in order to address issues such as variability in signals.
- Wearable EEG systems will gain immense popularity due to their portability and comfort. They are not intrusive. Since these systems are more mobile, it will allow the use of BCIs both in clinical and home environments, thereby reducing the impact of multiple hospital visits. The lack of invasiveness will also increase comfort, thereby increasing accessibility.
- Seamless integration with AI and virtual reality (VR) and EEG-based BCIs is another promising direction. AI can optimize neurofeedback with personalized treatment protocols, while the use of VR will help immerse the patient in rehabilitation procedures and aid their recovery in the case of motor im-

pairments. Remote monitoring through BCIs will allow continuous tracking of brain activity and potential early intervention for neurological disorders.

- The EEG-based BCIs will break free from their traditional application and break into cognitive enhancement, education, and entertainment. Convergence of such technologies will define a future where BCIs lead to the personalized medicine and healthcare - more tailored and effective treatments for widespread disorders.

7. CONCLUSION

BCI technology based on EEG can change the healthcare by developing innovative solutions in neurorehabilitation, communication, and the intervention of mental health. BCIs, which directly link the brain to external devices, may facilitate loss of functions regained or improve the quality of life in patients with neurological conditions. They offer motor recovery in patients recovering from stroke or traumatic brain injury by using BCIs to give immediate feedback of brain activity during neurorehabilitation. The only avenue of communication for patients with paralyzed and locked-in syndrome is through BCIs, which convey thoughts and needs. In psychiatry, BCIs are used in neurofeedback training: patients can learn to control brain activity patterns related to depression or anxiety, for instance. Thus, developing such devices requires a strong multidisciplinary approach involving the bringing together of diverse expertise from neuroscience, engineering, and clinical medicine. With further research, EEG-based BCIs will be set to improve patient outcomes and to make better the quality of healthcare delivery.

REFERENCES

Birbaumer, N. (2006). Breaking the Silence: Brain–Computer Interfaces (BCI) for Communication and Motor Control. *Psychophysiology*, 43(6), 517–532. DOI: 10.1111/j.1469-8986.2006.00456.x PMID: 17076808

Blankertz, B., Müller, K. R., Curio, G., Vaughan, T. M., Schalk, G., Wolpaw, J. R., Schlögl, A., Neuper, C., Pfurtscheller, G., Hinterberger, T., Schröder, M., & Birbaumer, N. (2004). The BCI Competition 2003: Progress and Perspectives in Detection and Discrimination of EEG Single Trials. *IEEE Transactions on Biomedical Engineering*, 51(6), 1044–1051. DOI: 10.1109/TBME.2004.826692 PMID: 15188876

Lee, K., Ko, G. H., Lee, C. H., & Geong, Y. S. (2023). Detection Performance Analysis Based on EEG Signals for Visual BCI. *IEEE Access : Practical Innovations, Open Solutions*, 11, 2516–2526. DOI: 10.1109/ACCESS.2023.9887523

Medina, A. S. A., Bonilla, M. I. A., Giraldo, I. D. R., Palacios, J. F. M., Gutiérrez, D. A. C., & Liscano, Y. (2024). Electroencephalography-Based Brain-Computer Interfaces in Rehabilitation: A Bibliometric Analysis (2013–2023). *Sensors (Basel)*, 24(22), 7125. DOI: 10.3390/s24227125 PMID: 39598903

Millan, J. R., Renkens, F., Mourino, J., & Gerstner, W. (2004). Noninvasive Brain-Actuated Control of a Mobile Robot by Human EEG. *IEEE Transactions on Biomedical Engineering*, 51(6), 1026–1033. DOI: 10.1109/TBME.2004.827086 PMID: 15188874

Pfurtscheller, G., Neuper, C., Guger, C., Harkam, W., Ramoser, H., Schlogl, A., Obermaier, B., & Pregenzer, M. (2000). Current Trends in Graz Brain–Computer Interface (BCI) Research. *IEEE Transactions on Rehabilitation Engineering*, 8(2), 216–219. DOI: 10.1109/86.847821 PMID: 10896192

Värbu, K., Muhammad, N., & Muhammad, Y. (2022). Past, Present, and Future of EEG-Based BCI Applications. *Sensors (Basel)*, 22(9), 3331. DOI: 10.3390/s22093331 PMID: 35591021

Wang, Y., Luo, J., Guo, Y., Du, Q., Cheng, Q., & Wang, H. (2021). Changes in EEG Brain Connectivity Caused by Short-Term BCI Neurofeedback-Rehabilitation Training: A Case Study. *Frontiers in Human Neuroscience*, 15, 627100. DOI: 10.3389/fnhum.2021.627100 PMID: 34366808

Wolpaw, J. R., Heetderks, W. J., McFarland, D. J., Peckham, P. H., Schalk, G., Donchin, E., Quatrano, L. A., Robinson, C. J., & Vaughan, T. M. (2000). Brain–Computer Interface Technology: A Review of the First International Meeting. *IEEE Transactions on Rehabilitation Engineering*, 8(2), 164–173. DOI: 10.1109/TRE.2000.847807 PMID: 10896178

Chapter 5
Leadership and Performance Evaluation Strategies for Remote Healthcare Teams in the Digital Era:
Effective Leadership in Remote Healthcare

Bharti Singh
Christ University, India

ABSTRACT

This chapter provides a detailed exploration of effective leadership practices and performance assessment strategies critical to managing remote healthcare teams in the digital health era. It begins by analyzing leadership styles, such as transformational, servant, and transactional leadership, and how these can address unique challenges in virtual environments, such as communication gaps, security, and system integration. Through a review of various assessment frameworks and methods, the chapter highlights tools and metrics suited to evaluate remote healthcare team performance effectively. Real-world case studies from renowned institutions, including Cleveland Clinic, Mayo Clinic, and UCSF, showcase the successful deployment of leadership strategies and provide insights into design and deployment best practices, such as usability, scalability, and compliance. The chapter concludes with actionable recommendations for healthcare leaders and identifies areas for further research to support continuous innovation and effectiveness in remote healthcare delivery.

DOI: 10.4018/979-8-3693-8598-2.ch005

1. INTRODUCTION

In recent years, the rapid advancement of innovative medical devices has revolutionized healthcare delivery, enhancing diagnostic accuracy, therapeutic interventions, and patient monitoring. These devices, ranging from wearable health technologies to complex diagnostic tools, transform how healthcare professionals interact with patients, particularly in remote settings. Integrating advanced technologies into medical devices improves patient outcomes, reduces operational inefficiencies, and makes healthcare more accessible to a global population.

This chapter explores the importance of leadership in managing remote healthcare teams reliant on innovative medical devices. It addresses the need for innovative leadership practices to navigate the complexities of remote healthcare environments, where traditional management frameworks may fall short. Moreover, it emphasizes robust performance evaluation methods for these teams, given the unique dynamics of working in a digital healthcare ecosystem.

The chapter aims to:

- Explore effective leadership practices for managing remote healthcare teams.
- Analyse how leadership can navigate the complexities of remote healthcare environments.
- Assess remote healthcare team performance.
- Highlight case studies demonstrating real-world applications of leadership strategies in remote healthcare.

By outlining the current state and future trends in medical device innovation, this chapter offers valuable insights for healthcare leaders, practitioners etc, guiding them toward optimizing team performance and leveraging medical devices for better patient care.

2. EFFECTIVE LEADERSHIP PRACTICES FOR MANAGING REMOTE HEALTHCARE TEAMS

In healthcare, effective leadership is critical for guiding teams through the complexities of medical care, particularly in remote settings where face-to-face interactions are limited. Remote healthcare teams often operate in dynamic and high-pressure environments, requiring leaders to adapt their strategies for communication, motivation, and performance management. The characteristics of effective leadership in these scenarios emphasize empathy, communication, adaptability, and trust-building. Leaders must ensure that remote healthcare teams remain engaged, cohesive, and aligned with organizational goals despite physical distance.

Key Characteristics of Effective Leadership in Remote Healthcare:

- **Clear Communication:** In a remote setting, the leader's ability to communicate clearly and consistently is paramount. This involves using technology efficiently to maintain transparent communication channels and ensure all team members are aligned with organizational objectives.
- **Empathy and Emotional Intelligence:** Effective leaders in healthcare must possess emotional intelligence to understand and manage the emotional well-being of their team members. Remote settings can create feelings of isolation or burnout, so leaders need to be empathetic and provide support.
- **Adaptability to Technology**: Remote leadership in healthcare requires quick adaptation to emerging digital health technologies. Leaders should be proficient in telemedicine platforms, electronic health records (EHR) systems, and AI-driven healthcare tools, ensuring their team can operate efficiently.
- **Trust-Building Through Data Transparency**: Using data from digital health monitoring systems, remote leaders can foster trust by sharing performance metrics transparently, ensuring team members understand how their efforts contribute to broader healthcare goals.
- **Proficiency in Remote Work Tools**: Technical competency in using remote work tools like cloud-based EHR systems, remote diagnostics devices, and virtual collaboration platforms is essential. Leaders need to ensure that all team members are trained in the use of these systems and that they are integrated smoothly into the healthcare delivery workflow.

Leadership Styles Suited for Remote Healthcare Teams:

1. Transformational Leadership
    - **Key Focus**: This style emphasizes inspiring and motivating team members to work towards a shared vision, encouraging innovation and higher performance beyond self-interest. It fosters trust, enthusiasm, and creativity, which is essential in the dynamic, often challenging environment of remote healthcare.
    - **Real-World Example**: **Mayo Clinic** has been a pioneer in transformational leadership, especially in their virtual healthcare initiatives. Leaders there promote cross-functional collaboration among research and clinical teams. During the global pandemic, the leadership ensured that the remote teams had a unified purpose to deliver superior patient care, despite geographical distances. This motivated the teams to con-

tribute to innovation in telehealth services, enhancing patient engagement and outcomes through virtual care.

2. Servant Leadership
   - **Key Focus**: In this style, the leader focuses on serving the needs of their team members and helps them grow both personally and professionally. A servant leader fosters a supportive and nurturing environment, which can be especially helpful in remote healthcare teams, where individuals may feel isolated or disconnected from the organization.
   - **Real-World Example**: At **Cleveland Clinic**, servant leadership was embraced during the COVID-19 pandemic, where leaders made it a priority to check on the well-being of their remote workers, offering additional training and resources to help them transition smoothly to telehealth platforms. By putting the team's needs first and creating an empathetic culture, they ensured high morale and maintained high levels of patient care during a disruptive period.**3. Transactional Leadership**
   - **Key Focus**: This leadership style revolves around structured roles and responsibilities, where rewards and penalties are used to motivate team members. It is highly effective in maintaining discipline and accountability, which is crucial in remote healthcare settings where teams are spread out and need clear expectations.
   - **Real-World Example**: **Kaiser Permanente** has effectively used transactional leadership in its remote call centres and telemedicine operations. Healthcare workers are incentivized with rewards for hitting performance metrics, such as response time and patient satisfaction scores, which ensure consistent service quality even when the teams are geographically dispersed. Transactional leadership has helped maintain high standards of care by aligning clear objectives with measurable rewards.

4. Democratic Leadership
   - **Key Focus**: Democratic leadership involves team members in decision-making processes, allowing them to contribute ideas and solutions. This leadership style can create a sense of ownership and engagement among remote healthcare workers, encouraging collaboration and fostering a culture of shared responsibility.
   - **Real-World Example**: At **Johns Hopkins Medicine**, leaders apply democratic leadership by actively involving remote research and clinical teams in the decision-making process. Virtual meetings are set up to gather input from healthcare professionals on care strategies and innovations in telemedicine. By encouraging feedback from all levels of staff,

Johns Hopkins creates a highly collaborative environment, where each team member feels valued and connected, despite working remotely.

5. Situational Leadership

- **Key Focus**: Situational leadership is about adapting the leadership style based on the needs and readiness of the team members. For remote healthcare teams, this means that the leader can shift between being directive (e.g., when new technologies are being introduced) and supportive (e.g., during high-stress situations like patient crises).
- **Real-World Example**: **Partners HealthCare**, known for its cutting-edge telemedicine services, used situational leadership when rolling out new remote healthcare tools. In the early stages of adoption, leaders took a directive approach, providing clear guidelines and training. As the teams became more comfortable, the leadership adapted, providing less direct supervision and more emotional support as team members dealt with the emotional challenges of providing care remotely. This flexibility helped employees' transition smoothly and ensured ongoing productivity and patient care quality.

3. NAVIGATING COMPLEXITIES IN REMOTE HEALTHCARE ENVIRONMENTS

Navigating the complexities of remote healthcare delivery involves addressing several challenges that impact both the quality of care and the effectiveness of healthcare teams. The physical distance between team members, limited face-to-face interaction with patients, and reliance on technology for communication all create potential obstacles. Leaders in remote healthcare must be adept at managing these difficulties to ensure both operational success and patient safety.

Challenges in Remote Healthcare Delivery and Strategies for Overcoming Them

1. Technology Reliance and Technical Issues
    - **Challenge**: Remote healthcare depends heavily on digital tools such as telemedicine platforms, electronic health records, and communication apps. Technical difficulties, such as software failures or lack of reliable internet, can disrupt healthcare delivery.
    - **Strategy**: Invest in reliable, high-quality technology infrastructure, including secure telemedicine platforms and remote diagnostic tools. Provide technical support and training to healthcare professionals to

ensure they are comfortable using these tools. Regularly update systems and offer backup communication methods in case of technology failures.

2. Maintaining Team Cohesion and Engagement
    - **Challenge**: Remote teams can suffer from a lack of cohesion and engagement due to the absence of face-to-face interactions, leading to feelings of isolation, reduced morale, and lack of collaboration.
    - **Strategy**: Leaders should prioritize team-building activities, even in virtual environments. Schedule regular team check-ins, virtual coffee breaks, and recognize achievements publicly to maintain morale. Implement collaboration tools like Slack or Trello to keep the team connected on shared goals and projects.
3. Monitoring and Ensuring Quality of Care
    - **Challenge**: Remote healthcare makes it harder to directly oversee the quality of patient care, increasing the risk of errors or inadequate treatments. Without physical supervision, maintaining high standards of care can be difficult.
    - **Strategy**: Use performance monitoring tools such as electronic medical record audits, remote supervision technologies, and automated feedback systems to track the quality of care. Encourage regular performance reviews and provide continuous feedback loops to ensure that standards are met.
4. Data Privacy and Security Concerns
    - **Challenge**: Handling sensitive medical information over digital platforms increases the risk of data breaches or unauthorized access, threatening patient confidentiality.
    - **Strategy**: Implement robust cybersecurity measures, including data encryption, two-factor authentication, and adherence to regulatory compliance standards such as HIPAA (Health Insurance Portability and Accountability Act). Conduct regular security audits and train team members on best practices for data protection and privacy.
5. Work-Life Balance and Burnout
    - **Challenge**: The blurring of work and personal life boundaries can lead to burnout among healthcare workers, especially in high-stress remote healthcare environments where they may feel "always on call."
    - **Strategy**: Set clear expectations around working hours and encourage healthcare professionals to maintain a work-life balance. Promote wellness programs, offer mental health resources, and provide flexible work schedules to prevent burnout. Encourage team members to take regular breaks and vacation time.

Exemplary Leadership in Remote Healthcare

Dr. Vivian Lee: A Leader in Remote Healthcare

(Exemplary figure in the field of remote healthcare leadership is Dr. Vivian Lee, who has made remarkable contributions to advancing healthcare delivery, particularly through technology and innovative practices.)

Background: Dr. Vivian Lee is a prominent healthcare executive, author, and former president of Health Platforms at Verily Life Sciences (a subsidiary of Alphabet Inc.). She has also served as the Chief Executive Officer of University of Utah Health, where she significantly improved operational efficiency and patient care quality.

Remarkable Contributions:

1. **Transformational Leadership**: Dr. Lee is known for her transformational leadership style, which emphasizes inspiring and motivating her team to pursue innovative healthcare solutions. During her tenure at the University of Utah Health, she implemented a system of integrated healthcare services that streamlined operations and improved patient outcomes.
2. **Embracing Technology**: Under her leadership, the University of Utah Health invested in advanced telehealth solutions, enhancing access to care for remote patients. This approach proved crucial during the COVID-19 pandemic, as it allowed healthcare providers to continue delivering essential services while maintaining safety protocols.
3. **Fostering Collaboration**: Dr. Lee emphasized the importance of cross-disciplinary collaboration, bringing together physicians, engineers, and data scientists to develop cutting-edge health technologies. Her efforts resulted in the development of innovative programs that improved patient engagement and care coordination.
4. **Data-Driven Decision Making**: Dr. Lee's focus on leveraging data analytics in clinical decision-making helped improve treatment protocols and operational efficiency. By analyzing patient data, her team could identify trends and make informed decisions that enhanced patient care.
5. **Advocacy for Patient-Centred Care**: Throughout her career, Dr. Lee has advocated for patient-centred care approaches. She understands the significance of integrating patient feedback into service delivery and ensuring that healthcare solutions align with patient needs.

Example in Action

During the COVID-19 crisis, Dr. Lee's leadership was particularly notable. She quickly pivoted the healthcare services at the University of Utah to prioritize telehealth, ensuring that patients could receive care safely from their homes. This rapid transition not only safeguarded patients and healthcare workers but also provided an example of effective crisis management in remote healthcare environments.

4. DESIGN AND DEPLOYMENT OF REMOTE HEALTHCARE SYSTEMS

The design and deployment of remote healthcare systems are fundamental in ensuring that patients receive quality care outside traditional healthcare settings, especially in a digital-first world. The focus is on creating systems that are robust, efficient, and scalable while ensuring ease of access for healthcare professionals and patients alike. This section explores the key aspects of designing these systems, along with deployment strategies that meet the growing demands of remote healthcare.

4.1 Designing for Usability and Accessibility

Designing remote healthcare systems with usability and accessibility at the forefront ensures that they are intuitive and inclusive for a diverse range of users. This includes patients with varying levels of technical proficiency, healthcare professionals, and individuals with disabilities. Below are key principles for achieving usability and accessibility in remote healthcare systems:

1. User-Centred Design

A successful system begins with understanding the needs and limitations of its end-users—both healthcare providers and patients. User-centred design involves iterative testing and feedback to refine interfaces, making them easy to navigate and reducing the learning curve. Features such as simple navigation menus, clear instructions, and minimal clicks to complete tasks can make healthcare platforms more intuitive.

2. Inclusive Design for Diverse Populations

Patients come from various backgrounds, and some may have disabilities that require specialized accessibility features. Inclusive design ensures that systems accommodate users with:

- **Visual impairments**: Screen reader compatibility, colour contrast adjustments, and customizable text sizes.
- **Hearing impairments**: Subtitles for video consultations or visual alerts for important notifications.
- **Motor impairments**: Voice command options or simple touch navigation to accommodate individuals with limited dexterity.

By addressing these needs, healthcare systems can offer a wider range of patients access to care, minimizing exclusion and improving patient satisfaction.

3. Mobile Optimization

A significant number of patients use mobile devices to access healthcare services. Designing systems that work efficiently on smartphones and tablets is essential for broadening accessibility. Mobile optimization ensures that pages load quickly, information is easy to read on smaller screens, and features such as video consultations and appointment scheduling work seamlessly across all devices.

This also involves considering bandwidth limitations in rural or low-infrastructure areas and designing systems to perform well under different network conditions.

4. Simplified Interfaces

To enhance usability, particularly for older adults or less tech-savvy users, interfaces should avoid clutter and complex layouts. The focus should be on delivering key features—like appointment booking, access to medical records, or telehealth sessions—in a straightforward, easy-to-find manner. Icons, tooltips, and color-coding can guide users intuitively through the process.

5. Cultural and Language Considerations

Healthcare systems often cater to a diverse patient base, requiring localization to account for different languages and cultural nuances. Offering multilingual support, as well as ensuring that translated content is medically accurate and contextually appropriate, can prevent miscommunication and make healthcare more accessible to non-native speakers. Additionally, sensitivity to cultural preferences in design can help reduce friction and encourage broader adoption.

Example in Practice:

Platforms like **Teladoc Health** have incorporated these principles effectively. By offering a simple, mobile-friendly interface and multilingual support, they ensure that users can access telehealth services easily from any location. They also provide voice and video consultations with closed captioning, making the platform accessible for patients with hearing impairments.

By focusing on these design principles, remote healthcare systems can increase their usability and accessibility, ensuring that they are inclusive and practical for all patients, regardless of their tech skills or physical abilities.

4.2 Security and Compliance

Security and compliance are critical components of remote healthcare systems, ensuring that sensitive patient data is protected and that systems adhere to industry regulations. The shift to remote healthcare introduces unique challenges, such as the increased risk of cyberattacks and the need to comply with strict healthcare privacy laws like HIPAA (Health Insurance Portability and Accountability Act) in the U.S., GDPR (General Data Protection Regulation) in Europe, and other international standards.

1. Data Encryption

One of the most fundamental security measures is the encryption of data both in transit and at rest. Encrypting patient health information (PHI) ensures that even if data is intercepted during transmission (e.g., during a telehealth session) or accessed improperly from a server, it cannot be read or misused by unauthorized parties. Strong encryption protocols, such as AES (Advanced Encryption Standard) or TLS (Transport Layer Security), are crucial to securing communications between healthcare providers and patients.

2. Secure Authentication

Remote healthcare systems should enforce robust user authentication protocols to verify the identity of both healthcare professionals and patients. Multi-factor authentication (MFA), which requires users to provide two or more verification factors (e.g., a password plus a code sent to a mobile device), adds an extra layer of security. This minimizes the risk of unauthorized access to sensitive patient data, especially in environments where healthcare workers are logging in remotely from different locations.

3. Compliance with Healthcare Regulations

Healthcare providers and technology platforms must comply with specific laws and regulations that govern patient data privacy and security. Compliance involves maintaining detailed logs of data access, ensuring that systems are designed with security in mind, and regularly auditing systems for vulnerabilities. Regulatory standards like HIPAA, GDPR, and others require healthcare platforms to implement stringent data protection policies, including the secure storage of medical records and limitations on how and when this data can be shared.

4. Regular Security Audits and Vulnerability Assessments

Routine security audits and vulnerability assessments help identify and address potential weaknesses in the system. By continually testing their infrastructure, healthcare providers can pre-emptively fix vulnerabilities before they are exploited. These audits should cover everything from the system's software and hardware architecture to third-party integrations, as any weak link in the ecosystem can be exploited.

5. Incident Response Plans

In the event of a data breach or other security incident, remote healthcare systems must have a robust incident response plan in place. This plan should outline the steps to contain the breach, mitigate damage, notify affected patients and regulatory bodies, and restore normal operations. Having a clear and well-rehearsed response strategy minimizes the impact of security incidents and helps maintain trust between patients and healthcare providers.

6. Compliance Reporting and Documentation

Meeting regulatory compliance also means maintaining up-to-date records and reports that demonstrate adherence to privacy laws and standards. This includes documenting data access logs, encryption methods used, employee training records, and audit results. Proper documentation not only ensures compliance but also provides a clear trail of accountability in case of an investigation or audit by regulatory authorities.

7. Training and Awareness

One of the most significant vulnerabilities in any system is the human factor. Healthcare professionals and administrative staff must be trained to recognize potential security threats like phishing attacks, which are common in healthcare environments. Regular security awareness training ensures that all stakeholders are aware of the importance of safeguarding patient data and understand best practices in cybersecurity.

Example in Practice:

Cleveland Clinic, a leader in telemedicine, adheres to strict HIPAA guidelines to protect patient data in their remote healthcare systems. They implement strong data encryption, use multi-factor authentication for healthcare providers, and conduct regular security audits to ensure that their platform remains secure. This level of diligence not only protects sensitive patient information but also ensures compliance with regulatory bodies, which helps build patient trust in using remote healthcare services.

By prioritizing security and compliance, remote healthcare systems can protect sensitive patient data while providing convenient and effective care, ensuring that they are both trusted by users and compliant with relevant regulations.

4.3 Integration with Existing Systems

Integrating new remote healthcare systems with existing healthcare infrastructures is vital for creating seamless workflows, enhancing data accuracy, and improving overall patient care. This process involves aligning new technologies with current Electronic Health Records (EHR), practice management systems, and other health information systems. The challenges and best practices for successful integration are discussed below.

1. Interoperability

Interoperability refers to the ability of different systems to communicate and exchange information effectively. To achieve this, remote healthcare systems must adhere to established standards such as HL7 (Health Level 7) and FHIR (Fast Healthcare Interoperability Resources). These standards facilitate data sharing among various healthcare systems, enabling healthcare providers to access comprehensive patient records seamlessly.

For example, integrating telehealth platforms with EHR systems allows providers to view patient history, lab results, and treatment plans in real time, improving decision-making during virtual consultations.

2. Data Mapping and Migration

Data mapping is the process of translating data from one system to another. When implementing a new remote healthcare system, it is essential to accurately map and migrate existing patient data to ensure consistency and reliability. This process involves identifying which data fields in the new system correspond to those in the existing system.

Effective data migration not only preserves the integrity of patient information but also prevents disruptions in care delivery. Thorough testing during this phase can identify any discrepancies before the new system goes live.

3. User Training and Support

Successful integration requires adequate training for healthcare providers and staff on how to use the new system effectively. This training should cover not only the technical aspects of the system but also the workflow changes that may occur as a result of the integration.

Ongoing support is also essential, particularly in the early stages after implementation. Creating a dedicated support team can help resolve issues quickly and reinforce user confidence in the new system.

4. Stakeholder Engagement

Engaging all stakeholders—including healthcare providers, administrative staff, and IT personnel—during the integration process is crucial. By involving users in the planning and decision-making stages, healthcare organizations can better understand their needs and preferences.

Regular feedback sessions can help identify potential issues early and ensure that the integrated system meets the diverse requirements of all users.

5. Testing and Validation

Before full deployment, comprehensive testing of the integrated system is necessary to identify and rectify any potential issues. This includes performance testing, security testing, and user acceptance testing (UAT).

UAT involves end-users evaluating the system to ensure it meets their needs and operates as expected. This phase is critical for building user confidence and ensuring a smoother transition to the new system.

6. Data Security Considerations

Integrating new systems raises data security concerns, particularly regarding patient information. Healthcare organizations must ensure that data transfer between systems is secure and compliant with regulations like HIPAA.

Implementing robust encryption protocols and access controls during integration can help safeguard patient data. Additionally, conducting security assessments post-integration ensures that all systems remain secure.

7. Scalability and Futureproofing

When designing remote healthcare systems, it's essential to consider scalability to accommodate future growth and advancements in technology. Integrating systems that can easily adapt to new features, functionalities, or additional user loads will extend the lifespan and effectiveness of the investment.

Example in Practice:

Mount Sinai Health System in New York City has successfully integrated its telehealth services with its EHR system, allowing for seamless access to patient records during virtual visits. This integration has enhanced communication between primary care providers and specialists, improving care coordination and patient outcomes. Their approach included comprehensive stakeholder engagement, rigorous testing, and a strong focus on data security and privacy.

By prioritizing effective integration with existing systems, healthcare organizations can optimize their remote healthcare services, ensuring that they deliver high-quality care while maintaining patient safety and confidentiality.

4.4 Scalability and Flexibility

In the rapidly evolving field of healthcare, the ability to scale and adapt remote healthcare systems is crucial for meeting the diverse and changing needs of patients and providers. Scalability refers to a system's capacity to handle increased demand, while flexibility encompasses the system's ability to adjust to new technologies, workflows, and patient requirements. Below are key considerations for achieving scalability and flexibility in remote healthcare systems.

1. Cloud-Based Solutions

Adopting cloud-based infrastructure can significantly enhance the scalability of remote healthcare systems. Cloud technology allows healthcare organizations to quickly adjust resources based on patient demand without investing in physical hardware. As patient populations grow or fluctuate, organizations can increase their storage capacity and computing power on demand, ensuring that performance remains consistent.

For example, **Mayo Clinic** utilizes cloud-based telehealth platforms that can easily scale up to accommodate high patient volumes during peak times, such as flu season, without compromising service quality.

2. Modular Design

Implementing a modular design in remote healthcare systems promotes flexibility. Modular systems consist of independent components that can be added, removed, or modified without affecting the entire system. This approach enables healthcare organizations to adopt new technologies or functionalities as they become available.

For instance, a telehealth platform that allows for the integration of various modules—such as remote monitoring devices, video conferencing tools, and patient engagement apps—can adapt to the evolving needs of providers and patients.

3. Interoperability

Ensuring interoperability with existing systems allows remote healthcare technologies to function seamlessly alongside current infrastructures. Systems that adhere to industry standards (like HL7 and FHIR) enable different applications and devices to communicate effectively, fostering a more integrated healthcare environment.

By prioritizing interoperability, healthcare organizations can implement new solutions without overhauling their existing systems, allowing for a more scalable approach to remote healthcare delivery.

4. User-Centric Design

Designing remote healthcare systems with the end-user in mind—patients and healthcare providers—enhances flexibility. Systems should be intuitive, user-friendly, and adaptable to varying user needs and preferences. User-centric design allows for quick updates and modifications based on feedback, improving user satisfaction and engagement.

Cleveland Clinic employed a user-centric approach when developing its telehealth platform, ensuring it could cater to the diverse needs of both patients and healthcare professionals.

5. Continuous Improvement and Upgrades

Remote healthcare systems should incorporate mechanisms for continuous improvement and regular upgrades. This approach ensures that the technology remains current, secure, and aligned with best practices. Continuous monitoring of system performance and user feedback can guide necessary upgrades, keeping the system scalable and flexible.

Regularly scheduled updates can also address emerging security threats, ensuring compliance with healthcare regulations and maintaining patient trust.

6. Training and Support

Providing ongoing training and support for healthcare staff is essential for maintaining scalability and flexibility. As systems evolve, so do workflows and processes. Regular training sessions can equip staff with the knowledge to utilize new features effectively, ensuring smooth transitions and minimizing disruptions.

For example, **Teladoc Health** emphasizes continuous education for its providers on new technologies and updates to ensure their teams remain adaptable in a fast-paced environment.

7. Data Analytics for Forecasting

Utilizing data analytics can enhance scalability by enabling organizations to forecast demand and plan accordingly. Analysing patient data and usage patterns can help healthcare organizations identify trends, allowing them to scale resources up or down based on anticipated needs.

By leveraging analytics, organizations can make informed decisions regarding staffing, technology investments, and resource allocation, thereby optimizing their remote healthcare services.

Example in Practice:

Mount Sinai Health System implemented scalable telehealth solutions that allowed for rapid expansion during the COVID-19 pandemic. By leveraging cloud technology and maintaining interoperability with existing EHR systems, Mount Sinai effectively scaled its virtual care offerings to meet increased patient demand. The organization emphasized user-centric design and provided continuous support and training to its staff, ensuring smooth transitions and high-quality care delivery.

By focusing on scalability and flexibility, healthcare organizations can create remote healthcare systems that are resilient, adaptable, and capable of meeting the evolving needs of the healthcare landscape. This proactive approach not only enhances patient care but also positions organizations for long-term success in a dynamic environment.

4.5 Deployment Strategies

Deploying remote healthcare systems effectively requires strategic planning and execution. Successful deployment ensures that the technology is integrated seamlessly into existing workflows, maximizes user adoption, and ultimately improves patient outcomes. Here are key deployment strategies to consider:

1. Phased Rollout

Implementing a phased rollout strategy allows organizations to deploy their remote healthcare systems gradually, which minimizes disruption and facilitates user feedback. By piloting the system in select departments or with specific patient groups, organizations can identify potential issues, make necessary adjustments, and build a case for wider adoption.

Example: The **University of California San Francisco (UCSF) Health** initially piloted its telehealth program in a few specialties before expanding it organization-wide. This phased approach allowed them to gather valuable insights and refine processes before a full-scale implementation.

2. Comprehensive Training Programs

Training is critical to the successful deployment of remote healthcare systems. A comprehensive training program should be designed to address the diverse needs of users, including clinicians, administrative staff, and patients. Training sessions should include hands-on practice, access to user manuals, and ongoing support to ensure proficiency.

For instance, **Mount Sinai Health System** developed targeted training initiatives for their staff, which were tailored to different user roles and included simulations to enhance comfort with the technology.

3. Change Management Strategies

Change management is vital for addressing resistance and ensuring a smooth transition to new technologies. Organizations should communicate the benefits of the new system clearly and involve staff in the decision-making process. This can be achieved through regular updates, feedback sessions, and by highlighting success stories from early adopters.

Teladoc Health effectively managed change during its deployment of remote health services by actively engaging its staff in discussions about the benefits of telehealth, thus increasing buy-in and reducing resistance.

4. Stakeholder Engagement

Engaging stakeholders—ranging from healthcare providers to patients—is crucial for successful deployment. Their input can inform system design and functionality, ensuring the technology meets user needs. Regular stakeholder meetings can provide a platform for ongoing feedback and collaboration.

Example: Cleveland Clinic conducted extensive stakeholder engagement sessions prior to deploying its telehealth services, which helped tailor the system to address the specific needs of various departments and patient populations.

5. Robust Technical Support

Providing robust technical support is essential during the deployment phase. Organizations should ensure that users have access to timely assistance through help desks, online resources, and troubleshooting guides. This support can help resolve issues quickly and enhance user confidence in the new system.

Case in Point: Mayo Clinic established a dedicated support team for its telehealth services, ensuring that users could receive immediate help during the initial rollout, which significantly improved adoption rates.

6. Continuous Evaluation and Feedback Loops

Establishing mechanisms for continuous evaluation and feedback is critical to refining remote healthcare systems post-deployment. Collecting user feedback through surveys, focus groups, and performance metrics can provide insights into areas needing improvement.

For example, **Dignity Health** implemented regular feedback loops after launching their telehealth services, allowing them to identify and address pain points swiftly, ensuring ongoing improvement and satisfaction.

7. Integration with Existing Workflows

To maximize the effectiveness of remote healthcare systems, it is crucial to ensure they are integrated with existing workflows and processes. This means aligning the new technology with current practices, such as electronic health records (EHRs) and billing systems, to reduce redundancy and streamline operations.

Example: Kaiser Permanente successfully integrated its remote monitoring tools with its EHR system, allowing for seamless data sharing and improved coordination of care, which enhanced both clinician efficiency and patient experience.

By employing these deployment strategies, healthcare organizations can navigate the complexities of introducing remote healthcare systems, ensuring successful implementation and long-term sustainability. These approaches not only enhance user adoption but also contribute to improved patient outcomes and overall organizational efficiency.

Case Study: Telehealth Implementation at Health First

Background: Health First is a healthcare organization based in Florida that sought to enhance its patient care through the implementation of a comprehensive telehealth system. Recognizing the growing demand for remote healthcare services, they aimed to design a solution that would not only improve accessibility for patients but also streamline operations for healthcare providers.

1. Designing for Usability and Accessibility

Health First conducted extensive user research to ensure that the telehealth platform was user-friendly and accessible to all patients, including those with disabilities. They involved end-users—patients and providers—in the design process through focus groups and usability testing. Feedback from these sessions led to features such as large text options, screen reader compatibility, and intuitive navigation, enhancing overall usability.

2. Security and Compliance

Given the sensitive nature of health information, Health First prioritized security and compliance with HIPAA regulations. They implemented end-to-end encryption for all patient communications and data storage, along with multi-factor authentication for users accessing the system. Regular security audits and employee training on data protection protocols were established to mitigate risks.

3. Integration with Existing Systems

To ensure a seamless transition and enhance workflow, Health First integrated the telehealth platform with its existing Electronic Health Records (EHR) system. This integration allowed providers to access patient histories during virtual consultations, improving the quality of care. Additionally, the system enabled automatic billing processes, reducing administrative burdens.

4. Scalability and Flexibility

Health First designed the telehealth platform to be scalable, accommodating a growing number of users without compromising performance. The cloud-based infrastructure allowed for flexible expansion, enabling the organization to add new features and services as demand increased. This adaptability was crucial during the COVID-19 pandemic, when patient volume surged, requiring quick adjustments to the platform.

5. Deployment Strategies

Health First opted for a phased rollout of its telehealth services, starting with primary care and gradually expanding to specialty services. They provided comprehensive training for healthcare providers, emphasizing hands-on practice with the new system. To facilitate user adoption, Health First also implemented a robust technical support system, offering 24/7 assistance during the initial launch period.

Outcomes

The implementation of the telehealth system at Health First resulted in significant improvements in patient access to care. Following the rollout, the organization reported a 200% increase in virtual visits within the first six months. Patient satisfaction scores also rose, as indicated by post-consultation surveys that highlighted the convenience and effectiveness of remote appointments.

5. ASSESSING REMOTE HEALTHCARE TEAM PERFORMANCE

In the evolving landscape of healthcare, the effectiveness of remote healthcare teams is crucial for delivering high-quality patient care. As telehealth becomes more prevalent, evaluating team performance poses unique challenges and opportunities, essential for maintaining operational efficiency, fostering collaboration, and driving continuous improvement. Effective assessments require a multifaceted approach that balances qualitative and quantitative metrics, as traditional evaluations may overlook the complexities of remote work, including communication dynamics and technology use. To navigate this landscape, healthcare leaders should implement strategies promoting transparency, feedback, and professional growth, focusing on key performance indicators (KPIs) and utilizing comprehensive assessment frameworks. This section will explore methods for evaluating remote healthcare team performance, including KPIs, 360-degree feedback, and self-assessment tools, while also examining existing frameworks that support this evaluation process to enhance the quality of care in remote healthcare settings.

Methods for Assessing Remote Healthcare Team Performance

1. **Key Performance Indicators (KPIs)**
   - **Description**: KPIs are specific, measurable metrics that help organizations evaluate their success in achieving essential objectives. For remote healthcare teams, relevant KPIs can include patient satisfaction scores, response times to patient inquiries, adherence to clinical protocols, and the number of successful telehealth consultations.
   - **Implementation**: Identify and tailor specific KPIs to match the individual roles within the team, such as metrics for physicians, nurses, and administrative staff. Establish a system for regular data collection and reporting to track these indicators. Incorporate KPI discussions into team meetings to assess performance trends and identify areas needing improvement. Utilizing software tools can help automate this process and provide real-time insights.
2. **360-Degree Feedback**
   - **Description**: This method gathers performance feedback from a variety of sources, including peers, supervisors, and patients, offering a holistic view of an individual's contributions and behaviour within the team.
   - **Implementation**: Design and distribute anonymous surveys that assess various competencies, such as communication skills, teamwork, and problem-solving abilities. Ensure that the feedback is constructive and focuses on actionable improvements. Conduct follow-up discussions with team members to review the feedback and collaboratively develop personal development plans that focus on growth areas.
3. **Self-Assessment Tools**
   - **Description**: Self-assessment encourages team members to critically evaluate their performance against established criteria, fostering personal accountability and professional growth.
   - **Implementation**: Create structured self-assessment questionnaires that prompt team members to reflect on their contributions, challenges faced, and areas where they can improve. Schedule regular intervals (e.g., monthly or quarterly) for team members to complete these assessments, followed by discussions in one-on-one or team meetings to

encourage open dialogue about self-identified challenges and development opportunities.

4. **Regular Performance Reviews**
    - o **Description**: Scheduled performance reviews provide formal opportunities for team members and managers to discuss individual contributions, set future goals, and address performance issues in a constructive manner.
    - o **Implementation**: Conduct biannual or quarterly reviews that focus on both individual performance and overall team dynamics. Utilize a structured framework to guide these reviews, which includes discussing achievements, areas for improvement, and setting goals for the upcoming period. Encourage team members to prepare for these sessions by gathering feedback from peers and self-assessments to facilitate a more in-depth conversation.
5. **Patient Outcome Metrics**
    - o **Description**: Evaluating patient outcomes is crucial for determining the effectiveness of remote healthcare teams. Metrics may include recovery rates, patient adherence to treatment plans, and overall health improvements over time.
    - o **Implementation**: Establish a system for tracking these outcomes systematically. This may involve setting specific goals for patient outcomes linked to team performance. Regularly analyse these outcomes in conjunction with team performance data to identify correlations between team effectiveness and patient health results. Share these findings with the team to highlight successes and areas for continued focus.
6. **Technology Utilization Metrics**
    - o **Description**: The effectiveness of technology usage in remote settings can be assessed by monitoring usage statistics and gathering feedback on telehealth platforms, communication tools, and other digital resources employed by the team.
    - o **Implementation**: Regularly review technology utilization data to ensure that team members are maximizing the tools available to them. Conduct surveys to assess user satisfaction with these technologies and identify any barriers to effective use. Provide additional training or support as needed to enhance technology proficiency and streamline workflows.

In the context of assessing remote healthcare team performance, several frameworks and tools can enhance the evaluation process, improving the quality of care. Here are some key frameworks and tools that can be utilized:

Frameworks for Assessment

1. **Balanced Scorecard (BSC)**: o This strategic planning and management system translates organizational goals into measurable outcomes across financial, customer, internal processes, and learning perspectives. It helps healthcare teams align their performance with strategic objectives, thus enhancing overall service delivery (Kaplan & Norton, 1996).
2. **Team Performance Assessment Framework (TPAF)**: o The TPAF focuses on assessing team dynamics, processes, and outcomes. It provides a structured approach to evaluate communication effectiveness, collaboration, and individual contributions within remote teams, making it particularly relevant in a virtual environment (Salas et al., 2004).
3. **Key Performance Indicators (KPIs)**: o Utilizing KPIs allows teams to set specific, measurable objectives related to their performance. Common KPIs in remote healthcare include patient satisfaction scores, response times, and adherence to clinical guidelines, which provide a clear framework for monitoring and improving team effectiveness (Gonzalez & Rodriguez, 2020).
4. **360-Degree Feedback**: o This method collects feedback from multiple sources, including peers, supervisors, and patients, to provide a comprehensive view of team performance. It encourages open communication and continuous improvement, which are essential in remote healthcare settings (Baker et al., 2013).
5. **Agile Performance Management**: o Agile methodologies emphasize flexibility and iterative assessment processes, which are beneficial in remote healthcare environments. This approach facilitates quick adaptations based on feedback and changing circumstances, thus improving team dynamics and patient care outcomes (Denning, 2018).

Tools for Assessment

1. **Surveys and Questionnaires**:
   - o Tools like Gallup Q12 or the Team Engagement Survey can assess team dynamics and individual contributions. These instruments gather data on employee engagement and satisfaction, which are crucial for evaluating remote teams' performance.
2. **Performance Management Software**:
   - o Platforms such as 15Five or BambooHR enable real-time performance tracking, goal setting, and feedback collection, supporting ongoing evaluations of team effectiveness in remote settings.
3. **Data Analytics Tools**:

- Using data analytics tools like Tableau or Power BI allows healthcare teams to visualize performance metrics, track trends, and make data-driven decisions to enhance service quality.

Real-World Example: Assessing Remote Healthcare Team Performance at MD Anderson Cancer Center

MD Anderson Cancer Center, one of the leading cancer treatment and research centers in the world, implemented a comprehensive performance assessment strategy for its remote healthcare teams, especially during the COVID-19 pandemic. The center adopted a variety of methods to evaluate team performance effectively in a remote setting.

1. **Key Performance Indicators (KPIs)**: MD Anderson tracked metrics such as patient wait times for virtual appointments, adherence to clinical guidelines, and patient satisfaction scores. By analysing these KPIs, the center identified areas for improvement in telehealth services and ensured that quality care was maintained despite the shift to remote consultations.
2. **360-Degree Feedback**: The center employed a 360-degree feedback process for its healthcare professionals, collecting insights from peers, supervisors, and patients regarding their performance in virtual environments. This feedback loop allowed team members to gain valuable perspectives on their communication skills and patient interactions, fostering continuous improvement.
3. **Self-Assessment Tools**: Healthcare professionals were encouraged to engage in self-reflection through structured self-assessment tools, evaluating their performance against established benchmarks. This practice not only promoted accountability but also empowered team members to identify their development needs.
4. **Regular Performance Reviews**: MD Anderson conducted regular virtual performance reviews, allowing healthcare providers to discuss their progress, set future goals, and receive constructive feedback. These reviews helped maintain a sense of connection and accountability among team members despite physical separation.
5. **Patient Outcome Metrics**: The center closely monitored patient outcomes related to remote care, such as treatment adherence and overall health improvements. This data was essential in assessing the effectiveness of remote care strategies and informing future practices.

By implementing these assessment methods, MD Anderson Cancer Center not only ensured the delivery of high-quality patient care during challenging times but also strengthened team dynamics and engagement among its remote healthcare professionals.

6. TECHNOLOGICAL INNOVATIONS IN REMOTE HEALTHCARE LEADERSHIP

Incorporating cutting-edge technology into healthcare has significantly influenced leadership practices, especially in remote environments. Leaders in the healthcare sector are now required to understand, adapt, and integrate new tools such as artificial intelligence (AI), virtual reality (VR), and wearable devices into their decision-making processes and team management strategies.

1. **Artificial Intelligence (AI):** AI is transforming the healthcare industry by automating administrative tasks, improving diagnostic accuracy, and enhancing patient monitoring. For healthcare leaders managing remote teams, AI can assist in predictive analytics to forecast patient needs and optimize resource allocation. It also helps streamline communication and coordination among team members by automating scheduling, task assignment, and follow-ups. Leaders can leverage AI to identify performance trends and flag potential issues within the team before they escalate.
2. **Virtual Reality (VR):** VR is gaining traction in training and education for remote healthcare teams. Leaders can use VR to simulate clinical scenarios, allowing team members to practice and improve their skills without being physically present in a medical facility. This enhances learning and preparedness for real-world situations. Additionally, VR fosters collaboration in remote settings, enabling healthcare teams to visualize complex medical procedures and treatment plans together, regardless of their geographical location.
3. **Wearable Devices:** Wearable technology such as smartwatches and health trackers provides real-time data on patient health metrics, enabling remote monitoring of patients with chronic conditions. Leaders overseeing remote healthcare teams can use wearable devices to enhance patient care by allowing team members to track vital signs and intervene promptly when abnormalities are detected. This technology supports continuous patient care, improving outcomes while reducing the need for frequent in-person visits.
4. **Telemedicine Platforms:** Telemedicine platforms have revolutionized the way healthcare is delivered, especially in remote areas. Effective leadership in remote healthcare teams requires a deep understanding of these platforms to ensure

smooth communication between patients and providers. Leaders must ensure that their teams are proficient in using telemedicine tools for consultations, diagnosis, and treatment. They also need to manage data privacy and compliance with healthcare regulations like HIPAA (Health Insurance Portability and Accountability Act).

5. **Cloud-Based Collaboration Tools:** Cloud technology has made it easier for remote healthcare teams to collaborate and share information securely. Leaders can utilize cloud-based platforms to store and access patient data, manage workflows, and facilitate real-time communication between team members. This enhances coordination, ensuring that all healthcare professionals involved in a patient's care have the necessary information to make informed decisions.

Real-World Example: Integration of AI at Mount Sinai Health System

Mount Sinai Health System launched its Hospital-at-Home program to provide hospital-level care to patients in their homes, particularly those with chronic conditions needing close monitoring. The leadership prioritized creating a comprehensive virtual care model that enables the delivery of acute care services such as IV therapy, remote monitoring, and virtual consultations. They invested in advanced remote technology to ensure timely, safe, and efficient care from home. The outcome of this initiative included a significant reduction in hospital readmission rates, improved patient satisfaction, and lower healthcare costs. Mount Sinai's leadership exemplifies how healthcare institutions can effectively scale remote care by focusing on patient-centred solutions and leveraging telemedicine, demonstrating resilience and adaptability, especially during crises like the COVID-19 pandemic.

Intermountain Healthcare's Virtual Hospital (Connect Care Pro)

Intermountain Healthcare launched Connect Care Pro, a virtual hospital that offers a wide range of remote healthcare services across the U.S., including emergency services, specialty consultations, and remote patient monitoring in smaller hospitals. The leadership at Intermountain prioritized integrating telemedicine into their care model, ensuring robust support for both patients and healthcare professionals. They provided extensive training for remote staff and established leadership structures that allowed for quick decision-making and high-quality care, even in rural areas. As a result, Intermountain's leadership successfully reduced patient transfer rates from smaller hospitals and improved access to specialists for patients in underserved regions. Their innovative model of remote care, paired with effective leadership, has set a standard for other healthcare organizations aiming to expand their telehealth services.

Kaiser Permanente's Remote Behavioural Health Initiative

Kaiser Permanente implemented a remote behavioural health initiative to effectively address the growing mental health needs through virtual care. The leadership team prioritized enabling mental health professionals to engage with patients remotely while ensuring high-quality care and confidentiality. During the COVID-19 pandemic, they quickly adapted to meet the surge in demand for remote mental health services by leveraging innovative technology platforms and telemedicine tools. As a result, the initiative achieved significant success, with improvements in patient satisfaction, reduced wait times, and increased overall access to mental health services. Kaiser Permanente's leadership showcased agility and resilience in overcoming challenges, ultimately delivering comprehensive mental health care in a remote setting.

7. CASE STUDIES: SUCCESSFUL EXAMPLES OF LEADERSHIP IN REMOTE HEALTHCARE

In the dynamic landscape of healthcare, effective leadership is critical, especially within the context of remote healthcare delivery. As the demand for telehealth services continues to rise, it is essential to examine successful models that exemplify strong leadership in this realm. This section will present case studies of leading healthcare organizations that have effectively navigated the challenges of remote care delivery through innovative leadership practices.

The following case studies will explore the leadership strategies implemented by renowned healthcare organizations, including UCSF Health, Cleveland Clinic, Mayo Clinic, and Teladoc Health. Each of these organizations has demonstrated a commitment to enhancing patient care through innovative solutions and effective team management, providing a wealth of knowledge for healthcare leaders and practitioners alike.

Cleveland Clinic Case Study

Overview

The Cleveland Clinic, a renowned healthcare institution, faced significant challenges in providing care during the COVID-19 pandemic. With a need to adapt to remote healthcare delivery, they implemented innovative leadership practices to manage their remote teams effectively. This case study examines the strategies employed by the Cleveland Clinic and the outcomes of their leadership initiatives.

Challenges Faced

1. **Increased Demand for Telehealth Services**: The pandemic led to a surge in patients seeking remote consultations, which required a rapid scaling of telehealth services.
2. **Employee Morale and Engagement**: Physical separation from colleagues resulted in feelings of isolation among healthcare staff, potentially affecting morale and productivity.
3. **Technological Integration**: There was a need for seamless integration of telehealth platforms and training for staff to ensure effective virtual care delivery.

Leadership Strategies Implemented

1. **Transformational Leadership**: Leaders at the Cleveland Clinic focused on inspiring their teams by creating a shared vision for telehealth. They communicated the importance of adapting to new technologies to ensure continuous patient care.
2. **Supportive Work Environment**: The leadership prioritized mental health and well-being by providing resources for staff to manage stress and work-life balance during challenging times.
3. **Regular Feedback Mechanisms**: Implementing regular check-ins and feedback loops allowed leaders to gauge employee sentiment, address concerns, and adjust strategies accordingly.

Outcomes

1. **Rapid Telehealth Expansion**: The Cleveland Clinic successfully increased its telehealth visits from approximately 1,000 per week before the pandemic to over 60,000 per week by April 2020. This shift significantly improved access to care for patients.
2. **Improved Employee Engagement**: Surveys indicated that employees felt more supported and engaged due to the initiatives put in place by the leadership. Staff reported feeling more connected despite physical distancing.
3. **Enhanced Patient Satisfaction**: Telehealth services led to higher patient satisfaction scores, as patients appreciated the convenience and accessibility of virtual visits.

Mayo Clinic Case Study

Overview

Mayo Clinic, a leading healthcare organization known for its integrated clinical practice, education, and research, faced significant challenges during the COVID-19 pandemic. With a surge in patients requiring remote consultations, the organization needed to quickly adapt its operations and implement effective leadership strategies to manage its remote healthcare teams. This case study highlights Mayo Clinic's innovative approaches and the outcomes of their leadership initiatives.

Challenges Faced

1. **Shift to Remote Consultations**: The pandemic necessitated a rapid transition from in-person visits to telehealth services, posing logistical and operational challenges.
2. **Maintaining Patient Care Quality**: Ensuring high-quality care while shifting to remote delivery required adjustments in workflows and training for healthcare providers.
3. **Workforce Adaptation**: The sudden need for remote work created challenges in communication, collaboration, and team cohesion among healthcare professionals.

Leadership Strategies Implemented

1. **Transformational Leadership**: Mayo Clinic's leaders focused on inspiring their teams through a shared vision of providing continuous, high-quality patient care, even in a remote setting. They emphasized the importance of adaptability and innovation during the crisis.
2. **Comprehensive Training Programs**: To address the shift to telehealth, the organization implemented training sessions for staff to familiarize them with virtual care technologies and best practices.
3. **Enhanced Communication Channels**: Leaders established regular virtual meetings and forums to facilitate open communication, allowing team members to share experiences, challenges, and solutions.

Outcomes

1. **Successful Telehealth Implementation**: Mayo Clinic quickly ramped up its telehealth capabilities, reporting a 1,000% increase in virtual visits within the first few months of the pandemic. This shift allowed the clinic to continue providing care while ensuring patient safety.

2. **Positive Employee Feedback**: Surveys conducted among staff indicated that the majority felt supported by leadership during the transition. The emphasis on communication and collaboration helped maintain team morale and cohesion.
3. **High Patient Satisfaction Rates**: Patient satisfaction scores remained high during the pandemic, as many patients expressed appreciation for the convenience and accessibility of telehealth services.

Teladoc Health's Leadership During Crisis

Overview

Teladoc Health, a pioneer in virtual healthcare services, experienced unprecedented growth and demand for its telehealth solutions during the COVID-19 pandemic. As healthcare systems worldwide faced the challenges of a rapidly evolving crisis, Teladoc's leadership played a pivotal role in navigating this period of uncertainty and disruption. This case study examines Teladoc Health's leadership strategies, their implementation, and the outcomes achieved during this critical time.

Challenges Faced

1. **Surge in Demand**: The onset of the pandemic led to an exponential increase in demand for telehealth services as patients sought safe and accessible healthcare options.
2. **Scalability of Services**: Rapidly scaling operations to accommodate the surge in patient consultations posed logistical challenges, including technology infrastructure and staffing.
3. **Patient and Provider Education**: Ensuring that both patients and healthcare providers were comfortable and knowledgeable about telehealth processes was essential for effective service delivery.

Leadership Strategies Implemented

1. **Agile Leadership**: Teladoc's leaders employed agile decision-making to adapt quickly to changing circumstances. This flexibility allowed the organization to respond effectively to new healthcare regulations and patient needs.
2. **Investment in Technology**: Teladoc significantly enhanced its technology infrastructure to support increased usage. This included improving its platform's capabilities and ensuring robust cybersecurity measures to protect patient data.

3. **Proactive Communication**: Leadership maintained open lines of communication with both employees and clients. Regular updates about service changes, best practices, and available resources helped foster a sense of community and support.

Outcomes

1. **Remarkable Growth**: Teladoc reported a substantial increase in its user base, with millions of virtual visits conducted during the pandemic. This growth solidified its position as a leader in telehealth.
2. **Enhanced Patient Experience**: Feedback from users indicated high satisfaction rates with telehealth services. The company's focus on user-friendly technology and effective communication helped build trust among patients.
3. **Recognition and Partnerships**: Teladoc established partnerships with various healthcare organizations, expanding its service offerings and solidifying its reputation as a dependable telehealth provider.

University of California San Francisco (UCSF) Health's Remote Care Program

Overview

The University of California San Francisco (UCSF) Health has been at the forefront of innovation in telehealth and remote patient care, particularly through its Remote Care Program. Launched to enhance patient engagement and improve access to healthcare, this program leverages technology to deliver high-quality care to patients in their homes. This case study delves into the leadership strategies employed by UCSF Health, the challenges encountered, and the positive outcomes achieved through the Remote Care Program.

Challenges Faced

1. **Transitioning to Telehealth**: The rapid transition from in-person visits to virtual consultations posed significant logistical and technological challenges for UCSF Health.
2. **Patient Compliance and Engagement**: Engaging patients and ensuring compliance with treatment plans in a remote setting was a concern, especially for those unfamiliar with technology.
3. **Integration with Existing Systems**: Ensuring that the Remote Care Program integrated seamlessly with existing healthcare systems and workflows was vital for operational success.

Leadership Strategies Implemented

1. **Collaborative Leadership**: UCSF Health's leadership adopted a collaborative approach, bringing together interdisciplinary teams from various specialties to design and implement the Remote Care Program effectively.
2. **Training and Support**: Comprehensive training programs were developed for both staff and patients to facilitate the transition to telehealth. This included user-friendly guides and technical support to assist patients during virtual visits.
3. **Data-Driven Decision Making**: Leadership utilized data analytics to monitor program effectiveness, patient satisfaction, and engagement levels. This data-driven approach allowed for continuous improvements and adaptations to the program.

Outcomes

1. **Increased Patient Access**: The Remote Care Program successfully expanded access to healthcare services, particularly for patients in underserved areas, ensuring timely interventions and improved health outcomes.
2. **High Patient Satisfaction Rates**: Patient feedback indicated a high level of satisfaction with the Remote Care Program, with many patients appreciating the convenience and accessibility of virtual consultations.
3. **Operational Efficiency**: The integration of telehealth into UCSF Health's operations led to improved workflow efficiency, allowing healthcare providers to manage more patients effectively without compromising care quality.

8. CONCLUSION

In summary, integrating effective leadership practices in managing remote healthcare teams is crucial in today's healthcare landscape. This chapter emphasizes the need for adaptable leadership styles and strategies to navigate the complexities of physical distance. Key leadership characteristics such as emotional intelligence, communication skills, adaptability, vision, and accountability are essential for fostering engagement and a cohesive team culture. Leadership styles like transformational, servant, and transactional leadership, illustrated through real-world case studies, provide insights into motivating and supporting remote teams. The chapter identifies challenges in remote healthcare delivery, including communication barriers, technology adoption, and performance monitoring, offering practical strategies to address these issues through regular communication, technical support, and team-building activities. Assessment methods for evaluating remote team performance, including 360-degree feedback and patient satisfaction surveys, provide a comprehensive view of team dynamics. Case studies from organizations like Cleveland Clinic, Mayo Clinic, Teladoc Health, and UCSF Health reinforce the importance of adaptability and patient-centred approaches, ensuring sustainable and effective solutions for remote healthcare challenges.

Recommendations

Considering these findings, several recommendations can be made for both practitioners and researchers in the field of remote healthcare:

1. **Invest in Leadership Development Programs**: Organizations should prioritize training programs that focus on developing leadership qualities specific to remote team management. This will help cultivate leaders who are skilled in navigating the unique challenges posed by virtual environments.
2. **Promote a Culture of Inclusivity and Support**: Leaders should foster an organizational culture that values diversity and inclusion. Regular team-building activities, both virtual and in-person, when possible, can strengthen team cohesion and improve morale.
3. **Leverage Data-Driven Decision-Making**: Utilizing data analytics tools to monitor team performance and patient outcomes can provide insights that inform better leadership decisions and strategic planning.
4. **Focus on Continuous Improvement**: Organizations should establish feedback mechanisms to gather insights from team members and patients alike. This feedback can guide ongoing improvements in team dynamics, technology adoption, and patient care practices.
5. **Adapt to Technological Advancements**: Leaders must stay abreast of emerging technologies and be willing to integrate them into their practices. Continuous education on new tools and methodologies will enhance the team's capability to adapt to changes.

By leveraging these recommendations, healthcare organizations can enhance the effectiveness of their remote teams, leading to improved patient care and more resilient healthcare systems. As the healthcare landscape evolves, integrating effective leadership practices, designing robust healthcare systems, and fostering continuous improvement will be paramount. The goal is to enhance patient outcomes and improve the overall quality of care delivered through remote healthcare systems.

REFERENCES

Aadahl, M., & Bjerre-Nielsen, A. (2019). Leadership in remote teams: The case of a Danish healthcare organization. *Journal of Health Organization and Management*, 33(2), 125–140. DOI: 10.1108/JHOM-09-2018-0268

Arora, V. M., & Kachalia, A. (2016). Leadership in healthcare: The importance of leadership for high-quality healthcare delivery. *Journal of the American Medical Association*, 316(10), 1063–1064. DOI: 10.1001/jama.2016.9472

Bach, S. (2021). Managing remote teams in healthcare: Strategies and challenges. *Health Services Management Research*, 34(1), 24–31. DOI: 10.1177/0951484820917712

Cleveland Clinic. (2020). **Telemedicine: A virtual visit for patients**. *Cleveland Clinic Newsroom*. https://newsroom.clevelandclinic.org/2020/03/31/telemedicine-a-virtual-visit-for-patients/

Davis, M., & Kohn, L. T. (2019). Leadership strategies in remote healthcare environments: A review of the literature. *International Journal of Healthcare Management*, 12(3), 205–211. DOI: 10.1080/20479700.2019.1630481

Mayo Clinic. (2020). **Virtual care: Patient-centered remote healthcare services**. *Mayo Clinic Social Media Network*. https://socialmedia.mayoclinic.org/2020/05/12/virtual-care-patient-centered-remote-healthcare-services/

Meyer, M., & Schaeffer, J. (2019). Challenges in remote healthcare delivery: Perspectives from healthcare leaders. *Health Affairs*, 38(8), 1346–1354. DOI: 10.1377/hlthaff.2019.00412

Mount Sinai Health System. (2021). *The Mount Sinai Health System's telehealth initiative: Expanding access to care*. Mount Sinai Health System News.

Teladoc Health. (2020). **Leadership during crisis: Adapting to remote healthcare delivery**. *Teladoc Health Blog*. https://www.teladochealth.com/leadership-during-crisis/

Wong, C., & Laschinger, H. K. (2019). The influence of authentic leadership on nurses' outcomes in a remote healthcare setting. *Journal of Nursing Management*, 27(6), 1095–1102. DOI: 10.1111/jonm.12786

ADDITIONAL READING

González, M., & Montalvo, J. (2021). Telemedicine and remote patient management: A new era for healthcare leaders. *Journal of Health Management*, 23(4), 451–462.

Khan, H. A., & Altun, A. (2020). The role of telemedicine in the healthcare system: A comprehensive review. *International Journal of Health Sciences*, 14(2), 73–80.

Wang, H., & Liu, Y. (2021). Remote healthcare during the COVID-19 pandemic: Insights from a systematic review. *Health Care*, 9(1), 10. PMID: 35052174

Chapter 6
Managing Capital Allocation for Better Technology Integration Outcomes in Healthcare Companies

Diogo Modesto
ISLA Santarém, Portugal

Ricardo Marcão
https://orcid.org/0000-0003-3277-3078
ISLA Santarém, Portugal

ABSTRACT

This paper explores the key strategies and frameworks for optimizing capital allocation to enhance technology integration outcomes, showing the importance of aligning financial investments with long-term strategic goals in technology. Effective capital allocation is mandatory in achieving successful technology integration outcomes. The process requires an understanding of both short and long-term value creation, ensuring that short-term financial decisions align with the organization's long-term strategic goals.

DOI: 10.4018/979-8-3693-8598-2.ch006

1. INTRODUCTION TO CAPITAL ALLOCATION IN TECHNOLOGY

Effective capital allocation is crucial for achieving successful technology integration outcomes. In today's rapidly evolving digital landscape, businesses must embrace technology not merely as a tool for growth but as a core pillar of their survival. The digital transformation is not just a trend—it is an essential step for businesses to remain relevant, competitive, and resilient in an increasingly tech-driven world. Whether it's a small marketing campaign on social media or implementing advanced digital tools to open new sales channels, every business must leverage technology. A non-digital business risks obsolescence. Without a deep commitment to technology and innovation, businesses may find themselves outpaced by competitors or unable to meet the evolving needs of customers. However, simply investing in technology is not enough. Capital must be allocated strategically, not just to acquire the latest technological tools, but also to build and sustain the broader ecosystem of innovation that supports long-term growth. This ecosystem includes the development of new skills, the creation of digital infrastructure, and the nurturing of a culture of continuous learning and adaptability. It's not just about adopting new tools, but about ensuring that the workforce is equipped to use those tools effectively and that the organization as a whole is capable of leveraging technology to drive value across all functions. The capital allocation process must consider both short-term and long-term value creation. While immediate financial returns are important, short-term decisions must always align with the organization's broader, long-term strategic goals. In this context, the challenge lies in balancing short-term financial performance with long-term innovation objectives. This requires a deep understanding of how investments in technology will not only pay off in the near term but will also position the organization for future success in an increasingly digital economy. This paper explores key strategies and frameworks for optimizing capital allocation in the context of technology integration. It emphasizes the importance of aligning financial investments with the organization's overarching strategic vision, ensuring that the pursuit of innovation and digital transformation is not just a series of tactical moves, but a cohesive, long-term strategy. From prioritizing investments that will yield the greatest impact to assessing risk and ensuring the integration of technology is seamless, this paper provides actionable insights for leaders looking to maximize the impact of their technology investments. (Martínez-Peláez et al.2023; Nwosu, 2024; Adebayo et al.2024)

2. THEORETICAL FRAMEWORKS IN CAPITAL ALLOCATION

Three outstanding frameworks reinforce the best practices in capital Allocation. Strategic capital budgeting, Investment project selection, and Investment governance. Strategic Capital Budgeting, Companies that exercise superior budgeting discipline invest in businesses rather than projects, translate portfolio roles into capital allocation guidelines, and strive for balanced investment portfolios. Invest in businesses rather than projects. Capital allocation is about looking at the forest and the trees, and top performers look at the forest first. The outperformers in BCG's capital allocation database invest systematically in businesses that create value from a strategic as well as a financial point of view, whereas underperformers invest too much in value-destroying growth. A business potential-based approach to capital budgeting helped IBM, for example, reorient its portfolio from hardware to cloud-based services. Similarly, Tata Consultancy Services divested its call center operations, even though the business was still booming, to free up management capacity and resources for a push into value-added services, which the company believed to be much more promising in the future. Today, many companies in the energy and automotive industries are shifting their investments away from their past cash cows and towards renewables and green technology. Naturally, the magnitude and speed of the shift depend on the perceived size of the concrete green business potential. Investment Project Selection, Outperformers work to understand the financial profile of projects being considered fully. They look beyond the internal rate of return, apply criteria relevant to the investment type, and work to obtain a true understanding of potential risks. In theory, there is a simple rule for choosing among competing investment projects: sort the list of projects based on their expected internal rate of return and select those with the highest IRRs until the budget is fully committed. In practice, however, the effectiveness of this approach is constrained by the quality of the assumptions that go into the valuations and by the influence of additional criteria that are not transparent or explicit in selection decisions. At many companies, criteria beyond financial returns also come into play in making investment decisions. However, if such factors are not made explicit and predefined upfront, they can distort the decision-making process and encourage political behavior. One European industrial conglomerate addresses this challenge by evaluating investment projects based on four explicit criteria that are summarized in a simple scoring model: strategic profile (growth potential and fit with the strategy of the underlying business), financial profile (expected project return and short-term impact on EBIT), risk profile (payback time and assessment of market risks), and resource profile (fit with existing capabilities and required management attention). Depending on the structure of a company's investment portfolio, decision-makers may need to apply different sets of criteria for the different types of investment.

For example, a strict focus on the internal rate of return and payback time may systematically favor incremental improvement investments at the expense of larger breakthrough or growth investments that tend to have longer-term and uncertain payoffs. Understanding the underlying risks should be a particular focus in project selection. Research has shown time and again that human beings are weak at risk assessment, but some techniques can help. A good starting point can be to frame the discussion in terms of a base question: What do we need to believe in to make this an attractive investment? This framing can help uncover the implicit business assumptions behind a proposal and the key risks hidden in the business plan. For very uncertain investments, the critical assumptions of an investment may even be tested in systematic validation experiments through a "discovery-driven planning" approach. Investment Governance High performers apply robust governance mechanisms to choose, support, and track major investments. They address cognitive biases, establish accountability, and institute effective feedback loops. Research and experience have shown that capital allocation decisions are prone to several cognitive biases, such as framing decisions too narrowly, relying too heavily on readily available information, anchoring (that is, being reluctant to adapt to new information), and falling into "groupthink" (making decisions as a group in a way that discourages individual dissent). In the end, successful capital allocation is the result of strong judgment skills, which are built through learning and adaptation. Effective feedback loops are essential. In M&A, which often requires a very large allocation of capital, this type of rigor and commitment to continued learning is one of the reasons that frequent dealmakers consistently outperform less experienced companies. While post-completion audits for large projects are common in many companies, the feedback into decision-making typically happens only sporadically. Advanced companies review not only projects but also past decisions. The head of corporate strategy at a large industrial conglomerate puts it this way: "We made our biggest losses from moves not made. So, we also explicitly review opportunity cost mistakes." Capital is only one scarce corporate resource requiring careful allocation. Executive time and management talent, IT capacity, and operating budgets are others. However, capital often has the biggest impact, which is easy to measure. The three basic disciplines of capital allocation—strategic budgeting, project selection, and investment governance—provide a powerful framework, and the best practices within each discipline give any company a good set of guidelines to follow. (Nilashi et al.2023; Ajiga et al., 2024; Zheng et al.2024)

3. TECHNOLOGY INVESTMENTS

The cornerstone of any technology investment is its alignment with the overall business strategy. Companies need to view technology not just to keep up with trends but as a strategic tool that enhances operational efficiency, drives innovation, and contributes to the achievement of business objectives. However, businesses must ensure that they don't just merely integrate tech into existing strategies. The pace of technological innovation often requires a fundamental re-evaluation or a complete redefinition of the business strategy itself. Businesses must adapt to a tech-centric world, reshaping their models and customer experiences. Technology should be seen not just as a tool but as a strategic driver, shaping and guiding the business direction. This new paradigm requires companies to continuously align their tech investments with their evolving business objectives, ensuring that they are not just keeping pace with technological advancements but are actively leveraging them to redefine their market presence, innovate their offerings, and sustain competitive advantage in a dynamically shifting business landscape. When looking at the technology market worldwide, its reach is almost untouchable — the 10 largest tech firms have a massive combined market capitalization of more than US$27 trillion. Deloitte posits that the drive-by enterprises to embrace digital transformation is pushing the growth of emerging technologies such as cloud computing, artificial intelligence, and cybersecurity. "Analysts estimate that public cloud spending will grow by more than 20%, and they foresee stronger demand for cybersecurity. AI investment (not specifically generative AI) is also seen as contributing to overall spending growth. Economists have projected that AI-related investments could reach $200 billion globally by 2025, led by the United States," Deloitte notes in its technology industry outlook. With exciting and profound advancements in natural language processing and prediction, AI adoption is beginning to pick up, particularly with the advent of OpenAI's ChatGPT. The evolution of AI is projected to influence and shape society, and analysts estimate that revenues from AI will grow at a CAGR of 37.3 percent to reach more than US$1.81 trillion in 2030. The mobile gaming market will also see growth in the years ahead, rising at a CAGR of 10.39 percent to reach an estimated US$164.81 billion by 2029. "The development of mobile games has resulted in scalability for the gaming industry. Platforms like Facebook and Instagram have also started to develop innovative mobile games to ensure high product differentiation and benefit from engaging games to enhance their advertisement strategies," states Mordor Intelligence in a recent report on the industry. As for the future of 3D printing, Grand View Research projects a CAGR of 23.5 percent, which would create a market worth US$88.28 billion by 2030. According to the firm, that growth will be driven by increasing prototyping applications from industries like healthcare, aerospace, and defense, as well as "aggressive research and development" on 3D printing. Blockchain is one of the most promising sectors in the future of the tech space. Grand View Research is forecasting a CAGR of 87.7 percent between 2023 and 2030 to reach a market value of more than US$1.43 trillion. Blockchain's use in the healthcare sector is expected to experience the fastest growth during the period mentioned, driven by the demand for digitization in the industry and an increasing number of regulations aimed at protecting patient data. Investing in cutting-edge technologies, while potentially rewarding, carries its own set of risks. As an investor, it's crucial to be aware of these challenges to make well-informed decisions. Here are key risks to consider: Uncertainty: Many emerging technologies are still in developmental stages, making their market success unpredictable. This unpredictability can pose significant risks. Regulatory changes: The tech sector can be subject to sudden regulatory changes, which can impact emerging technologies, creating uncertainty and potential liabilities. Future growth predictions: Predicting future growth in the realm of new technologies is challenging. Striking a balance between the potential for high returns and the risk of significant losses is crucial. Management team: The success of a tech company often hinges on its leadership. The ability of the team to navigate the complexities of the tech industry can greatly impact investment outcomes. Competitive Landscape: The tech industry is fiercely competitive. The success of your investment could largely depend on the strategies and strength of competing companies. (Wood & Sacks, 2023; Parlindungan et al.2021; Kastner et al., 2025)

4. TECHNOLOGY INVESTMENT TO COVER BUSINESS NEEDS

Ambitious digital transformations that promise the moon usually to crash spectacularly. Most companies are dismayed to learn that their recent digital investments are delivering less than a third of the impact they were aiming for. The reasons? Lack of skills, weak leadership support, poorly defined objectives, and unrealistic timelines. This wide gap between what businesses need and the tech they implement is a wake-up call. Preparing a solid business case for technology investments will help match your technology needs and budgets. By "business case" we mean not only budget approval but also demonstrating how the technology will meet stakeholders' expectations, align with company goals, and deliver tangible business outcomes. A well-crafted business case for technology investments paints a clear picture of the overall value of the investment, weighing the costs, benefits, and risks. Setting upfront objectives about what needs to be achieved is the first step. The second is ensuring there's transparency around financial metrics and the return on investment the team is working toward while maintaining focus on the consumer pain point the team is solving. All parties must agree on the metrics and how they are captured.

From there, you can begin to measure before launch and then monitor how the situation evolves. When creating a roadmap of digital priorities, it's essential to align closely with business goals. Without that alignment, investments may focus on delivering technology rather than meeting business objectives. Stakeholders do not perceive quantifiable value in IT production elements. Measure digitalization's impact on company outcomes, avoiding metrics that emphasize effort or technical output. Building a strong business case necessitates an appraisal of how the technology investment will help reduce costs. The success of technology investments heavily relies on the collaboration between IT and business units. The PWC report indicates that only 10% of business representatives felt that the collaboration with IT during the technology transition was effective. This disconnect often leads to incomplete project delivery and missed deadlines. Businesses who invest in technology and digital that align with a sustainable strategy, and in providing the training and skills needed to effectively transform, will gain a competitive advantage and the opportunity to add real value throughout the business or over a project's life cycle. Investments in digital transformation help businesses improve efficiency by using technology such as cloud computing, artificial intelligence, and app integrations. Enabling automation and data analytics makes a huge impact by allowing businesses to be increasingly agile and responsive. Investments in technology can also support sustainability transformation by enabling energy-saving practices and in reducing carbon footprint. Technology can support the automating, capturing, and reporting of ESG KPIs. This can help overcome issues like inconsistent data, information management, and workflow silos on projects. For these, it is vital to curate a suitable investment model for example an integrated digital platform best suited to the sustainable business plans of the company. As technology persists as the best global connectivity tool, customers are beginning to demand a more customized, effortless experience from brands they trust. Regardless of your industry, it's important to adopt technology that helps automate responsibilities and gives insight into customer behavior to move prospects along the pipeline faster, all while making more sales and offering a unique customer experience. (Wolf-Fordham, 2020; Ziervogel et al., 2022; Tuan, 2023)

5. ALIGN SHORT-TERM DECISIONS TO LONG-TERM STRATEGY IN CAPITAL ALLOCATION

Businesses concerned only with short-term goals overcome immediate challenges but fail to prevent their recurrence. Alternatively, businesses with only long-term goals may not last long enough to see them reached. CFOs should align with short-term goals like revenue or expense targets, cash flow management, and expense control, many critical for company survival, especially for early-stage startups. However, while focusing on the short term, they must consider the risks to delivering long-term value. To do that, they must plan for scenarios like market changes, economic fluctuations, and industry disruptions. Long-term value is built on understanding and supporting the strategic vision, which is the only way to drive sustainable growth. It requires technology investments, market expansion, new products or channels, and skills development. However, investment opportunities must be evaluated rigorously to ensure that capital is allocated efficiently and aligned with the strategy. Sometimes, that might require prioritizing growth initiatives even while trying to optimize costs. Short-term financial planning is about solving immediate problems and developing strategies that will lead to results, usually within one year. Short-term goals should be achievable and adaptable to emerging circumstances. Long-term and short-term financial planning are two sides of the same coin. When it comes to achieving financial stability and growth, it is essential to create a comprehensive financial plan that incorporates both long-term and short-term goals. A well-designed financial plan serves as a roadmap to guide businesses toward their desired financial outcomes. One of the fundamental aspects of a financial plan is budgeting. It involves tracking and managing your income and expenses to ensure that you have allocated your money most efficiently. By creating a budget, you gain better control over your finances, allowing you to allocate resources towards achieving both your short-term and long-term financial goals. The plan should outline specific strategies for saving and investing. This includes determining how much you want to save or invest regularly, as well as selecting appropriate investment vehicles that align with your risk tolerance and goals. By setting aside a portion of your income for savings or investments, you can make progress toward both short-term and long-term financial aspirations. Managing risk is an important aspect of any financial plan. This involves analyzing potential risks, such as unexpected events or emergencies, and devising strategies to mitigate them. By incorporating risk management measures, such as insurance policies or emergency funds. Overemphasizing short-term operations can lead to missed opportunities for innovation and growth, inability to adapt to market changes, and loss of competitive advantage. However neglecting short-term needs in favor of long-term goals can result in cash flow problems, decreased employee morale due to constant pressure without immediate gratification or rewards, and loss of market share to more agile competitors. Most companies' long-term financial plans include too many line items. This kind of detail slows down the process, makes iteration difficult, and can obscure the true drivers of value. To be effective, a long-term financial plan needs to be concise. For example, there is no need for ten or more items under general and administrative (G&A) expenses; the G&A line can stand alone. In most cases, income statements for each business should include only revenues, cost of goods sold, sales and marketing, R&D, and overhead costs

- without disaggregating detail. An enterprise runs on value drivers, not accounting items. An effective financial plan lays out the most important value drivers for each business unit, surfacing the few key elements that are most important for profitable growth, return on capital, and other company imperatives. What do key value drivers look like? Consider a filmmaking company: there is a lot that goes into creating successful movies over a multiyear period. But cut to the chase (as they say in Hollywood), and its model can be simplified to producing three blockbusters and five smaller films. Its most impactful value drivers are the average budgets for large and small films, marketing costs, and overhead expenses. A music subscription business, for its part, would have similarly compact but completely different key drivers: the number of subscribers, revenue per customer, and customer churn. A better approach is to be clear on targets and have the long-range financial plan highlight the specific resources that are allocated to the highest-priority initiatives, whether they are enterprise-wide or within a particular business unit, to make sure those targets are met. This typically requires the company to allocate resources among its business units differently from how it had in prior years, regardless of legacy spending or "fairness." For example, one major consumer-packaged-goods company took away the "base" level of spending for some of its legacy European operations because of their lack of growth and relatively low returns on capital. Instead, the company allocated those resources to three specific initiatives in Latin America. At one leading retailer, the CEO personally ensures the full funding and management of the company's top six enterprise initiatives, in addition to spending almost one day per week on those initiatives. (Sjölin & Sjölin, 2024; Fenech, 2024; Schechowiz, 2021)

6. TECHNOLOGY BUSINESS INVESTMENT RISKS

Personal devices on company networks. There has been a recent push to allow employees to use their mobile devices and laptops for company business. The issue for businesses then becomes how to manage these devices. Personal devices may not be up to date on the latest security patches. They also can download suspect material that company-owned devices block and they are at an increased risk of being lost or stolen. To fight against these issues, companies can create a set of mobile technology risk management policies that employees must follow. These help employees remain cognizant of the risks of using their mobile technology on a company's network. When an organization's technology system goes down, the business grinds to a halt. That is why businesses need to have a continuity plan in place with their IT service providers. The plan should map out how a business will get back online if service drops. This plan should include several factors. Chief among them is a list of emergency contact information for a company's MSP. Customers need to know who they can contact when service goes offline at 3 a.m., and there is nothing more frustrating for a client than having to hunt for the right person to contact. As a result, MSPs need to take every precaution to avoid these types of risks. While risk cannot be removed completely, companies want to know their MSP is taking every step imaginable to keep systems running and in working order. The most obvious benefit of technology risk management is that your organization can reduce its vulnerabilities. Active risk management plans reduce the likelihood that an anticipated risk will occur. That said, technology risk management has other benefits too, such as Reduced costs. Every risk has an associated cost, and technology risk is no different. By reducing the likelihood of risks, your organization saves on the costs associated with financial and reputational losses. Improved agility. Technology risks cause disruptions that delay business processes and scatter daily operations. A successful technology risk management strategy helps your business respond to risk events in a more agile way, allowing for briefer disruptions and improved business continuity. The first step in the technology risk management process is a technology risk analysis. At this stage, the risk management team uses tools to identify and prioritize the technology risks so they can assess and resolve those issues. Identifying technology risks should be an ongoing effort. Consequently, it makes sense to impanel a group of people to identify the sources of technology risks. These risk committee members should combine their knowledge and experience to scan the full range of possible technology risks, identifying which risk management frameworks are appropriate for each. The best technological investments require maintenance and regular upkeep to function at their best. Remember to back up your computer system and update its software each time there's a new update. IT experts have seen an increased number of hackers and those committing data theft. Remember to install malware protection on your technology devices and keep an eye out for online scams or security breaches. Make efforts to protect your intellectual property. While it may seem like a good idea to buy a cheaper piece of equipment, it's important to do your homework beforehand to see if this will be the best investment for your business. When business owners cut corners on equipment, they usually end up paying more long-term with replacements and costly repair services. (Weichbroth & Łysik, 2020; Thomasian & Adashi, 2021; Shafiq et al.2022)

7. CHANGE MANAGEMENT WITH NEW TECHNOLOGIES

Change management generally adopts controls, and implements change. Technology change management identifies new technology and then implements it for improved productivity and profitability. It reduces resistance, improves communication, and addresses the challenges inherent in major change. According to McKinsey & Company, a whopping 70% of digital transformations fail. A recent BCG survey reveals that 75% of transformation efforts don't deliver the anticipated results. Why? Technology project goals are often improperly defined and poorly communicated. This frightens and frustrates employees. Instead of adoption, you get resistance, misalignment across departments, and competing interests without common goals. New technology often disrupts established routines and workflows, leading to resistance among employees who are comfortable with existing systems. The fear of the unknown, coupled with concerns about job security and increased workload, can hinder the adoption of new tools. 38% of employees cite fear of the unknown as their reasoning behind opposing change. Implementing and embracing new technology may require a set of skills that employees currently lack. This gap can slow down the adoption process and lead to inefficiencies in utilizing the new tools. According to a report by the World Economic Forum, 60% of workers will require training and reskilling by 2027 to catch up with the changing nature of the workplace. New technology often requires a shift in organizational culture to align with its principles and benefits. A long-established culture, an unseen yet powerful force, might fuel the resistance to change, hindering the adoption of technology-driven practices. That's why 59% of change management practitioners name cultural awareness as a significant driver of successful change implementation. When a company invests in new technology, it typically does so with the expectation of improved productivity, streamlined processes, or enhanced competitive advantage. However, the success of any technological implementation heavily relies on how well it is embraced by the employees. Often, companies overlook the human element of change and underestimate the impact it can have on their technology initiatives. Supporting a technology implementation with an extensive, clear, and educational dialogue with the employees can turn caution and reluctant engagement into change acceptance and even genuine excitement about new tools and skills that come with it. To avoid common mistakes in change management during a technology implementation, here are some key notes: Poor or No Communication, A common mistake is the lack of clear and consistent communication about the change process. This can lead to confusion, resistance, and low motivation among employees. Leaving Out Employees, while change is often decided higher up, it impacts all employees, and you need their buy-in to make it a success. Involving them earlier in the process can ensure smoother transitions. Not Retiring Legacy Programs, change management should also determine how you handle previous systems. This complex topic involves culture, fear, and trying new things. Staff should be moved to new programs to help sunset legacy ones and get on the same page. Provide training and support to help employees adapt to the new system. Not Testing, launching in a test environment allows users to master the new way of working before the official launch, where misunderstandings and mistakes can be costly. Use pilot testing, user acceptance testing, and dry runs to identify and address issues before the full-scale implementation. CAB Bottlenecks, and Change Advisory Boards (CABs) are essential for reviewing and approving changes. However, they can often cause bottlenecks just by a lack of understanding of the process or available documentation. Be intentional with who attends these meetings, ensure details are addressed beforehand, and ensure the session is kept on point. Not Updating Your Method Over Time, Often, change management is done in one way without ever changing it. AI tools, personnel, tech, goals, or vendors change, so should the change management process. Regularly review and update your change management strategies to meet evolving business needs and market trends. (Viswa et al.2024; Karekla et al.2021; Velyako & Musa, 2024)

8. PERFORMANCE AND OUTCOME EVALUATION

Outcome evaluation is a type of evaluation that focuses on measuring the results or outcomes of a program or intervention. It is a systematic and objective process that involves collecting and analyzing data to determine whether the program is achieving its intended goals and objectives and whether the outcomes are meaningful and beneficial to the target population. Demonstrating accountability: Outcome evaluation provides evidence-based information on the effectiveness and impact of programs and interventions, which can be used to demonstrate accountability to stakeholders, such as funders, policymakers, and program participants. Improving program performance: Outcome evaluation can help to identify areas where the program can be improved and to make changes to program design or implementation to achieve better results. Informing decision-making: Outcome evaluation provides information that can be used to inform decision-making about program design, implementation, and resource allocation, by identifying programs and interventions that are achieving their intended outcomes and providing the greatest benefits to the target population. Generating new knowledge: Outcome evaluation can generate new knowledge and insights about what works and what doesn't work in programs and interventions, which can be shared with other stakeholders and used to inform future program design and implementation. Ensuring program sustainability: Outcome evaluation can help to ensure the sustainability of programs and interventions by providing evidence of their effectiveness and impact, which can be used to secure funding and support from stakeholders. The type of outcome evaluation used will depend on the specific goals and objectives of the program or intervention, as well as the research questions being asked. By using the appropriate type of outcome evaluation, program managers, policymakers, and other stakeholders can gain valuable insights into the effectiveness and impact of their programs and make informed decisions about resource allocation and program improvement. Technology investments are often substantial and can have a profound impact on an organization's operations, productivity, and competitive positioning. Proper evaluation of these investments is essential for several reasons: Maximizing ROI and evaluating technology investments helps organizations assess the potential return on investment (ROI). By understanding the financial and operational benefits of a technology solution, businesses can make informed decisions that lead to higher returns and better financial outcomes. Effective ROI analysis involves considering both tangible and intangible benefits, such as increased revenue, cost savings, and improved customer satisfaction. Minimize Risks, thorough evaluation helps identify potential risks and challenges associated with new technologies. By proactively addressing these risks, organizations can develop strategies to mitigate them and avoid costly pitfalls. This includes evaluating technical, operational, and financial risks that may impact the successful implementation and use of the technology. Ensure alignment with goals, a technology investment should align with an organization's strategic goals and objectives. Evaluating how well a technology supports key initiatives ensures that it contributes to long-term success and enhances overall business performance. This alignment helps prioritize investments that drive growth and achieve desired outcomes. Enhance Competitive Advantage, Effective evaluation helps identify technologies that provide a competitive edge. By selecting solutions that drive innovation and improve operational efficiency, organizations can differentiate themselves in the marketplace and gain a strategic advantage over competitors. Also evaluating the scalability and flexibility, whether the technology can scale with your business as it grows and adapts to changing needs and market conditions. Scalable and flexible technologies offer long-term value by supporting future expansion and evolving requirements without requiring a complete overhaul. (Juba, 2024; Almasri, 2024; Rositch et al., 2020)

9. TECHNOLOGY PROCUREMENT AND OUTSOURCING

At its core, technology procurement outsourcing involves delegating the responsibility for acquiring IT products and services to external vendors. This can include everything from hardware and software purchases to contract negotiation and vendor management. By outsourcing procurement tasks, businesses can leverage the expertise and resources of third-party providers, freeing up internal resources to focus on core business activities. Technology procurement plays a crucial role in ensuring that companies obtain the necessary resources at the right price, quality, and quantity to meet their operational needs. Technology procurement providers source, purchase, and acquire technology goods or services for a business or organization. Their scope of activities usually includes supplier selection, negotiation, contract management, and inventory control. Cost Saving, Businesses outsourcing procurement can save on training and labor costs, purchasing procurement software and tools, and managing databases, whilst avoiding incurring extra costs due to poor planning or procurement errors. The extensive knowledge of procurement service providers means that they know how to negotiate competitively with suppliers. It also means that they can identify the best options in the market for their clients so that they not only get the best prices but also the best quality of a technology product or service. On top of that, technology procurement providers might take advantage of bulk purchasing opportunities and discounts that are simply not available to regular buyers. Time efficiency with streamlined processes, by centralizing sourcing and standardizing their procedures, as well as using professional procurement software and tools, technology procurement providers can streamline the acquisition processes for their clients. Better control and visibility, Expertise leads to efficiency. Procurement experts handle several tasks (from supplier selection to contract management), reducing the administrative workload of your internal teams. Having access to procurement automation tools also means that fewer errors are made during the process, improving its effectiveness and reducing costs. Improved compliance and procurement services establish robust vendor selection criteria, ensuring suppliers meet legal and ethical requirements. They also monitor supplier performance to ensure adherence to quality and regulatory standards and provide regular audits and assessments to identify and rectify any non-compliance issues promptly. Procurement companies stay updated on industry regulations, adjusting strategies accordingly. Through proactive risk management and comprehensive documentation, they can mitigate compliance risks, safeguarding their clients' reputations and operational integrity. Thanks to these practices procurement services enhance compliance for their clients. Access to deep procurement expertise, Procurement service providers typically have extensive experience within the industry they work in, an asset that makes them successful in effective supplier selection, contract negotiation, and overall process management. With a keen understanding of market dynamics, they offer invaluable insights into emerging trends and industry benchmarks, empowering businesses to maintain a competitive edge.10. Sustainability and Green Technology Investments Green tech is a group of technologies that seek to reduce or eliminate the negative impacts of human activity on the natural environment. This can include anything from exploring new clean and renewable sources of energy to pioneering new and clean materials and finding ways to recycle waste and used materials. There are many ways to invest in green technology, from installing wind turbines and solar arrays to supporting electric vehicle research. Both private and government actors can contribute to green technology. Governments invest in green technology by giving subsidies or tax credits to green technology companies, while private individuals can support them by financing green technology enterprises. The global green technology and sustainability market size was valued at USD 17.21 billion in 2023. The market is projected to grow from USD 20.90 billion in 2024 to USD 105.26 billion by 2032, exhibiting a CAGR of 22.4% during the forecast period. Green technologies and sustainability include advanced environmental solutions that are deployed to secure natural resources and atmosphere, mitigate or minimize undesirable impacts from human-made actions on the surroundings, and increase sustainable development. In addition, the main aim of the solution is to secure and maintain the environment and repair past damages. The market is growing with a positive trajectory due to the increasing investment by key players in developing customized solutions and services. Key players are integrating their green technology solutions with emerging technologies, such as generative artificial intelligence (AI), advanced analytics, the Internet of Things (IoT), blockchain, cloud, cybersecurity, big data, and others. These technologies assist end-users in gathering, integrating, and analyzing data from numerous real-time data sources, such as sensors, a global positioning system (GPS), and cameras. Green technology refers to eco-friendly technologies and tools that enhance business operations. This technology also facilitates consumer applications such as charging systems, electric vehicles, smart homes, and other applications powered by IoT sensors. The Internet of Things (IoT) is an important aspect of the green technology and sustainability industry. IoT in green tech enables sensor-based solutions, minimizes the need for human intervention, and provides rich data insights to enable service providers to constantly improve their services. The combination of IoT and green technology has been facilitating the use of renewable energy in recent years. Green networks in IoT are likely to deliver a reduction in emissions and pollution, exploiting surveillance and conversation and minimizing operational costs and consumption. The Green Internet of Things (G-IoT) is projected to initiate significant changes that will support to realization of the idea of green ambient intelligence. In general, traditional technologies are less expensive than green technology solutions. The high costs of green technology solutions are constituted by the environmental expenses that are externalized in many conventional production procedures. In addition, as the technology is still new, the associated training and development costs are expected to be higher in comparison with existing technologies. High initial deployment costs are likely to restrict the adoption of green technologies among enterprises. Conclusion and future work. In conclusion, managing capital allocation for technology integration is not only a strategic imperative but also an operational challenge that demands a balanced and thoughtful approach. Leaders must consider how to prioritize investments in a way that maximizes value while minimizing potential risks. This involves evaluating the costs and benefits of each technological investment, understanding its long-term impact, and ensuring alignment with the organization's overarching goals. A clear framework for capital allocation allows companies to maintain flexibility, adapt to evolving technological landscapes, and leverage innovations as they emerge. Moreover, effective management of capital allocation for technology integration requires fostering a culture of collaboration between departments, including IT, finance, and operations, to ensure that all stakeholders are aligned in their vision for the future. Leaders must also remain vigilant in monitoring the performance of their technology investments, making necessary adjustments to stay ahead of market trends and technological advancements. When executed effectively, optimized capital allocation not only drives smoother technology integration but also positions a company to innovate at scale, respond agilely to competitive pressures, and ensure long-term sustainability. This process enables businesses to future-proof themselves, ensuring that they not only survive in a digital-first world but excel in it. By making informed, strategic decisions today, organizations lay the foundation for continuous growth, technological advancement, and market leadership tomorrow. (Massonini et al.2023; Devkota et al.2024; Güldürek & Esenboğa, 2024; Xu et al., 2024)

REFERENCES

Adebayo, Y. A., Ikevuje, A. H., Kwakye, J. M., & Esiri, A. E.Yetunde Adenike AdebayoAugusta Heavens IkevujeJephta Mensah KwakyeAndrew Emuobosa Esiri. (2024). Driving circular economy in project management: Effective stakeholder management for sustainable outcomes. *GSC Advanced Research and Reviews*, 20(3), 235–245. DOI: 10.30574/gscarr.2024.20.3.0351

Ajiga, D., Okeleke, P. A., Folorunsho, S. O., & Ezeigweneme, C. (2024). Methodologies for developing scalable software frameworks that support growing business needs. DOI: 10.1016/j.apenergy.2024.123789

Almasri, F. (2024). Exploring the impact of artificial intelligence in teaching and learning of science: A systematic review of empirical research. *Research in Science Education*, 54(5), 977–997. DOI: 10.1007/s11165-024-10176-3

Devkota, S., Karmacharya, P., Maharjan, S., Khatiwada, D., & Uprety, B. (2024). Decarbonizing urea: Techno-economic and environmental analysis of a model hydroelectricity and carbon capture based green urea production. *Applied Energy*, 372, 123789. DOI: 10.1016/j.apenergy.2024.123789

Fenech, M. (2024). The business development role of Maltese listed entity CFOs. DOI: 10.3390/su16135800

Güldürek, M., & Esenboğa, B. (2024). Assessment of Corporate Carbon Footprint and Energy Analysis of Transformer Industry. *Sustainability (Basel)*, 16(13), 5800. DOI: 10.3390/su16135800

Juba, O. O. (2024). Impact of workplace safety, health, and wellness programs on employee engagement and productivity. International Journal of Health. *Medicine and Nursing Practice*, 6(4), 12–27.

Karekla, M., Pollalis, Y., & Angelopoulos, M. (2021). Key drivers of digital transformation in greek businesses: Strategy vs. technology. *Central European Management Journal*, 29(2), 33–62. DOI: 10.7206/cemj.2658-0845.45

Kastner, F., Escamilla, E. Z., Langenberg, S., & Ng, M. S. (2025). Adoption of Life Cycle Thinking: Impact-driven comparative assessment of Japanese construction corporations' trends in practices. *Building and Environment*, 267, 112131. DOI: 10.1016/j.buildenv.2024.112131

Martínez-Peláez, R., Ochoa-Brust, A., Rivera, S., Félix, V. G., Ostos, R., Brito, H., Félix, R. A., & Mena, L. J. (2023). Role of digital transformation for achieving sustainability: Mediated role of stakeholders, key capabilities, and technology. *Sustainability (Basel)*, 15(14), 11221. DOI: 10.3390/su151411221

Massonini Ngoma, R. G. T., Abraham Mahanga Tsoni, C. G., Meng, X., & Bashiru Danwana, S. (2023). The impact of the mining equipment, technological trends, and natural resource demand on climate change in Congo. *Sustainability (Basel)*, 15(2), 1691. DOI: 10.3390/su15021691

Nilashi, M., Keng Boon, O., Tan, G., Lin, B., & Abumalloh, R. (2023). Critical data challenges in measuring the performance of sustainable development goals: Solutions and the role of big-data analytics. *Harvard Data Science Review*, 5(3), 3–4. DOI: 10.1162/99608f92.545db2cf

Nwosu, N. T. (2024). *Reducing operational costs in healthcare through advanced BI tools and data integration*. World Journal of Advanced Research and Reviews.

Parlindungan, H. H., Masatip, A., & Manurung, H. (2021). Tourism investment and financial digital. European Journal of Science. *Innovation and Technology*, 1(4), 30–44.

Rositch, A. F., Unger-Saldaña, K., DeBoer, R. J., Ng'ang'a, A., & Weiner, B. J. (2020). The role of dissemination and implementation science in global breast cancer control programs: Frameworks, methods, and examples. *Cancer*, 126(S10), 2394–2404. DOI: 10.1002/cncr.32877 PMID: 32348574

Schechowiz, R. (2021). Contributions of chief financial officers working as interim managers to organisation success in small and medium-sized companies. DOI: 10.1155/2022/8669348

Shafiq, M., Gu, Z., Cheikhrouhou, O., Alhakami, W., & Hamam, H. (2022). The Rise of "Internet of Things": Review and Open Research Issues Related to Detection and Prevention of IoT-Based Security Attacks. *Wireless Communications and Mobile Computing*, 2022(1), 8669348. DOI: 10.1155/2022/8669348

Sjölin, E., & Sjölin, S. (2024). Navigating Corporate Venture Capital: A Framework for Strategic Success. DOI: 10.1155/2022/8669348

Thomasian, N. M., & Adashi, E. Y. (2021). Cybersecurity in the internet of medical things. *Health Policy and Technology*, 10(3), 100549. DOI: 10.1016/j.hlpt.2021.100549

Tuan, L. H. A. (2023). The entrepreneurial pathway of Vietnamese super-rich. The sources of their successful business performance. *International Journal of Entrepreneurship and Small Business*, 10, 1–17.

Velyako, V., & Musa, S. (2024). The relationship between digital organizational culture, digital capability, digital innovation, organizational resilience, and competitive advantage. *Journal of the Knowledge Economy*.

Viswa, C. A., Bleys, J., Leydon, E., Shah, B., & Zurkiya, D. (2024). *Generative AI in the pharmaceutical industry: Moving from hype to reality*. McKinsey & Company.

Weichbroth, P., & Łysik, Ł. (2020). Mobile security: Threats and best practices. *Mobile Information Systems*, 2020, 1–15. DOI: 10.1155/2020/8828078

Wolf-Fordham, S. (2020). Integrating government silos: Local emergency management and public health department collaboration for emergency planning and response. *American Review of Public Administration*, 50(6-7), 560–567. DOI: 10.1177/0275074020943706

Wood, B., & Sacks, G. (2023). The influence of share buybacks on ill-health and health inequity: An exploratory analysis using a socio-ecological determinants of health lens. *Globalization and Health*, 19(1), 3. DOI: 10.1186/s12992-023-00905-0 PMID: 36631805

Xu, W., Yang, L., Niu, Z., Wang, S., Wang, Y., Zhu, Z., & Cui, P. (2024). Thermodynamic and economic analysis of a novel DME-power polygeneration system based on the integration of biomass gasification and alkaline electrolysis of water for hydrogen production. *Energy*, •••, 134185.

Zheng, H., Wu, J., Song, R., Guo, L., & Xu, Z. (2024). Predicting financial enterprise stocks and economic data trends using machine learning time series analysis. *Applied and Computational Engineering*, 87(1), 26–32. DOI: 10.54254/2755-2721/87/20241562

Ziervogel, G., Enqvist, J., Metelerkamp, L., & van Breda, J. (2022). Supporting transformative climate adaptation: Community-level capacity building and knowledge co-creation in South Africa. *Climate Policy*, 22(5), 607–622. DOI: 10.1080/14693062.2020.1863180

Chapter 7
Managing Emotions:
Ecological Validation of Stimulus-Videos

Hugo Miguel Carvalho
ISCIA, Portugal

Vasco Santos
Instituto Politécnico de Tomar, Portugal

Lara Bacalhau
https://orcid.org/0000-0001-9674-4167
CEOS.PP Coimbra, Portugal

Ricardo Marcão
https://orcid.org/0000-0003-3277-3078
ISLA Santarém, Portugal

Stéphanie Monteiro
Institute for Systems and Robotics, Portugal

ABSTRACT

This study develops an ecologically validated video stimulus system targeting Izard's ten emotions, exploring whether there is an intersubjective agreement regarding the most salient emotion in dynamic VS and if these stimuli can form a "battery" for use in research and practice. We hypothesize that different genders will exhibit varying responses to these stimuli. Two studies were conducted with Portuguese participants. Study included 19 individuals who evaluated 150 video excerpts, leading to the selection of 50 "effective" stimuli with high emotional salience. Study II involved 175 participants who assessed these VS across dimensions of "valence" and "arousal" using the SAM and DES scales. Results showed agreement for

DOI: 10.4018/979-8-3693-8598-2.ch007

emotions such as surprise, joy, sadness, and fear, with notable gender differences in responses. In both genders, VS mapped along the axes of intensity and valence deviated from the expected circumplex model. These findings suggest that gender plays a significant role in emotional perception, but further validation with psychophysiological variables is necessary.

1 INTRODUCTION

Emotions play a decisive role in human communication and behavior by serving as intrinsic motivators that shape decision-making processes and influence individual actions and social interactions (Panksepp, 2003, 2004), helping human beings avoid danger (Chanel, 2009), and, for some theorists and philosophers (psychologists and naturalists), supporting values (Hessen, 2001). These emotional responses affect several cognitive functions, including perception, attention, and judgment, which together influence how individuals perceive, interpret, and respond to their environment (Arangüena & Dorado, 2001; Correia, 2023). Therefore, the study of emotions is critical, not only for understanding everyday human experiences and decision-making processes but also for gaining insights into psychopathological conditions like emotional lability, apathy, and anxiety (Correia, 2023).

Despite extensive research, accurately capturing emotional responses in a manner that replicates the complexity of real-world interactions remains challenging. Traditional approaches have typically relied on static stimuli, such as photographs or facial expressions, that, while insightful, often suffer limited ecological validity (EV) of the stimuli used to evoke emotions, as they fail to replicate the dynamic nature of emotional interactions experienced in everyday real-world contexts (Ekman, 1999). EV refers to the extent to which experimental findings can be generalized to real-life settings (Christensen, 2007), making it essential in psychological and medical assessments of patients. Increasingly, researchers advocate the need to develop stimuli that more accurately reflect everyday emotional experiences, since emotions are rarely static or isolated; instead, they are frequently triggered by complex, time-evolving stimuli, such as social interactions or environmental changes. The use of ecologically valid stimuli, such as dynamic video-based stimuli (VS), can enhance the development of therapeutic tools, diagnostic methods, and emotion recognition technologies, advancing research on how emotions impact cognitive processes (Barrett & Wager, 2006; Bradley & Lang, 1994; Christensen, 2007). The EV of these stimuli depends on their capacity to evoke consistent emotional responses across diverse participant groups, aligning closely with real-life emotional encounters and enabling insights into the effects of emotions on cognitive processes like attention, perception, and judgment (Barrett & Wager, 2006; Panksepp, 2003).

In light of these challenges of accurately capturing emotional responses using static stimuli, video-based stimuli have emerged as a promising alternative in bridging this gap, offering a richer, more ecologically valid representation of emotional experiences by accurately simulating the temporal flow and context of real-world interactions. These VS can potentially transform the assessment and therapeutic applications in psychological and medical contexts. This study develops and validates 50 video stimuli (VS) aimed at eliciting Izard's ten basic emotions, establishing an ecologically valid resource for emotion research.

The specific research questions guiding this study are as follows:

(1) Can a set of VS reliably elicit intersubjective agreement (IA) on the most salient emotion?
(2) Are these VS effective across different dimensions, such as "arousal" and "valence"?
(3) Are there significant gender differences (GD) in the perception and rating of emotions?

To address the first two research questions, the present study investigates whether a series of dynamic VS can elicit an intersubjective consensus about the most salient emotion also evaluating "arousal" and "valence" dimensions (Bradley & Lang, 1994; Ekman, 1999). These dimensions are central in the circumplex model of emotion, which maps emotions across a continuum of pleasure-displeasure (valence) and high-low activation (arousal) (Russell, 1980). The circumplex model and Izard's discrete emotions theory collectively offer a robust framework for categorizing emotional responses, potentially enhancing the accuracy and applicability of emotion research in clinical settings. Furthermore, previous research suggests that men and women may exhibit different physiological reactions and behavioral responses to emotional stimuli (Bradley & Lang, 1994), due to a combination of biological predispositions and sociocultural influence (Mendes et al., 2014). These differences, however, are rarely accounted for in the validation of emotion-eliciting stimuli, and this study seeks to fill that gap by testing gender-specific responses to various emotions across a large sample of participants. Therefore, the third research question of the present study focuses on gender-based differences in emotional responses. Recognizing that gender may influence the perception and intensity of emotional experiences, leading to differences in emotional response, is particularly relevant for the development of emotion-sensitive medical devices and therapeutic tools based on accurate emotional feedback, which can be used to improve personalized treatments and interventions. To explore these questions, two studies were conducted with Portuguese participants, as described in the methodology section of this chapter.

In conclusion, the validation of these ecologically valid emotional VS represents a critical step toward bridging the gap between laboratory-based emotional assessments and real-world experiences allowing advances in both theoretical and applied research in the field of nature of emotions, providing a robust framework for future investigations. This study not only addresses the methodological limitations of previous research but also offers a comprehensive approach to understanding the complexities of emotional experience across genders, which can be used as groundwork for integrating emotion-sensitive technologies into medical devices, thereby enhancing their capacity for accurate, responsive, and personalized patient care.

2 LITERATURE BACKGROUND

2.1 Defining Emotions and Their Role in Human Behavior

Emotions are complex, short-lived but intense responses to stimuli, involving subjective experiences, physiological reactions, and behavioral expressions that influence cognition, motivation, interpersonal dynamics, and even survival mechanisms (Ekman, 1999; Panksepp, 2003). The complexity of the emotions makes them difficult to define, therefore, there isn't a universal definition for "emotion". Theorists from multiple fields like philosophy, computer science, and neuroscience, tried since immemorial times to present a concept of emotion (Bota et al., 2019).

From a cognitive perspective, emotions guide various processes, including perception, memory, attention, and judgment. Panksepp (2003) argues that affective or emotional processes provide intrinsic values, which serve as organic pressures and drive effects on how a given behavior will be performed at a certain moment, impacting immediate responses and shaping longer-term decision-making patterns by influencing, how tends to change over a longer period. Research indicates that emotions are essential in organizing cognitive activities, as affective states influence how individuals evaluate situations, comprehension of complex social interactions, and moral judgments (Arangüena & Dorado, 2001; Barrett & Wager, 2006). The influence of emotions on cognitive processing is illustrated by theories such as the Yerkes-Dodson Law, which suggests that arousal, an emotional component, can improve the performance on cognitive tasks to only to a certain level, beyond which it will lower the performance (Yerkes & Dodson, 1908).

In addition to their cognitive functions, emotions have a very important role in psychological well-being and psychopathology. Prior research has shown that dysregulated emotional responses can contribute to various mental health disorders, including anxiety, depression, and bipolar disorder, highlighting the need for a nuanced understanding of emotional mechanisms in clinician's practice contexts

(Correia, 2023; Mendes et al., 2014). Negative emotions such as apathy, lability (mood changes that are rapid and exaggerated), and ambivalence are commonly linked to psychiatric conditions, suggesting that emotions are not only simple reactions to external stimuli but also reflections of internal states and personal life experiences (Barrett & Wager, 2006).

Two primary perspectives dominate emotion research: Darwin's evolutionary approach, which emphasizes emotions as adaptive responses, and the constructivist view, which frames emotions as culturally shaped phenomena (Cornelius, 2000; Panksepp, 2004). The evolutionary perspective, widely popularized by Ekman and Izard, highlights the universality of emotions, as they reflect evolutionary adaptations common to all humans, such as fear in response to threats or disgust to avoid toxins (Ekman, 1972; Ekman, 1999, 2008; Ekman & Friesen, 1971; Ekman et al., 1987; Izard, 1977), suggesting that basic emotions such fear, joy, anger and sadness are innate and serve as core components of human nature, and therefore, universally experienced across cultures (Panksepp, 2004). In contrast, social constructivist theories challenge the notion of universality, arguing that emotions are shaped by cultural norms, social contexts, and personal experiences, which influence their expression and interpretation (Marsh et al., 2003). According to this approach, emotions are not purely biological but are constructed through language, socialization, and interpersonal interactions, resulting in variability across cultures in how emotions are perceived, expressed, and valued (Barrett & Wager, 2006). For instance, while expressions of anger may be discouraged in certain collectivist cultures to maintain social harmony, the same emotion might be openly displayed in individualistic societies where self-assertion is valued (Markus & Kitayama, 1991).

However, despite these divergent views, there is a consensus that emotions can be understood both as biologically grounded responses and as phenomena influenced by sociocultural factors, in other words, the evolutionary and constructivist perspectives must be integrated to obtain a comprehensive understanding of emotions as both universal and context-dependent phenomena, underscoring the importance of studying emotions in diverse cultural and social settings (Pio Abreu, 2015). This multifaceted understanding of emotions forms the basis for their study in various applied fields, including clinical psychology, educational psychology, and human-computer interaction, where accurate emotional assessment and management are crucial (Arangüena & Dorado, 2001).

2.2 Theoretical Models of Emotions: Discrete vs. Dimensional Approaches

Two primary theoretical approaches dominate the study of emotions: the discrete emotions theory and the dimensional model.

Discrete Emotion Theories

Discrete emotion theories suggest that emotions are biologically rooted and consist in distinct, universally recognizable states that evolved to support survival and correspond to unique specific facial expression patterns, physiological patterns, or behavioral tendencies that are largely consistent across cultures and individuals (Ekman, 1999; Izard, 1977) and recognize that emotions are the key motivators of human behavior. Izard (1977) proposed a system of ten fundamental emotions that are thought to be innate, observable in the first months of life, and universally expressed but may vary in the intensity or the manner of their expression. Ekman identified six basic emotions (anger, disgust, fear, joy, sadness, and surprise), each with distinct facial expressions, as shown in Figure 1, that are observable across cultures, supporting their evolutionary role in communication (Ekman & Cordaro, 2011).

Figure 1. Ekman's 6 basic emotions and corresponding facial expressions

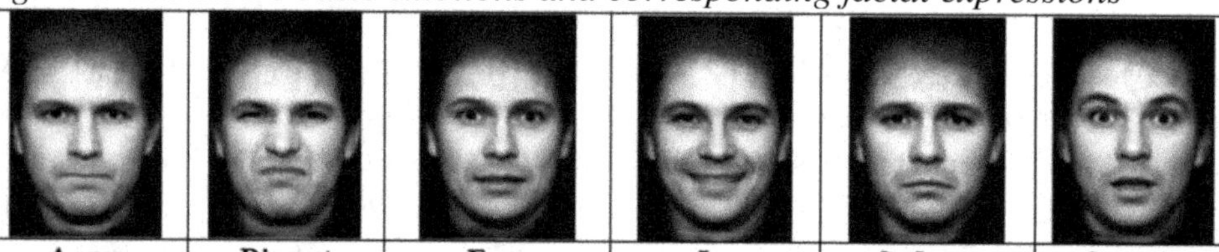

Anger	Disgust	Fear	Joy	Sadness	Surprise
Eyebrows drawn together and downwards; eyes fixed and glare; narrowing of the lips	*Nose wrinkling; upper lip raised; tongue pushed outward*	*Eyebrows raised and pulled together; raised upper eyelids; tensed lower eyelids; lips slightly stretched horizontally back to ears; mouth corners retracted*	*Crow's feet wrinkles; cheeks lifted; movement from muscle that orbits the eye; mouth forming smile*	*Eyebrows inner corner raised; dropping upper eyelids; losing focus in eyes; slight pulling down of lip corners*	*Eyebrows raised; eyes widened; mouth open and rounded in oval shape*

Source: Adapted from Atanassov et al. (2024, p. 730).

Dimensional Models of Emotion

On the other hand, dimensional models of emotion, such as the circumplex model proposed by Russell (1980), conceptualize emotions along two primary axes: valence (ranging from pleasant to unpleasant) and arousal (ranging from calm to excited). According to this approach, emotions are not discrete entities but rather points within a continuous space defined by these dimensions, so they can be represented in the two-dimensional space according to their affective quality and intensity (Russell, 1980). This approach is advantageous for its flexibility in describing complex, blended emotions that do not fit neatly into discrete categories (Russell & Barrett, 1999).

To visually represent the valence-arousal (VA) space and enable participants to rate their emotional responses along these dimensions, it could be used, for example, the Self-Assessment Manikin (SAM), which provides a nonverbal, intuitive tool for emotion assessment and has been widely used in research involving affective stimuli. This tool will be explained in detail later.

By cross-referencing the V-A self-assessments of various individuals, and even though multiple studies aim to identify a wide range of emotions using audiovisual content, it can be seen that the affective responses identified in Russell's (1980) circumflex model tend to be concentrated around a parabolic region, as can be seen in Figure 2 the orange shadow area (Kim & Jo, 2019).

Figure 2. Mapping emotions through Russell's (1980) Circumplex Model and SAM

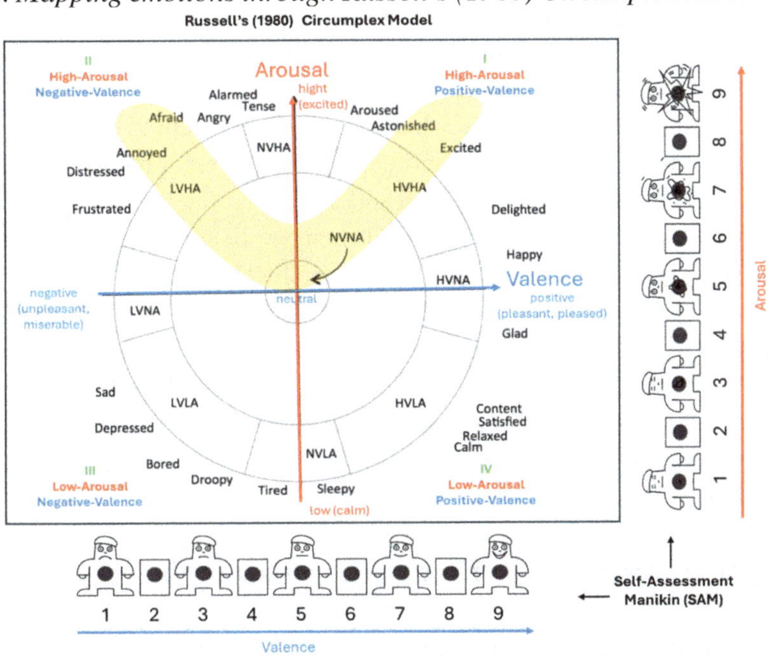

Source: Self Elaborated.

Recent advances in affective computing and emotion recognition systems increasingly utilize dimensional models to capture continuous fluctuations in emotional states, particularly when analyzing real-time data from physiological measures like EEG and heart rate (Dai et al., 2018; Yu et al., 2016). Dimensional models are also more adaptable in cross-cultural research, as they allow for differences in emotional expression without prescribing specific categories. The VA framework is culturally robust and commonly used in AI for emotion classification (Kim et al., 2020; Probst et al., 2016).

2.3 Ecological Validity and the Use of VS in Emotion Research

One of the major problems in emotion research is the need to make sure that the emotion-eliciting stimuli are ecologically valid which means they use the sort of emotional stimuli that are encountered in everyday situations. As it has been referred, the traditional research employing static images or isolated facial expressions to study emotional responses has been criticized for limited ecological validity as they fail to capture the dynamic and context-dependent nature of emotional experiences that occur in everyday life (Christensen, 2007; Ekman, 1999). The shift toward using VS represents an important development in the field of emotion research, as video clips offer a more naturalistic and dynamic means of eliciting emotions. The VS incorporates contextual and temporal elements, facial expressions, voice cues, and body language, among other stimuli, which are more representative of natural social interactions, so the provide a richer, more ecologically valid medium for eliciting emotions (Christensen, 2007). Research indicates that such stimuli can enhance the accuracy of emotional assessments and their applications in both clinical and therapeutic settings (Bradley & Lang, 1994; Marsh et al., 2003).

The present study builds on the work of Christensen (2007) and others by developing a system of ecologically validated VS aimed at eliciting the ten emotions outlined by Izard (1977). By using video excerpts from daily life, this research seeks to replicate the complexity of emotional experiences more accurately than static stimuli, offering a more robust tool for emotion research in both experimental and clinical settings.

2.4 Gender Differences in Emotional Responses

There has been a great deal of research documenting the differences in emotional expression and perception between the genders. Most studies show that men's and women's emotional intonation and demonstration vary about factors of time and severity. Often these explanations are believed to be the result of both biological, especially hormonal, and sociocultural, particularly regarding expectations of behavior in one's sex, influences (Bradley & Lang, 1994; Mendes et al., 2014).

For instance, the available literature indicates that women easily show emotions such as sadness, fear, or even compassion, while men are likely to show anger or superiority at various emotional triggers (Bradley & Lang, 1994). Such tendencies are believed to mirror the general culture which prescribes the types of emotions suitable for either gender. In addition to these, gender has been reported to influence physiological responses to emotional stimuli as well. For example, it has been found in studies that women react to emotional imagery with more profound physiological responses measured in heart rate variability, in comparison to men (Bradley & Lang, 1994).

As a consequence of that, within the framework of this project, we determine that differences in VS perception and evaluation according to gender will appear. More precisely, we predict that men and women will exhibit varying tendencies when rating emotional intensity (arousal) valence implication as it has been established in the existing literature previously.

2.5 Measuring Emotions: The Self-Assessment Manikin Scale and Differential Emotions Scale

Over the years, a variety of approaches have been adopted to study human emotions. These methods are often grouped into three broad categories, these being: questionnaires and self-reports, physical signs, and physiological signs, as can be seen in Figure 4.

Figure 4. Emotion sensing techniques

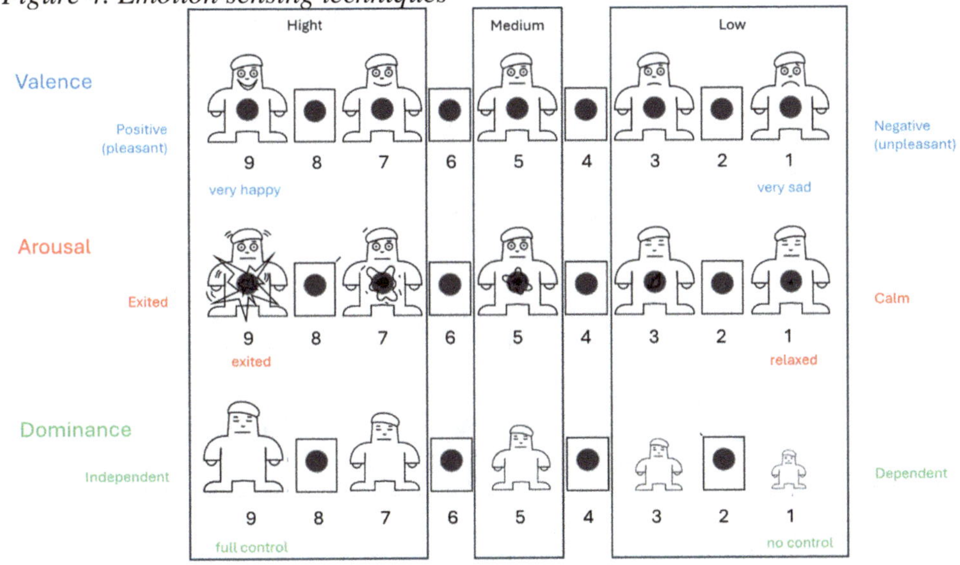

Source: Self elaborated based on Bradley and Lang (1994), Cacioppo and Gardner (1999), Cacioppo et al. (2017), Csikszentmihalyi and Larson (1987), Ekman and Friesen (1971), Fordson et al. (2022), Kang et al. (2022), Larradet et al. (2020), Picard (2000), Pollak and Adams (2011), Scherer (2003), Scherer et al. (2001), Shu et al. (2018)Tran (2020) and Watson et al. (1988).

Figure 1 highlights the fact that several tools and techniques have been developed to recognize and measure emotions. Continuous comparing these techniques regarding their advantages and disadvantages and possible ways of use, the authors of this paper believe that the SAM) technique and Differential Emotions Scale (DES) would best provide for evaluation of emotional aftereffects elicited by moving images and therefore those two tools are explained in detail.

Self-Assessment Manikin

SAM is a non-verbal emotion self-reports assessment tool that, through a pictogram, measures the emotional impact of a stimulus according to the dimensions of **affective valence, arousal, and dominance**. This tool enables individuals to rate their emotional reactions on a continuous scale where each of the dimensions is assessed on a nine-point scale with five images and four intermediate points, as shown in Figure 5 (Bradley & Lang, 1994). The simplicity of this visual scale, ease of use, ability to be applied quickly, and reliability in measuring the emotional impact of a stimulus in different populations because it reduces the potential linguistic or literacy biases, make this instrument one of the most widely used in emotion research to self-capture immediate emotional reactions to stimuli, particularly in studies involving large samples or cross-cultural comparisons (Bradley & Lang, 1994; Lang et al., 1997a, 1997b).

Figure 5. SAM scale

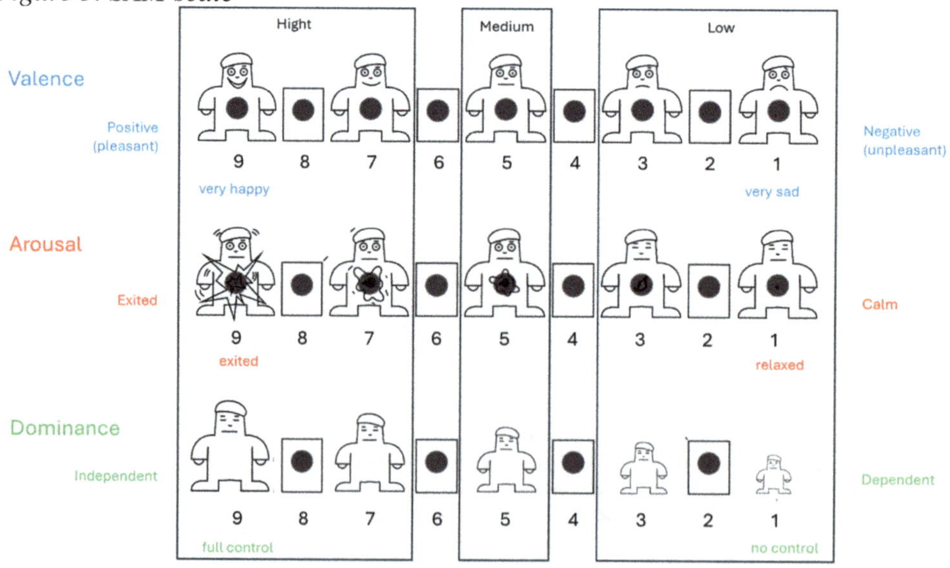

Source: Self elaborated, adapted from Bradley and Lang (1994)

The **affective valence dimension** refers to the **pleasantness or unpleasantness** of an emotional experience and its scale is made up of five figures that range from **a very happy**, smiling expression (positive affective valence: pleasure, happiness) **to** a **very unhappy** expression (negative affective valence: displeasure, unhappiness) (Bradley & Lang, 1994), so the study participant can be asked, after the VS, to rate how much the video presented generates pleasant or unpleasant emotions. **The 10 Izard's (1974)emotions can be classified through the affective valence as follows: seven have negative valence (anger, sadness, contempt, disgust, fear, shame, and guilt), two have positive valence (interest and joy) and one (surprise) can have negative or positive valence**.

The **arousal dimension** reflects the **intensity or activation level** of an emotional state. This dimension has its extremes from wide-open eyes looking figure indicating maximum **excitement** (great agitation / high activation) to another extremity whose figure is eyes closed, indicating a **calm** expression (relaxed/asleep /no activation) (Bradley & Lang, 1994). It can be done by asking the research participant after the sustained VS to rate how arousing the stimulus was. Strong feelings evoke high degrees of arousal, such as excitement, anger, or fear, while calmer feelings, such as relaxation, boredom, or sadness, tend to result in lower degrees of arousal.

The **dominance dimension**, not used in this study, assesses the **degree of control or power** that a person feels over a given emotional situation and varies between a pole represented by a **figure much larger** than the midpoint (independent: control of the situation, high dominance, low dominance) to a **figure much smaller** than the midpoint (dependent: lack of control of the situation) (Bradley & Lang, 1994). For example, emotions like anger or pride may be associated with high dominance, while emotions like fear or submission may be associated with low dominance.

Differential Emotions Scale

Based on the theory presented by Izard et al. (1974), the second instrument selected to assess emotions is the DES, which categorizes emotions into ten distinct primary emotions, including **surprise (neutral), joy (positive), interest (positive), fear (negative), anger (negative), disgust (negative), sadness (negative), contempt (negative), shame (negative) and guilt (negative)**, of which considered as innate, universals, and correlate with certain expressive and physiological features. According to the same authors, the approach can be described from five basic points:

- The ten fundamental emotions constitute the main motivational system of human beings.
- Each emotion has unique motivational and phenomenological properties.
- Each emotion is associated with its experience and its behavioral effect.

- There are interrelations between emotions and one emotion can induce, amplify, or attenuate another emotion.
- Emotional processes interact with and influence a person's cognitive processes.

In light of the above, Izard et al. (1974) set a **five-point self-report Likert scale (1 = very weak emotion, 5 = very strong emotion) to measure the intensity of each emotion**. In this way, within the DES those who watched the film were asked how they felt each emotion when watching the movie and graded that emotion on a scale of 1-5 providing a finer picture of the emotional states generated by each clip. Thus, in DES, participants were asked to indicate how each emotion related to their feelings while watching the movie, rating that emotion between 1 and 5, thus providing a detailed profile of the emotional states elicited by each clip. Unlike the SAM, which measures broader dimensions of emotion, the DES was specifically designed to capture the subjective experience of distinct emotions. This makes it particularly useful for studies that aim to capture specific emotional states in addition to general affective dimensions (Boyle, 1984).

The SAM scale has high correlation coefficients with the DES, both in the affective valence dimension and in the arousal dimension. The SAM has a high internal consistency (0.94) determined by the split-half method. The test-retest analysis revealed values of 0.99 and 0.97 for the affective valence and arousal (V&A) dimensions, respectively (Lang et al., 1997). The use of SAM and DES in combination in this study, the authors aimed to obtain a comprehensive means of measuring emotion through continuous dimensions and specific emotional categories through discrete measurements. While SAM focused on the overall affective tone and intensity, DES provided a multi-dimensional assessment of the specific emotions triggered by the VS. This dual-method approach allowed a more nuanced analysis of the data captured, helping the researchers to understand the emotional landscape evoked by the ecologically valid VS and explore potential GD in robust and reflective real-world emotional responses.

3 METHODOLOGY

In this section it will be described the tow-step study made with Portuguese participants. Study I used 19 participants to evaluate the emotional salience of 150 video clips. Those VS were used in Study II to select the final 50 VS ecological validated.

3.1 Study I: Initial Selection of Emotionally Effective VS

Participants

In study I, 19 Portuguese individuals aged 18 or overtook part, with a mean age of 23.47 years (SD = 5.67), distributed by gender and educational level as described in Table 1, using a convenience sample in which the participants were selected through the researchers' personal networks and social media.

Table 1. Descriptive characterization of the participants of Study I.

		Gender		Total
		Male	Female	
Educational background	Equal or less than 12 of education	3	2	**5**
	Complete higher education	9	5	**14**
	Total	**12**	**7**	**19**

Source: Self Elaboration

For this sample, the **inclusion criteria** stated that participants had to be fluent in Portuguese, without any reported cognitive impairments nor any diagnosed psychological disorders, and be able to provide written informed consent. No exclusions were applied based on gender, socioeconomic status, or other demographic factors.

Materials

The emotional stimuli consisted of video excerpts taken from the Internet, from platforms such as YouTube, where the videos were available for free under public licenses or where licenses for use had been requested and explicitly granted to the holders of the respective copyrights. An initial pool of 200 videos was constructed by a panel of 3 experts (Christensen, 2007) in a double-blind format, considering that this selection of videos was intended to induce one of Izard's (1977) ten discrete emotions - surprise, joy, interest, fear, anger, disgust, sadness, contempt, shame and guilt. The main aim of selecting these videos was to include a minimum of 10 videos for each of the emotions. These videos were then classified into one of the following genres: drama, humor, horror, suspense, romance, police, animation, sports, fantasy, traffic, events, social activity, mystery, music, biomedicine, science, urban legend, "viral", implicit and explicit sex, to have a significant sample of what could fulfill the induction of the most diverse emotions by the participants during viewing.

From this initial pool of 200 videos, 150 videos were randomly selected. For this purpose, each " VS was assigned a number from 1 to 200, numbers recorded on small rolls of paper, and each of the 3 experts took 50 of these rolls of paper from a bag at random, thus building the group of 150 final films. The 150 VS selected by judges made it possible to identify VS for all the emotions in Izard's model (Table 2). The percentages suggest a preponderance of positive valence videos.

Table 2. Number of effective videos per emotion and percentage of IA.

Emotion	Number of VS	IA Defined by Judges
Interest	33	22%
Joy	24	16%
Positive Surprise	21	14%
Negative Surprise	15	10%
Disgust	12	8%
Anger	12	8%
Contempt	9	6%
Shame	9	6%
Sadness	6	4%
Fear	6	4%
Guilt	3	3%

Source: Self Elaboration

As all the videos selected had different durations and sound and light intensities, they were edited according to specific methodological standards:

1. **Length:** Each video clip was precisely 90 seconds long. This duration was chosen to balance engagement with the stimuli and to avoid participant fatigue.
2. **Calibration:** Sound levels were normalized, and lighting levels were adjusted uniformly using Adobe Premier. The goal was to maintain consistency across all videos to minimize the influence of technical factors on emotional responses.

For the study were also selected **two evaluation tools:** the **SAM** (valence, activation, and dominance) for the subjective evaluation of the emotional impact of the SV, and the **DES** was used to evaluate the SV in terms of inducing emotions.

Procedure

The 19 participants in the study were selected individually through a convenience sample. They were then invited individually to a controlled environment where they watched the 150 videos. No more than 5 subjects were allowed to take part in each session of viewing and evaluating the VS stimuli. These participants, although in the same room, were separated by at least 2 meters, at different tables and chairs to minimize distractions, and did not influence each other in their emotional responses. The viewing setup included a standard video projector with controlled lighting conditions, as well as headphones to ensure uniform listening experiences.

1. **Instructions:** Before each session, the objectives, procedures, and stages of the research were explained to the participants. Then the participants decided whether to take part in the study by filling in the informed consent form. At the beginning of each section, the participants were instructed to watch each of the 150 videos and focus on how it made them feel, to meet the objective of the study. After each video, they immediately completed two evaluations: (1) they used the SAM to rate the video's (V&A) dimensions, and (2) they used the DES to identify the most salient emotion elicited by the video.
2. **Randomization:** The order of the video clips was randomized for each participant to control for order effects.
3. **Response Recording:** After each video, participants had approximately 1 minute to self-complete the two scales. Responses were collected on paper and later entered into a database for analysis.

Data Analysis

According to Maroco (2007) and Segurado (1980), the measures of intersubjective dispersion, the degree of Cartesian proximity of the coordinates of the different VS, and the number of participants who evaluated each VS in both dimensions ("number of views") guarantee a selection of VS that is consistent from the point of view of content. These criteria were therefore considered when analyzing the data. First, in the assessment of each video clip was used on two main criteria:

1. **Intersubjective Agreement:** For each video, was calculated the percentage of respondents who agreed on the same "most salient" emotion (as measured by the DES). Videos with more than 60% agreement were qualified as "effective".
2. **Valence and Arousal Scores:** Mean scores of V&A dimensions (obtained using SAM) for each video clip were computed to understand its general emotional tone and intensity.

For all dimensions (V&A) were computed descriptive statistics (means (M), standard deviations (SD)). A cut-off of 50 video clips was set based on IA (>60%) and the films with the lowest SD in both dimensions were chosen. This measure of dispersion was calculated using the sum of the variances of the two dimensions for each film, considering the coordinates given by the medians of the individual responses. The definition of the number of 50 VS (around one-third of the original pool) was made considering that it was intended to identify a pool of 5 videos for each of the 10 emotions in order not to overload the subsequent evaluation activity in the second study and at the same time increase the probability of finding two VS for each emotion. The aim of obtaining at least 2 VS for each emotion has to do with the learning effects to be avoided in experimental studies in which VS might be used (Christensen, 2007). The application of the criteria of 50 VS with the highest IA and minimum SD, defined the "number of views" as the number that each VS was evaluated simultaneously in the two dimensions "valence" and "arousal". The application of this procedure led to a 17 number of views as the cut-off point to eliminate the 100 VS. These selected videos were carried forward into Study II for validation purposes.

3.2 Study II: Validation of Emotionally Effective Stimuli

Participants

For Study II were selected 175 Portuguese individuals over the age of 18 (adults), whose distribution by gender and educational level can be seen in Table 3 (Before ER80, MMSE, BSI). Using a convenience sample technic, participants were recruited through Portuguese universities and professional networks, aiming to diversify the sample in terms of age, education, and background. Ethical requirements regarding participation in the study were respected by the men and women in the sample.

Table 3. Descriptive characterization of the participants of study II.

		Before ER80, MMSE, BSI			After ER80, MMSE, BSI		
		Gender		Total	Gender		Total
		Male	Female		Male	Female	
Educational background	Equal or less than 12 of education	46	64	**110**	42	50	**92**
	Complete higher education	29	36	**65**	25	31	**56**
Total		**75**	**100**	**175**	**67**	**81**	**148**

continued on following page

Table 3. Continued

	Before ER80, MMSE, BSI			After ER80, MMSE, BSI		
Age Average			**26,91**	**28,15**	**25,99**	**26,91**
Age SD			**9,76**	**8,87**	**10,58**	**9,76**

Source: Self Elaboration

The **inclusion criteria** used in Study I was also followed in Study II: the participants should be fluent in Portuguese and present no cognitive impairments, and no diagnosed psychological disorders. Screening for possible cognitive impairments or psychological disorders was carried out by a clinical team using the ER80, MMSE, and BSI methodologies. Participants who failed the cognitive screening or showed signs of psychological distress were excluded from the study. At the end of this inclusion/exclusion process, 148 individuals were included in Study II with distribution as illustrated in Table 3 (After ER80, MMSE, BSI).

A brief explanation can be given for the ER80, MMSE, and BSI methodologies as follows:

- **Revision Scale 80 (ER80):** is used in clinical and epidemiological studies to carry out a global psychological assessment of psychopathologies and mental well-being in the population, measuring factors such as depression, anxiety, somatic problems, and other psychological symptoms. The 16-item scale is intended to measure a generalized disturbance in the body's homeostasis associated with the overall disruption of intrapersonal and interpersonal communication systems that characterize psychiatric illness. Developed by Pio Abreu and Vaz Patto (1981), this scale was used in the context of the present study as a screening tool to ensure that the participants had no mental health problems that could influence their emotional responses to stimuli. Every participant that had positive scores for Females$\geq$ 7 and Males$\geq$ 6 was excluded.
- **Brief Symptom Inventory (BSI):** is a self-report measure of psychological distress (Canavarro, 1999, 2007). This instrument consists of 53 items from the Symptom Checklist-90 (SCL-90), grouped into various symptomatologies, such as somatization (7 items); obsessions-compulsions (6 items); interpersonal sensitivity (4 items); (d) depression (6 items); (e) anxiety (6 items); (f) hostility (5 items); (g) phobic anxiety (5 items); (h) paranoid ideation (5 items); and (i) psychoticism (5 items) and other relevant symptomatologies (4 items). Each of these items should be rated on the degree to which it has affected the individual in the last week on a 5-point Likert scale: "Never" (0), "A few times" (1), "Sometimes" (2), "Often" (3) and "Very often" (4). This

scale, validated for the Portuguese population by Canavarro (1999), reveals a cut-off point for the Positive Symptoms Index, considering that there is a greater likelihood of finding emotionally disturbed individuals in subjects with scores ≥ 1.7. The participants with scores exceeding cutoff points were excluded to maintain a normative sample.

- **Mini-Mental State Examination (MMSE):** is a screening instrument that assesses the specific cognitive functions of temporal and spatial orientation, retention and recall of memory, attention and calculation, language, and two-dimensional constructive praxis. The respondent is given a questionnaire with 30 items to which they have to assign a score of zero or one, with the sum of the scores being analyzed at the end (Folstein et al., 1975). Given that the level of education influences the results of this instrument, this study used a scale validated for the Portuguese population by Guerreiro et al. (1994), where three cut-off points are considered according to education level: (a) illiterate: 0 to 15 points (with dementia); 16 to 30 points (without dementia); (b) 1 to 11 years of schooling: 0 to 22 points (with dementia); 23 to 30 points (without dementia); and (c) more than 11 years of schooling: 0 to 27 points (with dementia); 28 to 30 points (without dementia). This tool was used in the present study to ensure that the participants did not suffer from cognitive disorders (it excluded all individuals with less or equal to 25 points).

Materials

The 50 VS selected from Study I, based on their high IA in eliciting emotions, judges' evaluation, and 17 minimum number of visualizations, were used in Study II for further validation. The videos were evaluated using the same tools as in Study I: SAM and DES.

Procedure

The 175 volunteer participants were invited to a controlled environment (day, time, and place duly identified). On arrival, they were informed of the objectives, procedures, and stages of the study, and the informed consent form was given to those who agreed to take part in the study. After reading and signing the consent form, it was coded to guarantee the anonymity of the data collection. They were asked to fill in a sociodemographic data sheet and answer the MMSE, BSI, and ER-80 to validate their eligibility to take part in the study. This stage resulted in the exclusion of 27 individuals for having cognitive or psychological disorders. The remaining 148 participants were divided into groups of 10. For each group, the participants were randomly assigned to individual stations without visual or physical contact with other participants, in rooms equipped with personal computers and headphones to ensure the controlled viewing of stimuli. Each participant viewed the 50 video clips in random order to control for order effects.

1. **Viewing Setup:** The videos were displayed on a standardized computer screen with equalized sound, and participants were instructed to avoid distractions. Each video was played once, followed by immediate completion of the SAM and DES for that video.
2. **Instructions:** Participants were instructed to focus on how each video made them feel and to provide honest, spontaneous responses using the SAM and DES.
3. **Response Recording:** After each video, participants had approximately 1 minute to **SELF**-complete the two scales (SAM and DES). At the end of the visualization of the 50 VS, the participant should leave the room, handing the notebook with the answers of SAM and DES to a researcher who then records the data in an Excel document for later analysis and export to an SPSS document.
4. **Randomization:** The order of video presentation was randomized to reduce the likelihood of sequence effects influencing emotional responses.
5. **Timing:** After each video, participants were given a 90-second window to complete both the SAM and DES scales before the next video began.

Data Analysis

The effectiveness of the 50 selected video clips was analyzed based on two main criteria:

1. **Intersubjective Agreement:** The percentage of participants who agreed on the most salient emotion (measured using the DES) was calculated for each video. Based on the data recorded in Excel of the agreement values for each of the 50 SVs and Izard's ten emotions, the SVs with the highest agreement values and with a maximum of 2 emotions were selected (one of which is always "Interest") - not only because it appeared in all the items but also because, conceptually, interest would always be an emotion present due to the novelty of the stimuli. Thus, a threshold of 60% agreement was maintained to confirm the reliability of the emotional elicitation.
2. **Gender Differences**: GD in emotional perception was explored by comparing male and female ratings across the SAM and DES scales using t-tests and chi-square tests. The primary focus was on identifying any statistically significant differences in valence, arousal, and the intensity of specific emotions.

To assess potential GD, separate descriptive statistics (means, SD) were calculated for males and females across the two dimensions of V&A. Correlational Pearson analyses were also conducted to explore the relationship between the two dimensions and the intensity of specific emotions. Alfas were used as follows: .05 (significant), .01 (highly significant), and .001 (highly significant).

So, the analyses carried out respected the requirements such as the data, the size of the samples and the hypothesis to be tested (Maroco, 2007; Murteira, 2004; Oliveira, 2009; Reis, 2006).

4 RESULTS

In this section, we detail the methodology employed in the study, outlining the participant selection, stimuli preparation, procedural steps, and data analysis techniques used to investigate the emotional responses elicited by the VS across dimensions of V&A, while accounting for potential gender-based differences.

4.1 Study I

Selection of Emotionally Effective VS

Participants were invited individually to a controlled environment where they watched 150 videos across several sessions to elicit one of the ten basic emotions identified by Izard (1977). Each video was assessed for V&A using the SAM and for emotional salience using the DES. The viewing setup included a standard video projector with controlled lighting conditions, as well as headphones to ensure uniform auditory experiences. Participants sat alone in a room to minimize distractions and the influence of social factors on their emotional responses. Considering the 150 VS being evaluated in this phase, the 50 VS that had a number greater than or equal to 17 views went on to the next phase in both dimensions (V&A). This criterion was determined empirically from the data on the coordinates and dispersion values of perceived V&A, evaluated by SAM, and the IA (to choose those with the greatest consensus) by DES.

The number of views of the 50th VS of the video clips is serialized in descending order of number of views. The VS that had at least 60% of participants agreed on the most salient emotion evoked by each video clip (IA across participants) and had the lowest SD in the V&A dimensions were chosen (classified as "effective"). Table 4 summarizes the selected 50 videos, the corresponding emotions, and the level of agreement among participants. The remaining 100 VS either had a lower number of views or only had evaluations in one dimension.

Table 4. Number of effective videos per emotion and percentage of IA.

Emotion	Number of VS	IA (Mean) by DES
Interest	11	78%
Joy	8	72%
Positive Surprise	7	75%
Negative Surprise	5	66%
Sadness	7	68%
Fear	6	65%
Disgust	4	64%

Source: Self Elaboration

SAM: Valence and Arousal Ratings

V&A ratings were collected using the SAM scale for each video. The SAM scale revealed that there were differences in both the intensity and the emotional tone of the VS as can be seen in Table 5. VS associated with positive emotions like joy and positive surprise (interest), tended to score higher on the valence (pleasure) scale (M = 6.5, SD = 0.8), while those linked to negative emotions such as sadness, fear, and disgust stimuli received lower valence scores (M = 2.3, SD = 1.1), indicating displeasure. The arousal dimension, which reflects the intensity of emotional activation, rated high with fear, surprise (positive and negative), and disgust VS (M = 7.5, SD = 0.9), while lower ratings applied for sadness and joy (M = 5.0, SD = 0.7).

Table 5. Mean V&A ratings for emotionally effective VS by SAM test.

Emotion	Mean Valence	Mean Arousal
Interest	5.5	6.0
Joy	6.5	5.0
Positive Surprise	6.0	7.5
Negative Surprise	2.0	7.5
Sadness	2.5	5.0
Disgust	2.3	7.5
Fear	3.0	7.5
Anger	3.5	6.5

Source: Self Elaboration

DES Ratings

As reported, the 50 VS that have at least 60% of participants agreed on the most salient emotion evoked by each video clip (**IA** across participants) and had the lowest SD in the V&A dimensions were chosen (classified as "effective"). Then, a group of three university researchers in the field of emotions, in this study referred to as "experts" or "judges", evaluated the selected VS to identify the salient emotion of each VS. The salient emotion had to be indicated by at least 2 of the 3 experts - the judges' method (Christensen, 2007). The judges (2 female and 1 male) assessed the salient emotion (from (Izard, 1977; Izard et al., 1974) based on the objective indicators (sound, luminance, movements, facial expressions and postures of characters, contexts, and consequences, associated cultural values) in conjunction with their knowledge of studies in the field of experimental social psychology of emotions. They did not evaluate the VS in terms of their emotional impact on them. According to this method, the associations between each VS and a salient emotion were obtained and summarized in Table 6. When it came to identifying salient emotions, the judges agreed on 24 VS (48% of the total 50 VS). This VS were used in the Study II.

Table 6. Associations of emotions between judges.

Emotion	Number of VS	%	Number of Agreements between the 3 judges	
			3/3	2/3
Interest	11	22%	6	5
Joy	8	16%	4	4
Positive Surprise	7	14%	4	3
Negative Surprise	5	10%	2	3
Disgust	4	8%	2	2
Anger	4	8%	1	3
Contempt	3	6%	2	1
Shame	3	6%	1	2
Fear	2	4%	1	1
Sadness	2	4%	1	1
Guilt	1	2%	0	1
Total	50		24	26
Percentage		100%	48%	52%

Source: Self Elaboration

4.2 Study II

Validation of Emotionally Effective Stimuli

Study II involved a larger sample of 175 participants to evaluate if the 50 VS identified in Study I were validated as emotionally effective. The participants evaluated each video using the SAM and DES scales to assess emotional salience, valence, and arousal. The findings obtained from Study II validated the ability of those VS to evoke the desired emotion with a good degree of reliability. In fact, in the case of most of the video clips, 60% or more of the individuals agreed on the identified intended emotion for each video clip, confirming the emotional salience of the stimuli. **So, for six basic emotions: joy, fear, interest, sadness, disgust, and surprise (positive and negative),** significant IA was observed. The level of agreement for these emotions was at least or even greater than the stipulated 60% rule, which points to a good level of agreement among the respondents, as can be seen in Table 7. **No SVs were found for the emotions of anger, contempt, shame, and guilt**. This validation confirmed the reliability of the stimuli for use in emotion elicitation research.

Table 7. Percentage of the agreement for validated emotions.

Emotion	Number of VS	Percentage of Agreements (Mean)
Interest	10	80%
Joy	7	75%
Positive Surprise	8	72%
Negative Surprise	6	65%
Fear	6	68%
Sadness	6	66%
Disgust	5	64%

Source: Self Elaboration

Valence and Arousal Ratings

In Study II, for all emotions, participants provided V&A ratings through SAM self-evaluation tests. The scores confirmed the hypothesized patterns for each emotion, following the trends observed in Study I, revealing clear distinctions between positive and negative emotions. Videos related to positive emotions such as joy and positive surprise ($M = 6.3$, $SD = 0.9$) received higher valence scores, indicating pleasant emotional responses, while negative emotions such as fear, sadness, and disgust scored much lower valence (M = 2.4, SD = 1.2), signifying negative emotional reactions. Arousal ratings were highest for videos eliciting fear, surprise, and disgust (M = 7.4, SD = 0.8), which indicates these emotions are theoretically associated with higher emotional intensity. On the other hand, the arousal levels of the joy and sadness videos (M = 4.8, SD = 0.9) were rated lower, reflecting a more subdued emotional activation.

One of the key objectives of Study II was the examination of the emotional reactions of participants belonging to different genders. The results of SAM mean scores indicated statistically significant GD (p-value < .05) in both V&A ratings for specific emotions, with women typically displaying heightened arousal for negative emotions and men showing stronger arousal for positive emotions suggesting that men and women process and express emotions differently. These findings are aligned with previous literature(Bradley & Lang, 1994). Specifically, in Study II, the principal results can be summarized as follows in Table 8:

Table 8. Mean V&A ratings by gender in study II

Emotion	Gender	Mean Valence	Mean Arousal	Comment
Interest	Male	5.5	6.5	Interest is rated with higher arousal by men than women. This aligns with existing research.
	Female	5.5	6.0	
Joy	Male	6.8	8.0	Joy elicited the highest arousal ratings for men and slightly lower arousal for women. Similarly, men rated joy higher in valence compared to women. This aligns with existing research indicating that men may exhibit stronger arousal and emotional responses to positive stimuli.
	Female	6.5	7.5	
Positive Surprise	Male	6.8	7.9	Men reported higher V&A for positive surprise compared to women. These results suggest that men may experience more intense positive emotional responses to surprising stimuli, consistent with gender-based differences in emotional reactivity.
	Female	6.0	7.6	
Negative Surprise	Male	3.5	7.4	Both genders reported similar arousal levels for negative surprise, suggesting it is perceived as a highly activating emotion across participants. However, the lower valence rating among female participants indicates that women may interpret negative surprises with a greater degree of emotional displeasure than men. This pattern aligns with findings that suggest women generally experience more intense negative affective responses to surprise, potentially due to heightened sensitivity to unexpected negative stimuli.
	Female	2.0	7.5	

continued on following page

Table 8. Continued

Emotion	Gender	Mean Valence	Mean Arousal	Comment
Sadness	Male	2.3	5.0	Women rated sadness higher in both V&A compared to males, reflecting a greater emotional sensitivity to sad stimuli, a finding consistent with GD in emotional processing.
	Female	2.5	7.5	
Disgust	Male	2.0	6.5	Disgust-related videos were rated similarly in valence by both men and women, indicating that both genders perceived disgust as a strongly negative emotion. However, women reported higher arousal compared to men, although the difference was not statistically significant. This trend supports previous findings that women may experience certain negative emotions with greater intensity.
	Female	2.0	7.5	
Fear	Male	3.5	7.0	Female participants rated fear videos as significantly higher in arousal compared to males. This suggests that women experience fear-related stimuli with more intensity than men, aligning with existing literature on GD in emotional sensitivity.
	Female	3.0	7.5	

Source: Self Elaboration

DES Ratings

Using the DES scale, it was possible to identify VS with an IA equal to or greater than 60% in identifying the most salient emotion, and six emotions were identified for both genders: In the Study, I successfully identified 50 effective VS-related with ix emotions (surprise (positive to negative), joy, interest, sadness, disgust and fear). No SV could be found for the emotions of anger, contempt, shame, and guilt. However, as can be seen in Table 9, only for the emotions of Positive Surprise and Fear do the evaluations made between the two genders coincide. It should be noted that VS44 was rated differently between women (negative surprise) and men (disgust). In addition, comparing the ratings given by the participants and the judges, they coincide for all the emotions, except for V138, which was rated as interest by the male participants, while it was rated as guilt by the male judges.

Table 9. VS by gender of participants and judges

Emotion	VS Sample		VS Judges	
	Female	Male	Female	Male
Interest	**VS24**	**VS138**	**VS24 ***	**VS24 ***
Joy	VS155	VS85	VS155	VS85

continued on following page

Table 9. Continued

Emotion	VS Sample		VS Judges	
Positive Surprise	**VS9**	**VS9**	**VS9**	**VS9**
Negative Surprise	**VS44**	VS132	VS44	VS132
Fear	**VS63**	**VS63**	**VS63**	**VS63**
Sadness	VS3	VS74	VS3	VS74
Disgust	VS93	**VS44**	VS93	VS44

Source: Self Elaboration

Table 10. Description of the battery of VS with a congruent classification by participants and judges

VS	Description
VS3	A man injured after a motorcycle accident without a helmet, people around him waiting for paramedics to help, and someone who looks like a friend/family member is crying and asking for help in great tears.
VS9	A "fakir" on a TV talent show, with levitation.
VS24	Traffic and a queue behind a truck, an oncoming car crashes into the truck, and other cars stop for the drivers to see the result of the accident.
VS44	Orthopedic surgery in which a muscle is separated from the tibia below the knee, with "bloody" images and whose operative acts appear "cold" (sic) and efficient.
VS63	Vaporous figures can be associated with spirits and in the final scene there are paintings banging and ashtrays levitating which seem to indicate the presence of a poltergeist.
VS74	A skydiver who had an accident while landing, with an open fracture of the right tibia and fibula, and in a selfie format he is recording the moment; seeming to control himself, he seems to be expecting to lose his leg, and the images are of pain and grief caused by the situation and the expectation of the outcome.
VS85	Three duck chicks interact with a cat with young, in which the cat welcomes and warms the chicks.
VS93	Explicit oral sex in the context of male homosexuality.
VS132	Artistic carving by removing skin to match the final design.
VS138	A prank carried out by "friends" on an individual locked in a truck container, informing him that the truck has broken down on a railway line and that they can't open the container, they play the sound of an approaching train with speakers next to the container and the individual is terrified at the prospect of the train colliding with the container.
VS155	Cooking Francesinha with a robot, with a female explainer in a professional but cheerful format.

Source: Self Elaboration

Valence and Arousal Ratings versus DES Ratings

The comparison of the valence of VS found for emotions evaluated by DES and SAM shows that 68.4% of the subjects who rated the videos with the positive valence on SAM also did the same on DES, and 82.2% for the negative valence. These results were proven statistically ((χ^2 = 264,136; gl = 1; p =.000; η^2 =.509) indicating that SAM and DES tend to be concordant in valence ratings, even though DES may be more suitable for some emotions than others. As can be seen in Table 11, for emotions like positive surprise, negative surprise, joy, disgust, and sadness, the valence ratings were as per the theoretical expectations which confirmed that for 4 out of 6 emotions, the valence of the VS is assessed in the same way by DES and SAM for both genders i.e. 66.7% of the emotions. In this Study II, differences were noted just for emotions such as fear (negative valence) and interest (positive valence). For the fear-evoking video, female participants rated it with negative valence while the male participants rated it with positive valence. In the case of 'interest,' males gave a negative rating for VS24, whereas females rated positive for VS138.

Table 11. Concordances between theoretical and assessed valences (SAM and DES)

SAM/DES "valence" concordances			
Theoretical validity of emotions			
Emotion		Gender	
		Female	Male
Positive	Interest	(VS24) 90.0% –	(VS138) 81.2% +
	Joy	(VS155) 93.8% +	(VS85) 80.0% +
	Positive Surprise	(VS9) 97.4% +	(VS9) 96.9% +
Negative	Negative Surprise	(VS44) 98.8% –	(VS132) 90.6% –
	Fear	(VS63) 55.6% –	(VS63) 55.4% +
	Sadness	(VS3) 76.5% –	(VS74) 93.8% –
	Disgust	(VS93) 71.6% –	(VS44) 73.8% –

Source: Self Elaboration

The comparison of the perceived arousal of VS found for emotions evaluated by DES and SAM when evaluated by each gender shows that less than half of the emotions are classified in the same way. Bearing in mind that the scale of perceived arousal in the SAM ranges from "1 (activated) to 9 (apathetic)" and in the DES it ranges from "1 (very weak) to 5 (very strong)", with the correlations expected to be negative and considering the results summarized in Table 12. Of the 14 correlations calculated, only 6 (42.9%) are statistically significant. The emotions evaluated congruently by the SAM and DES scales in terms of arousal were: "positive surprise" (only in women), "joy" (also only in women), "fear" (in both genders), "interest" (only in men) and "sadness" (only in men). The emotions "negative surprise" and "disgust" did not have a congruent evaluation between the two scales in either sex. That is, without considering gender, we found 5/6 (83.3%) emotions congruently assessed by both scales.

Finally, in the overall sample, the correlation between the perceived arousal assessed by the SAM and the DES was negative, as expected, and statistically significant ($r = -.218$; $p = .000$), but with a very low effect ($r^2 = .048$). In men, the correlation between arousal assessed by SAM and by DES was statistically significant ($r = -.235$; $p = .000$), but very low ($r^2 = .055$). In women, the correlation was also significant ($r = -.206$; $p = .000$), but also very low ($r^2 = .042$).

Table 12. Correlation between theoretical and assessed arousal (SAM and DES)

Correlations "perceived arousal" SAM/DES					
Theoretical validity of emotions					
Positive			**Negative**		
Emotion	**Gender**		**Emotion**	**Gender**	
	Female	**Male**		**Female**	**Male**
Interest	**(VS24)** **r – ; <.01**	(VS138) n.s.	Fear	(VS63) **r – ; <.001**	**(VS63)** **r – ; <.001**
Joy	(VS155) n.s.	(VS85) **r – ; <.001**	Sadness	(VS3) **r – ; <.01**	(VS74) n.s.
Positive Surprise	(VS9) n.s.	(VS9) **r – ; <.001**	Negative Surprise	(VS44) n.s.	(VS132) n.s.
			Disgust	(VS93) n.s.	(VS44) n.s.

Source: Self Elaboration

For individual emotions, the correlation between the two evaluations of perceived arousal assessed by SAM and DES can be summarized in the following way:

- **Interest:** For men, the correlation was statistically significant (r = -.370, p = .003), though very low (r^2 = .014). For women, the correlation was not significant (r = -.133, p = .239).
- **Joy:** The correlation was not statistically significant for men (r = -.145, p = .248), but was significant for women (r = -.445, p = .000, r^2 = .198).
- **Positive Surprise:** Among men, the correlation between arousal ratings for SAM and DES was not statistically significant (r = -.200, p = .107), but it was significant for women (r = -.446, p = .000), although the effect size was small (r^2 = .199).
- **Negative Surprise:** For both men (r = -.106, p = .406) and women (r = -.107, p = .343), the correlation was not statistically significant.
- **Fear:** Statistically significant correlations were found for both men (r = -.577, p = .000, r^2 = .330) and women (r = -.547, p = .000, r^2 = .300).
- **Sadness:** The correlation was significant for men (r = -.283, p = .022, r^2 = .080), but not for women (r = -.049, p = .662).
- **Disgust:** For both men and women, the correlation was not statistically significant (women: r = -.035; p=.755); men: r = -.153; p=.225).

Based on the above results, it can be presented the profiles of the VS in terms of V&A for both genders as follows in Table 13:

Table 13. V&A ratings for each emotion.

Emotion	Female			Male		
	Video ID	**Valence**	**Arousal**	**Video ID**	**Valence**	**Arousal**
Interest	VS138	3	5	VS24	7	4,5
Joy	VS85	2	5	VS155	5	9
Positive Surprise	VS9	3	5	VS9	3	5
Negative Surprise	VS132	7	5	VS44	7	3,5
Fear	VS63	5	5	VS63	6	5
Sadness	VS74	7	5	VS3	8	3
Disgust	VS44	7	5	VS93	8	5

Source: Self Elaboration

Table 13 shows that only for "positive surprise" do the ratings of both genders coincide (valence = 3, arousal = 5). There are differences between the other emotions:

- **Female participants:** the emotions associated with the videos all have the same arousal (5) and, in the "positive valence → negative valence" sense, are positioned as follows: joy (valence =2), interest and positive surprise (valence = 3), fear (valence = 5), disgust, sadness and negative surprise (valence = 7).

- **Male participants:** the emotions associated with the videos have arousal values between 3 (sadness) and 9 (joy) and, in the "positive valence → negative valence" sense, are positioned as follows: positive surprise (valence = 3), joy (valence = 5), fear (valence = 6), negative surprise and interest (valence = 7) and disgust and sadness (valence = 8).

In conclusion, the results demonstrated the reliability of VS in eliciting distinct emotional responses, with significant IA and notable GD in V&A ratings across a range of emotions, validating the VS set for use in future emotion-based studies and clinical applications.

5 DISCUSSION

The objective of this study was to develop a battery of ecologically valid VS, referred to as "video-stimuli" (VS), that could be used to assess emotional responses, with a particular focus on GD, across three dimensions: salience, perceived intensity (arousal), and valence. Two internationally recognized instruments were employed for this purpose - SAM and DES - to capture participants' subjective emotional experiences. In this context, four hypotheses were tested across two studies, each of which will be discussed considering the results.

5.1 Study I: Selection of Effective Emotional Stimuli

Study I aimed to identify a set of VS with high IA (≥ 60%) regarding the most salient emotion, tested using the DES and SAM. The objective was to create a battery of "ecologically valid" stimuli that could be used in both research and clinical settings.

Hypothesis 1: Intersubjective Agreement of ≥ 60% for Salient Emotions

The first hypothesis predicted that it is possible to find VS with a significant IA (≥ 60%) in the identification of the most salient emotion. This hypothesis was confirmed, as the results showed that 50 of the 150 videos, evaluated by both male and female participants, met the threshold for IA, with participants consistently identifying the most salient emotion. These findings indicate that a significant portion of the stimuli reliably triggered consistent emotional responses, as identified by both male and female participants, due to their evolutionary significance (Boyle, 1984; Ekman, 1999; Izard, 1977, 1991, 2009; Izard et al., 1974). Unlike static images or simple affective tasks, the use of ecologically valid VS that mimic real-life emotional experiences more closely (Christensen, 2007), likely contributed to this high level of agreement, as noted by Christensen (2004) regarding the importance of using dynamic stimuli for emotional elicitation. The **dynamic nature** of these stimuli, which include auditory and visual elements, makes them especially suitable for studying emotional processing in more naturalistic environments. Moreover, the 90-second duration of each video allowed for a fuller emotional experience, which is often not possible with shorter or less immersive stimuli. Specifically, emotions such as **joy**, **sadness**, **fear**, and **disgust** consistently exceeded the 60% threshold for agreement, which can be attributed to their strong behavioral and physiological markers that are easily discerned by participants (Ekman, 1999; Panksepp, 2003), demonstrating the validity and reliability of these videos in eliciting clear and distinct emotional responses. The fact that in the study I only obtained six of the ten emotions studied can be explained by the number of VS available, given the high inter-individual variability in the response to contents of great ecological value (Panksepp, 2003). From a conceptual point of view, some authors do not include guilt, shame, and contempt in the conceptual group of emotions (Ekman, 1972). For example, guilt is understood as a judgment that activates certain emotions (Guerreiro, 2011). For example, of the six Izard emotions for which we obtained EV, five correspond to the six basic emotions identified by Ekman (1972): surprise, joy, sadness, disgust, and fear. So, to test the induction of Eckman's six basic and cross-cultural emotions, we had EV for five. The only emotion we didn't get VS for was anger.

Limitations

While Study I successfully identified 50 effective VS, several limitations should be noted:

- **Sample Size:** The relatively small sample size (n = 19) may limit the generalizability of the findings because the sample may not be fully representative of broader population responses. This issue was addressed in Study II with a larger sample.
- **Cultural Specificity:** The videos were evaluated by Portuguese participants, and cultural differences in emotional expression and perception may influence the generalizability of the findings to other cultures. Future studies should consider cross-cultural validation.

- **Sample Selection Method:** the convenience sampling method could have introduced biases in emotional responses, as the participants were recruited from the researchers' personal networks.

Conclusion of Study I

Study I effectively identified a set of 50 VS that reliably elicited distinct emotions, with strong IA. These videos were validated in Study II, where a larger sample and more detailed analyses, including GD, were explored.

5.2 Study II: Validation and Gender Differences

The objective of Study II was to validate the emotionally effective VS identified in Study I with a larger sample of participants, examining how these stimuli elicited emotional responses among participants of both genders. This study employed two widely recognized instruments, SAM and DES, to assess the participants' emotional responses concerning the dimensions of V&A. The four hypotheses outlined in the study focused on IA, GD, and the consistency of V&A ratings across SAM and DES. This section discusses the findings of Study II under these hypotheses and compares them with previous literature.

Hypothesis 1: Intersubjective Agreement of ≥ 60% for Salient Emotions (Validation of Emotionally Effective Stimuli) using DES

The results confirmed the effectiveness of the VS, with 60% or more participants agreeing on the most salient emotion across the majority of the videos using DES. This replication of results from Study I across a much larger sample provides strong evidence for the robustness of these dynamic VS stimuli in evoking consistent emotional responses with high IA. This is consistent with prior literature that highlights the reliability of VS in evoking specific emotions that are recognized across individuals, genders, and cultures (Ekman, 1999; Izard, 1991; Izard et al., 1974; Lang et al., 1997a).

As has been seen, in Study II, six emotions - interest, joy, surprise (positive or negative), fear, sadness, and disgust - were identified by the participants of both genders (Table 7). The fact that this study only obtained six of the ten emotions of Izard et al. (1974) with a high IA can be explained by the number of VS available, given the high inter-individual variability in response to content of great ecological value (Panksepp, 2003). However, it is worth noticing that of these six emotions, five correspond to the six basic emotions identified by Ekman (1972) (all except interest). Also, the findings from the SAM ratings for V&A revealed patterns consistent with prior literature. Videos eliciting joy and interest were rated higher on valence (indicating more positive emotions), whereas fear and disgust videos were rated lower on valence, suggesting negative emotional reactions. Arousal ratings were highest for videos depicting fear, disgust, and surprise, indicating that these emotions were perceived as more intense or activating. These results support Russell's (1980) circumplex model of effect, which posits that emotions vary along dimensions of V&A, with emotions like fear and disgust often eliciting high arousal but negative valence (Tables 7 and 8).

In study II, it was not possible to find VS for the emotions anger, contempt, shame, and guilt, nor find identical VS between the sexes for four of the emotions, except for surprise (positive) and fear (Table 9). These findings are in line with previous research because some authors like Ekman (1972) don't include contempt, shame, and guilt in the group of basic emotions

Hypothesis 2: Gender Differences in Emotionally Effective Stimuli

The second hypothesis predicted that emotionally effective stimuli would differ between male and female participants for each emotion. The GD observed in Study II is particularly noteworthy. The results partially confirmed this hypothesis, as GD emerged in the intensity of emotional responses (arousal), although both genders agreed on the most salient emotions (valence), that is these results confirm that emotional experiences vary not only in terms of the type of emotion but also in the intensity of the emotional reaction based on gender. Female participants tended to rate videos eliciting negative emotions (e.g.: fear, sadness) as more intense (higher arousal) than males, whereas males rated disgust-related videos as more arousing, although this difference was not statistically significant. Male participants showed higher arousal ratings for positive emotions like joy and positive surprise (Table 8).

These findings align with previous research by Bradley and Lang (1994), which observed that women generally exhibit greater sensitivity (arousal) to negative emotional stimuli, particularly fear and sadness (Bradley & Lang, 1994; Fischer et al., 2004) and are generally more expressive of certain emotions, particularly in contexts involving vulnerability or empathy (Fischer et al., 2004), while men tend to respond more intensely to positive emotions. Such GD in emotional processing may be explained by both biological factors, such as hormonal influences, and social conditioning, where women are socialized to be more expressive and attuned to certain emotions (Mendes et al., 2014).

Additionally, was observed in study II that only VS9 (positive surprise) and VS63 (fear) were identified coincidentally by both sexes using valence, which corroborates previous studies indicating that these emotions do not involve GD, but rather that these emotions prepare and/or activate the defense system, which is essential for human survival and due to the explicit and unambiguous nature of the video content, which is often used in the television and film industries (Deleuze, 2004; Hayward, 2009; Lange & Houran, 1998; López, 2016; Otta & Fiquer, 2004)

These gender-based differences findings in emotional perception have important implications for emotion research, particularly in clinical settings. These differences suggest that gender may play a significant role in how emotional stimuli are processed and experienced, which could have practical applications in designing gender-sensitive therapeutic interventions (Fischer et al., 2004). For example, the heightened emotional responses to fear and sadness in females could be considered when designing emotional regulation therapies, while males' stronger responses to disgust may be useful in studying emotional responses related to aggression or aversion.

Hypothesis 3: Consistency of Valence Ratings Between SAM and DES

Hypothesis 3 suggested that, in each sex, SV valence would be evaluated consistently between SAM and DES. This hypothesis was partially confirmed since it was only possible to find significant agreement between the valence assessments on the SAM and DES scales (Tables 8 and 11) for four of Eckman's six basic emotions (Surprise, Joy, Disgust, and Sadness), i.e. 66.7%, which reinforces the convergent validity of these scales for specific emotions. The strong correlation between SAM and DES valence ratings (Table 12) corroborates previous findings by Lang et al. (1997a) regarding the reliability of these tools for measuring valence. These results further validate the use of SAM and DES in emotional research involving dynamic stimuli.

On the other hand, divergences were found for other emotions, such as fear and interest, and for the valence associated with negative surprise. These differences can be explained probably because both scales aim to measure a very subjective construct, associated with a subjective experience of watching films and analyzing them from an emotional point of view, analyzed by self-report (Ribeiro & Monteiro, 2015). Specifically, these differences can be explained by contextual factors or the idiosyncratic characteristics of the participants.

- **Negative Surprise:** The results suggested that DES may be more suitable than SAM for assessing the valence of negative surprise. This is possibly related to the theoretical basis of the DES, which was built on Izard's theory of differential emotions, which argues that primary emotions have a unique motivational tendency and a particular neuronal organization. This organization makes it easier for emotions to direct sensory and cognitive processes, allowing for a better evaluation of negative surprises through DES (Reis & Horta, 2015).

- **Fear:** There was a significant incongruity in the valence evaluations of the fear video, especially among the female participants. Although fear is classically considered a negative valence emotion, around 56% of women and 55% of men attributed positive valence to the fear stimulus. There is no clear explanation for this incongruity, and the results may reflect a "chance effect", or perhaps individual differences in the interpretation of the stimulus. These differences highlight the complexity of measuring emotions such as fear, which can be influenced by contextual or cultural factors.
- **Interest:** The video that generated responses related to interest also produced divergent results between men and women. 81.2% of men rated the video as having negative valence on both scales, due to the disturbing nature of the content (a car accident). On the other hand, 90% of women attributed a positive valence to the video of interest, even though the content was equally disturbing (an imminent accident involving a truck and a train). This divergence can be explained by the emotional context of the interest, which can be both positive and negative, depending on the situation. Interest, described by Nuttin (2014) as "alertness", can reflect a response to both dangerous situations and surrounding events, depending on the subjective interpretation of the participant. The differences found could be explained by the specific content of the videos, the idiosyncrasies of the participants (Smith & Mackie, 2008), and GD (Brody & Hall, 2008).

The results that confirmed the hypothesis for emotions such as joy, disgust, and sadness corroborate the studies by Ekman (1999) and Boyle (1984), who identified these emotions as universal and differentiated in terms of valence. However, the divergences observed for more complex emotions, such as fear and interest, highlight the role of the contextual specificities of the stimuli and GD in emotional interpretation, as described in studies such as Brody and Hall (2008) and Smith and Mackie (2008).

In general, the results suggest that both scales are valid tools for measuring valence, although the DES may be better suited to capturing the complexity of negative or ambiguous emotions.

Hypothesis 4: Consistency of Arousal Ratings Between SAM and DES

Hypothesis 4 predicted that, for both sexes, the perceived arousal of VS would be evaluated consistently between SAM and DES. However, this hypothesis was partially confirmed, since the correlations between the two scales, although statistically significant, were negative and of low value, suggesting an inverse relationship between the two instruments. That is, without considering gender, we found 5/6 (83.3%) emotions congruently assessed by both scales, which suggests a good convergent validity of the scales about these emotions. It should be remembered that the SAM and DES scales measure arousal in opposite directions, which explains the negative correlation between them. On the SAM scale, lower values indicate greater emotional activation (1 = very activated; 9 = not activated at all), while on the DES scale, the assessment is the opposite (5 = very strong; 1 = very weak). When the sample was analyzed as a whole (without considering GD), the correlation between the arousal perceived by the SAM and the arousal perceived by the DES was negative (as expected) and statistically significant, although with a very low effect size. This means that although the scales capture the same construct of arousal, the inverse nature of their scores contributes to the negative correlation, but the magnitude of this correlation is small, which suggests that the DES has a lower discriminative capacity than the SAM. This may be because the DES scale has a more limited response range, as pointed out byLarán and Rossi (2006), which hinders its ability to discriminate subtle variations in arousal compared to the SAM. The present study adds to the literature by exploring this relationship in a dynamic stimulus-video context, revealing how the interpretation of arousal can be influenced by both the content of the stimulus and the measuring instrument.

The analysis also revealed interesting differences in the dispersion of emotions in terms of V&A for men and women. Table 13 shows that, for women, all the emotions associated with the videos had the same arousal value (equal to 5), while for men the arousal varied between 3 (sadness) and 9 (joy). These results suggest that men experienced greater variation in emotional intensity (arousal) in response to the stimuli, while women showed a more stable emotional response in terms of activation.

As far as valence is concerned, in the sense of "positive valence → negative valence", the emotions are positioned as follows: joy, interest and positive surprise, fear, disgust, sadness, and negative surprise. In study II it was possible to identify some discrepancies concerning the Russell (1980) circumplex model in terms of valence, with some emotions positioned in a not conceptually congruent way(Arangüena & Dorado, 2001). For example: For women, the emotions of positive surprise and interest had similar positive valences, while emotions such as fear, sadness, and negative surprise were associated with negative valences. In men, there was greater variation in valence, with joy and positive surprise being the emotions with the most positive valence, and disgust and sadness as those with the most negative valence. Curiously, fear and interest were evaluated in a way that was incongruent with what was expected, with some participants considering them to have positive valences, which may reflect contextual factors or individual experiences with the videos. The variation in arousal response between men and women is also in line with studies by Bradley & Lang (1994), which highlighted the challenges of measuring arousal consistently across different scales and indicate that men tend to report greater variations in emotional intensity, while women can present more consistent emotional responses.

The partial confirmation of this hypothesis may reflect the subjective nature of arousal and the limitations of self-report measures.

Limitations of Study II

Although Study II involved a larger sample size compared to Study I, certain limitations remain:

- **Cultural Specificity:** The sample was drawn exclusively from Portuguese participants, and emotional responses may vary across different cultures. This suggests the need for cross-cultural validation in future research.
- **Sampling Bias:** The convenience sampling method used to recruit participants may limit the generalizability of the findings. Future studies should employ random sampling to ensure broader representation.
- **Variables analysis:** while GD was explored, other demographic factors such as age, socioeconomic status, and education were not thoroughly analyzed in this study. Future research could explore how these variables interact with emotional perception, as previous studies have shown that age and socioeconomic background can influence emotional regulation and experience (Carstensen et al., 2000; Lewis, 2007; Papalia et al., 2021; Wager et al., 2003)

Conclusion of Study II

Study II successfully validated the effectiveness of the 50 VS identified in Study I. The results confirmed that these videos reliably elicit specific emotions with high IA. GD in emotional perception was evident, particularly in the V&A dimensions for emotions like fear, sadness, and disgust. The validated VS offers a valuable tool for future research into emotion elicitation and the influence of gender on emotional experience.

6 CONCLUSION

This research had the objective of developing and validating a set of emotionally effective VS that could reliably evoke specific emotions and demonstrate high EV. Across two studies, the findings confirmed that these stimuli elicited strong IA on emotions such as joy, sadness, fear, interest, disgust, and surprise, providing a robust tool for future emotion research.

Study I successfully identified 50 effective VS from an initial pool of 150, demonstrating that dynamic, naturalistic video clips are capable of reliably inducing distinct emotions. The results highlighted the importance of both V&A dimensions in shaping emotional experiences and confirmed that certain emotions are more consistently recognized across participants due to their strong physiological and behavioral markers.

Study II validated these findings with a larger sample to increase the level of reliability in the stimuli eliciting the intended emotions. This study however showed that there were some significant differences between the genders in the perception of emotions, whereby females were more emotional towards sadness and fear while males were more emotional towards disgust. In other words, there are feelings associated with experiencing such emotions that differ between genders across populations, therefore, underscoring the need for personalized approaches in emotional regulation strategies and psychological treatments.

The implications of this research on emotional perception extend beyond the laboratory, they have real clinical, therapeutic, and even educational implications. Given the quality of the validation procedures, the stimuli will be useful during psychophysiological studies and clinical examinations as well as emotional regulation therapy, explaining how emotion is processed understood, and felt in various situations. Additionally, the findings on GD highlight the need for more gender-sensitive approaches in both research and practice, particularly in interventions aimed at emotional well-being.

Despite the strengths of this research, certain limitations must be acknowledged. The cultural specificity of the stimuli, which were tested Future research should aim to validate these stimuli across diverse cultural contexts to ensure broader applicability. In the same line of thought, GD has been addressed in the current study, but other demographic factors such as age and socio-economic status have not been looked at deeply leaving it for future research to find out how these factors shape emotional experiences.

In conclusion, this research provides a valuable set of tools for studying emotions in more naturalistic and ecologically valid contexts. By bridging the gap between laboratory-based emotional stimuli and real-world emotional experiences, this study offers significant contributions to the field of emotion research. Future studies should continue to refine and expand on these findings, exploring how cultural, gender and demographic differences influence emotional perception and experience.

ACKNOWLEDGEMENTS

Funding: This research received no funding.

Informed Consent Statement: Informed consent was obtained from all subjects involved in the study.

Conflicts of Interest: The authors declare no conflict of interest.

REFERENCES

Arangüena, L., & Dorado, J. (2001). *Psicofisiologia: fundamentos metodológicos*. Ediciones Pirâmide.

Atanassov, A., Pilev, D., & Tomova, F. (2024). MULTIMODAL SYSTEM FOR FACIAL EMOTION RECOGNITION BASED ON DEEP LEARNING. *Journal of Chemical Technology and Metallurgy*, 59(3), 729–740. DOI: 10.59957/jctm.v59.i3.2024.29

Barrett, L. F., & Wager, T. D. (2006). The structure of emotion: Evidence from neuroimaging studies. *Current Directions in Psychological Science*, 15(2), 79–83. DOI: 10.1111/j.0963-7214.2006.00411.x

Bota, P. J., Wang, C., Fred, A. L. N., & Placido Da Silva, H. (2019). A Review, Current Challenges, and Future Possibilities on Emotion Recognition Using Machine Learning and Physiological Signals. *IEEE Access : Practical Innovations, Open Solutions*, 7, 140990–141020. DOI: 10.1109/ACCESS.2019.2944001

Boyle, G. J. (1984). Reliability and validity of Izard's differential emotions scale. *Personality and Individual Differences*, 5(6), 747–750. DOI: 10.1016/0191-8869(84)90124-7

Bradley, M. M., & Lang, P. J. (1994). Measuring emotion: The self-assessment manikin and the semantic differential. *Journal of Behavior Therapy and Experimental Psychiatry*, 25(1), 49–59. DOI: 10.1016/0005-7916(94)90063-9 PMID: 7962581

Brody, L. R., & Hall, J. A. (2008). Gender and Emotion in Context. In M. Lewis, J. M. Haviland-Jones, & L. F. Barrett (Eds.), *Handbook of Emotions* (3° ed., pp. 309-408). The Guilford Press.

Cacioppo, J. T., & Gardner, W. L. (1999). Emotion. *Annual Review of Psychology*, 50(1), 191–214. DOI: 10.1146/annurev.psych.50.1.191 PMID: 10074678

Cacioppo, J. T., Tassinary, L. G., & Berntson, G. (2017). *Handbook of Psychophysiology* (t. ed., Ed.). Cambridge University Press.

Canavarro, M. C. S. (1999). Inventário de Sintomas Psicopatológicos (BSI). In Simões, M. R., Gonçalves, M. M., & Almeida, L. S. (Eds.), *Testes e provas psicologias em Portugal* (Vol. 2, pp. 95–109). APPORT/SHO.

Canavarro, M. C. S. (2007). Inventário de Sintomas Psicopatológicos (BSI): Uma revisão crítica dos estudos realizados em Portugal. In Simões, M. R., Machado, C., Gonçalves, M. M., & Almeida, L. (Eds.), *Avaliação psicológica: Instrumentos validados para a população portuguesa* (Vol. III). Quarteto Editora.

Carstensen, L. L., Pasupathi, M., Mayr, U., & Nesselroade, J. R. (2000). Emotional experience in everyday life across the adult life span. *Journal of Personality and Social Psychology*, 79(4), 644–655. DOI: 10.1037/0022-3514.79.4.644 PMID: 11045744

Chanel, G. (2009). *Emotion Assessment for Affective Computing Based on Brain and Peripheral Signals,* University of Geneve. https://theses.eurasip.org/theses/492/emotion-assessment-for-affective-computing-based/

Christensen, L. B. (2007). *Experimental Methodology* (10th ed.). Pearson / Allyn & Bacon.

Cornelius, R. (2000). *Theoretical approaches to emotion* ISCA Tutorial and Research Workshop (ITRW) on Speech and Emotion, https://www.isca-archive.org/speechemotion_2000/cornelius00_speechemotion.html#

Correia, D. T. (2023). *Manual de psicopatologia - Psiquiatria & Psicologia Clínica - De Acordo com o DSM-5 e o CID-11* (3rd ed.). LIDEL.

Csikszentmihalyi, M., & Larson, R. (1987). Validity and reliability of the experience-sampling method. *The Journal of Nervous and Mental Disease*, 175(9), 526–536. DOI: 10.1097/00005053-198709000-00004 PMID: 3655778

Dai, Y., Wang, X., Zhang, P., Zhang, W., & Junfeng, C. (2018). Sparsity constrained differential evolution enabled feature-channel-sample hybrid selection for daily-life EEG emotion recognition. *Multimedia Tools and Applications*, 77(17), 21967–21994. Advance online publication. DOI: 10.1007/s11042-018-5618-0

Deleuze, G. (2004). *A imagem-movimento: Cinema 1* (Godinho, R., Trans.). Assírio & Alvim.

Ekman, P. (1972). Universals and cultural differences in facial expressions of emotion. *Nebraska Symposium on Motivation*, Lincoln.

Ekman, P. (1999). Basic Emotions. In *Handbook of Cognition and Emotion* (pp. 45-60). https://doi.org/DOI: 10.1002/0470013494.ch3

Ekman, P. (2008). An argument for basic emotions. *Cognition and Emotion*, 6(3-4), 169–200. DOI: 10.1080/02699939208411068

Ekman, P., & Cordaro, D. (2011). What is Meant by Calling Emotions Basic. *Emotion Review*, 3(4), 364–370. DOI: 10.1177/1754073911410740

Ekman, P., & Friesen, W. V. (1971). Constants across cultures in the face and emotion. *Journal of Personality and Social Psychology*, 17(2), 124–129. DOI: 10.1037/h0030377 PMID: 5542557

Ekman, P., Friesen, W. V., O'Sullivan, M., Chan, A., Diacoyanni-Tarlatzis, I., Heider, K., Krause, R., LeCompte, W. A., Pitcairn, T., Ricci-Bitti, P. E., Scherer, K., Tomita, M., & Tzavaras, A. (1987). Universals and cultural differences in the judgments of facial expressions of emotion. *Journal of Personality and Social Psychology*, 53(4), 712–717. DOI: 10.1037/0022-3514.53.4.712 PMID: 3681648

Fischer, A. H., Rodriguez Mosquera, P. M., van Vianen, A. E., & Manstead, A. S. (2004). Gender and culture differences in emotion. *Emotion (Washington, D.C.)*, 4(1), 87–94. DOI: 10.1037/1528-3542.4.1.87 PMID: 15053728

Folstein, M. F., Folstein, S. E., & McHugh, P. R. (1975). "Mini-mental state". A practical method for grading the cognitive state of patients for the clinician. *Journal of Psychiatric Research*, 12(3), 189–198. DOI: 10.1016/0022-3956(75)90026-6 PMID: 1202204

Fordson, P., Xing, X., Guo, K., & Xu, X. (2022). Emotion Recognition With Knowledge Graph Based on Electrodermal Activity. *Frontiers in Neuroscience*, 16, 911767. DOI: 10.3389/fnins.2022.911767 PMID: 35757534

Guerreiro, M., Botelho, M. A., Leitão, O., Castro-Caldas, A., & Garcia, C. (1994). *Adaptação à população portuguesa na tradução do Mini Mental State Examination*. Reunião da Primavera da Sociedade Portuguesa de Neurologia.

Guerreiro, V. (2011). *Desenvolvimento moral: relações entre consistência do raciocínio moral, a atribuição de emoções e ação moral*. ISPA.

Hayward, P. (2009). *Terror tracks: music, sound and horror cinema*. Equinox.

Hessen, J. (2001). *Filosofia dos valores*. Almedina.

Izard, C. E. (1977). *Human Emotions*. Plenum Press. DOI: 10.1007/978-1-4899-2209-0

Izard, C. E. (1991). *The psychology of emotions*. Springer Science & Business Media. DOI: 10.1007/978-1-4899-0615-1

Izard, C. E. (2009). Emotion theory and research: Highlights, unanswered questions, and emerging issues. *Annual Review of Psychology*, 60(1), 1–25. DOI: 10.1146/annurev.psych.60.110707.163539 PMID: 18729725

Izard, C. E., Dougherty, F. E., Bloxom, B. M., & Kotsch, W. E. (1974). *The differential emotions scale: A method of surveying the subjective experience of discrete emotions*. Vanderbilt University Press.

Kang, S., Park, C. Y., Kim, A., Cha, N., & Lee, U. (2022). *Understanding Emotion Changes in Mobile Experience Sampling*. https://doi.org/DOI: 10.1145/3491102.3501944

Kim, B., & Jo, S. (2019). *An Affective Situation Labeling System from Psychological Behaviors in Emotion Recognition*. https://doi.org//arXiv.1911.01158DOI: 10.48550

Kim, B. H., Jo, S., & Choi, S. (2020). A-Situ: A computational framework for affective labeling from psychological behaviors in real-life situations. *Scientific Reports*, 10(1), 15916. DOI: 10.1038/s41598-020-72829-3 PMID: 32985534

Lang, P. J., Bradley, M. M., & Cuthbert, B. N. (1997a). *International Affective Picture System (IAPS): Technical Manual and Affective Ratings*. Center for the Study of Emotion and Attention.

Lang, P. J., Bradley, M. M., & Cuthbert, B. N. (1997b). Motivated attention: Affect, activation, and action. In *Attention and orienting: Sensory and motivational processes* (pp. 97–135). Lawrence Erlbaum Associates Publishers.

Lange, R., & Houran, J. (1998). Delusions of the paranormal: A haunting question of perception. *The Journal of Nervous and Mental Disease*, 186(10), 637–645. DOI: 10.1097/00005053-199810000-00008 PMID: 9788641

Larán, J. A., & Rossi, C. A. V. (2006). Surpresa e a formação da satisfação do consumidor. *RAE Eletrônica*, 5(1). Advance online publication. DOI: 10.1590/S1676-56482006000100002

Larradet, F., Niewiadomski, R., Barresi, G., Caldwell, D. G., & Mattos, L. S. (2020). Toward Emotion Recognition From Physiological Signals in the Wild: Approaching the Methodological Issues in Real-Life Data Collection. *Frontiers in Psychology*, 11, 1111. DOI: 10.3389/fpsyg.2020.01111 PMID: 32760305

Lewis, P. M. J. (2007). *Gendering emotions in organizations*. Palgrave Macmillan. DOI: 10.1007/978-1-137-07297-9

López, M. A. (2016). The Role of Emotions in the Consumer: Theoretical Review and Analysis of Components. *World Academy of Science, Engineering and Technology, International Journal of Social, Behavioral, Educational, Economic. Business and Industrial Engineering*, 10(3), 890–894.

Markus, H. R., & Kitayama, S. (1991). Culture and the self: Implications for cognition, emotion, and motivation. *Psychological Review*, 98(2), 224–253. DOI: 10.1037/0033-295X.98.2.224

Maroco, J. (2007). *Análise estatística: com utilização do SPSS (3ª Edição)*. Edições Sílabo.

Marsh, A. A., Elfenbein, H. A., & Ambady, N. (2003). Nonverbal "accents": Cultural differences in facial expressions of emotion. *Psychological Science*, 14(4), 373–376. DOI: 10.1111/1467-9280.24461 PMID: 12807413

Mendes, E., Timóteo, J., & Cabral, A. S. (2014). Aspetos médico-legais em psiquiatria. In C. B. Saraiva & J. Cerejeira (Eds.), *Psiquiatria fundamental* (Vol., pp. 507-520). LIDEL – Edições Técnicas, Lda.

Murteira, B. J. F. (2004). *Análise exploratória de dados: estatística descritiva*. McGraw-Hill.

Nuttin, J. (2014). *Future time perspective and motivation: Theory and research method*. Psychology Press. DOI: 10.4324/9781315802244

Oliveira, A. G. (2009). *Bioestatística, epidemiologia e investigação: teoria e aplicações*. LIDEL.

Otta, E., & Fiquer, J. (2004). Subjective well-being and emotional regulation. *Psicologia em Revista*, 10(15), 144–149. https://periodicos.pucminas.br/index.php/psicologiaemrevista/article/view/204

Panksepp, J. (2003). At the interface of the affective, behavioral, and cognitive neurosciences: Decoding the emotional feelings of the brain. *Brain and Cognition*, 52(1), 4–14. DOI: 10.1016/S0278-2626(03)00003-4 PMID: 12812799

Panksepp, J. (2004). *Affective Neuroscience: The Foundations of Human and Animal Emotions*. Oxford University Press.

Papalia, D. E., Martorell, G., & Feldman, R. D. (2021). *Desenvolvimento Humano* (14.ª ed.). McGraw Hill.

Picard, R. W. (2000). *Affective computing*. The MIT Press. DOI: 10.7551/mitpress/1140.003.0008

Pio Abreu, J. L. (2015). *Introdução à psicopatologia compreensiva*. Fundação Calouste Gulbenkian.

Pio Abreu, J. L., & Vaz Patto, M. L. (1981). A Utilização de uma Escala de Rastreio em Epidemiologia Clínica. *Psiquiatria Clínica*, 2, 119–133.

Pollak, J., & Adams, P. (2011). *PAM: A Photographic Affect Meter for frequent, in situ measurement of affect*. https://doi.org/DOI: 10.1145/1978942.1979047

Probst, T., Pryss, R., Langguth, B., & Schlee, W. (2016). Emotion dynamics and tinnitus: Daily life data from the "TrackYourTinnitus" application. *Scientific Reports*, 6(1), 31166. DOI: 10.1038/srep31166 PMID: 27488227

Reis, E. (2006). *Estatística multivariada aplicada* (2.ª ed.). Edições Sílabo.

Reis, M. A. B. M. N., & Horta, M. P. (2015). O papel das emoções na relação confiança-exatidão do testemunho. *Psicologia USP*, 26(2), 231–239. DOI: 10.1590/0103-656420140003

Ribeiro, A., & Monteiro, L. (2015). Induction affective scenarios virtual reality: Assessment of the sensation of presence. *Psicologia Clínica*, 27(1), 139–160. DOI: 10.1590/0103-56652015000100008

Russell, J. A. (1980). A Circumplex Model of Affect. *Journal of Personality and Social Psychology*, 39(6), 1161–1178. DOI: 10.1037/h0077714

Russell, J. A., & Barrett, L. F. (1999). Core affect, prototypical emotional episodes, and other things called emotion: Dissecting the elephant. *Journal of Personality and Social Psychology*, 76(5), 805–819. DOI: 10.1037/0022-3514.76.5.805 PMID: 10353204

Scherer, K. R. (2003). Vocal communication of emotion: A review of research paradigms. *Speech Communication*, 40(1-2), 227–256. DOI: 10.1016/S0167-6393(02)00084-5

Scherer, K. R., Schorr, A., & Johnstone, T. (2001). *Appraisal Processes in Emotion*. Oxford University Press., DOI: 10.1093/oso/9780195130072.001.0001

Segurado, M. A. P. (1980). *Biomatemática: matemática aplicada para estudantes de biologia, farmácia e medicina* (Vol. 1). Plátano Editora.

Shu, L., Xie, J., Yang, M., Li, Z., Li, Z., Liao, D., Xu, X., & Yang, X. (2018). A Review of Emotion Recognition Using Physiological Signals. *Sensors (Basel)*, 18(7), 2074. DOI: 10.3390/s18072074 PMID: 29958457

Smith, E., & Mackie, D. (2008). Intergroup Emotions. In M. Lewis, J. M. Haviland-Jones, & L. F. Barrett (Eds.), *Handbook of Emotions* (3ª ed., pp. 428-439). The Guildford Press. https://doi.org/DOI: 10.4324/9780203361993

Tran, V. (2020). Positive Affect Negative Affect Scale (PANAS). In Gellman, M. D. (Ed.), *Encyclopedia of Behavioral Medicine* (pp. 1708–1709). Springer International Publishing., DOI: 10.1007/978-3-030-39903-0_978

Wager, T. D., Phan, K. L., Liberzon, I., & Taylor, S. F. (2003). Valence, gender, and lateralization of functional brain anatomy in emotion: A meta-analysis of findings from neuroimaging. *NeuroImage*, 19(3), 513–531. DOI: 10.1016/S1053-8119(03)00078-8 PMID: 12880784

Watson, D., Clark, L., & Tellegen, A. (1988). Development and Validation of Brief Measures of Positive and Negative Affect: The PANAS Scales. *Journal of Personality and Social Psychology*, 54(6), 1063–1070. DOI: 10.1037/0022-3514.54.6.1063 PMID: 3397865

Yerkes, R., & Dodson, J. (1908). The relation of strength of stimulus to rapidity of habit-formation. *The Journal of Comparative Neurology and Psychology*, 18(5), 459–482. http://psychclassics.yorku.ca/Yerkes/Law/. DOI: 10.1002/cne.920180503

Yu, L.-C., Lee, L.-H., Hao, S., Wang, J., He, Y., Hu, J., Lai, K., & Zhang, X. (2016). *Building Chinese Affective Resources in Valence-Arousal Dimensions.*

KEY TERMS AND DEFINITIONS

Arousal: The condition of being awake and reactive to stimuli, both physiologically and psychologically. In emotion studies, arousal is an impulse that triggers a reaction in an organism and is the most affected by the stimulus of an emotion measured in its quiet and excited states.

Differential Emotions Scale (DES): A self-assessment by Carroll Izard that captures the extent of ten universal emotions such as joy and sadness, anger and fear, and disgust, among others. The DES is designed to assess the experience of the emotion evoked by a certain stimulus.

Ecological Validity: The degree to which the outcome of research projects is relevant to the environment outside experimental settings. In this specific study, it is limited to the extent to which the emotional material used in the study can evoke real-life emotions.

Emotion: Is the mental state constituted by three components: a subjective experience, a physiological response, and a behavioral or expressive response. Emotions are an important aspect of human interrelations as well as human decision-making.

Intersubjective Agreement: The extent to which a group of people achieves the same judgment concerning an emotion or a stimulus. High intersubjective agreement means that the different participants exhibit and feel similar emotions when they are subjected to exactly the same stimuli.

Self-Assessment Manikin (SAM): A nonverbal pictorial assessment device that gauges emotion in three dimensions, namely valence (pleasure-displeasure), arousal (intensity), and dominance (control).

Valence: It is the degree of attractiveness or satedness inherent in the emotional experience as it relates to the individual. Valence speaks to the emotional range available for inclusion in an experience from pleasant to unpleasant.

Chapter 8
Performance Evaluation in Anesthesiology: A Literature Review on Psychological and Organizational Factors Influencing Professional Performance

Stéphanie Monteiro
Institute for Systems and Robotics, Instituto Superior Técnico, Portugal

Ricardo Marcão
https://orcid.org/0000-0003-3277-3078
ISLA Santarém, Portugal

Vasco Santos
Polytechnic Institute of Tomar, Portugal & ISLA Santarém, Portugal & GOVCOPP, Portugal & CiTUR, Portugal

Patrícia David
ISLA Santarém, Portugal & TechnoPhage, Portugal

Maria José Sousa
https://orcid.org/0000-0001-8633-4199
ISCTE, University Institute of Lisbon, Portugal

Filipa Martinho
ISLA Santarém, Portugal

Marta Correia Sampaio
https://orcid.org/0000-0003-0004-601X
Polytechnic Institute of Santarém, Portugal

ABSTRACT

This chapter examines the evaluation of anesthesia professionals by focusing on the psychosocial and organizational factors that impact their performance. Traditional assessments tend to emphasize technical skills but often neglect critical influences such as job satisfaction, stress, and organizational support. Using Allen and Meyer's

DOI: 10.4018/979-8-3693-8598-2.ch008

Organizational Commitment Model, the review explores how affective, continuance, and normative commitment shape professional behavior in high-pressure environments like anesthesiology. The findings highlight that beyond technical competence, psychosocial well-being and organizational dynamics, including leadership and team culture, are crucial to ensuring optimal performance. The chapter suggests that pre- and post-intervention questionnaires can provide valuable insights into these factors, advocating for a more integrated approach to performance evaluation in anesthesiology.

1. INTRODUCTION TO ANESTHESIOLOGY AND PROFESSIONAL PERFORMANCE

Anesthesiology is a critically important medical discipline that involves the comprehensive management of perioperative care for patients, ensuring their utmost safety and facilitating the delivery of anesthesia during surgical procedures. The profession entails an exceptionally demanding nature, as it necessitates a fusion of advanced technical aptitude and the capacity to make swift decisions under immense pressure. Conventional performance assessments for anesthesiologists have primarily concentrated on clinical outcomes, encompassing elements such as patient safety, successful anesthesia administration, and recovery periods. However, these evaluations often disregard the vital psychosocial and organizational factors that substantially contribute to overall professional performance. (Gottumukkala et al., 2023; Su & Zeng, 2023) In the context of high-stress environments like operating rooms, where anesthesiologists must operate within deadlines and within the confines of immense pressure, it is imperative to broaden modern performance evaluation frameworks to encompass these aforementioned factors. Integrating psychosocial factors with organizational commitment is pivotal in adopting a holistic approach to evaluate the performance of anesthesiologists. Such an approach incorporates various factors, including but not limited to, effective communication and collaboration with the surgical team, empathy towards patients, and the ability to proficiently manage stress levels while maintaining optimal mental well-being. These psychosocial factors not only influence the delivery of anesthesia but also substantially impact the overall patient experience and subsequent outcomes. (NGUYEN et al., 2021; Weer & Greenhaus, 2020) Moreover, the advent of cutting-edge technological advancements, such as biomedical simulators, introduces a novel realm for enhancing the training and performance of anesthesiologists. These sophisticated simulators facilitate realistic practice scenarios that expertly replicate complex surgical procedures and critical events. By utilizing these simulators, anesthesiologists are able to augment their technical skills, heighten their ability to make informed decisions, and effectively manage crisis situations. The integration of simulators into training programs provides an opportunity for anesthesiologists to gain invaluable hands-on experience within a controlled and safe environment, thereby enabling them to refine their techniques and ultimately improve patient outcomes. (Chen et al.2022) In addition to bolstering technical competency, the utilization of biomedical simulators also presents a unique prospect to address the psychological and cognitive facets of anesthesiologists' performance. Simulators that incorporate virtual reality and augmented reality technologies provide truly immersive experiences that flawlessly replicate high-stress situations. By exposing anesthesiologists to challenging scenarios, simulators actively contribute to the cultivation of resilience, heighten situational awareness, and enhance the capacity to perform seamlessly under pressure. Furthermore, these simulators greatly facilitate the development of non-technical skills, including but not limited to effective teamwork, decision-making amidst uncertainty, and the art of clear communication during critical moments. (Haavik & Våpenstad, 2020; Abaalkhayl, 2024) Broadly speaking, this chapter definitively advocates for the adoption of a holistic approach to evaluate the performance of anesthesiologists by strategically integrating psychosocial factors with organizational commitment. Furthermore, it accentuates the paramount importance of incorporating biomedical simulators into the training and development of anesthesiologists to actively enhance their overall performance. This expanded framework fundamentally acknowledges the significance of non-clinical aspects in driving overall professional performance and lays much emphasis on the continual training and development within both the technical and psychological realms. By embracing such an approach, healthcare institutions are able to effectively equip anesthesiologists with the essential skills and unwavering resilience required to consistently provide high-quality care within demanding and high-stress environments. (Panditrao and Panditrao2024)

2. THEORETICAL FRAMEWORKS IN PERFORMANCE EVALUATION

The Allen and Meyer Organizational Commitment Model (1990) is a foundational framework for evaluating employee commitment across various professions. It defines commitment through three distinct dimensions: Affective Commitment: Emotional attachment to the organization and a strong desire to contribute meaningfully to its goals and objectives. This emotional attachment encompasses a deep sense of loyalty and passion towards the organization, fostering a strong sense of belonging and dedication. Continuance Commitment: The perceived cost of leaving the organization, both on a personal and professional level. This dimension encompasses the individual's assessment of the sacrifices they would have to make if they were to leave the organization, such as the loss of benefits, financial security, and career opportunities. It also takes into consideration the magnitude of potential negative consequences associated with leaving the organization, such as the difficulty of finding a new job or the impact it may have on personal relationships. Normative Commitment: A sense of moral or ethical obligation to remain with the organization. This dimension reflects the individual's belief in the social or ethical responsibility to stay with the organization, regardless of personal costs or benefits. It is grounded in a feeling of obligation and a desire to honor commitments and agreements made with the organization, colleagues, or clients. (Agegnehu et al.2022; Jonathan, 2020) These three components of commitment have been extensively studied and have shown to exert a significant influence on employee performance, particularly in high-stress professional environments. In anesthesiology, where decisions made under pressure can have life-or-death consequences, the emotional and organizational support provided by the workplace plays a critical role in an anesthesiologist's ability to function effectively. The unique challenges and demands of the field necessitate a high level of commitment from anesthesiologists, as their performance directly impacts patient safety and outcomes. (Kao et al.2022) By applying the Allen and Meyer model in the context of anesthesiology, we aim to better understand how commitment influences anesthesiologists' performance and ultimately enhance patient care. In this chapter, we propose a new version of the Allen and Meyer questionnaire, specifically adapted to evaluate the commitment levels and factors relevant to anesthesiologists. This modified questionnaire will encompass scenarios and challenges commonly faced by anesthesiologists and will be administered in conjunction with the use of biomedical simulators. Through this integrated approach, we aim to capture a comprehensive understanding of anesthesiologists' commitment and its impact on their performance in a realistic and controlled setting. (Mohadeseh et al.2021; Basarah et al.2022; Robinson, 2022) The findings of this study have the potential to contribute to the development of targeted interventions and strategies aimed at fostering commitment among anesthesiologists, ultimately improving patient outcomes and quality of care. As we delve deeper into the understanding of anesthesiologists' commitment levels, we can identify specific areas where support and resources can be allocated to ensure a positive work environment and maximize patient safety. The intricacies of anesthesiology require an unwavering commitment from healthcare professionals, as the decisions and actions taken during procedures can have far-reaching consequences. By nurturing commitment and providing adequate support, organizations can create an atmosphere that promotes excellence in patient care and overall organizational success. (Mcevoy & Abernathy, 2023) As research continues to shed light on the importance of commitment in the field of anesthesiology, we can anticipate the implementation of evidence-based interventions and practices that enhance commitment levels among anesthesiologists, leading to improved outcomes for patients and the healthcare system as a whole. This will require collaboration between healthcare institutions, policymakers, and researchers to create and implement strategies that support anesthesiologists in their commitment to delivering safe and high-quality care. By prioritizing commitment and actively working towards its enhancement, we can pave the way for a future where patient care in anesthesiology reaches new heights of excellence and effectiveness. (Parnikh et al.2022)

3. PSYCHOLOGICAL FACTORS IMPACTING ANESTHESIOLOGISTS' PERFORMANCE

Psychological factors play an exceedingly significant role in determining how anesthesiologists effectively perform their duties in high-pressure environments. The impact of stress, job satisfaction, burnout, emotional resilience, and the ability to cope with challenging situations directly influences their ability to function optimally and provide the best possible care for their patients. These highly skilled professionals often find themselves in situations where quick decision-making is of utmost importance for ensuring the safety of patients and delivering successful outcomes. (Alotaibi et al.2024; Fincher, 2023) Consequently, it becomes crucial to thoroughly comprehend and address these psychological factors to ensure the field of anesthesiology excels in terms of performance and outcomes. Anesthesiologists must possess the necessary skills and employ appropriate strategies to effectively manage stress levels, foster job satisfaction, prevent burnout, and fortify emotional resilience. By doing so, they can optimize their performance and best care for their patients at the highest level, achieving remarkable results that benefit both the healthcare professionals themselves and the patients they diligently serve. (Margolis & Ku, 2021) This endeavor not only benefits the well-being of anesthesiologists but also enhances patient outcomes and overall healthcare system efficiency. Recognizing the profound impact of psychological factors is crucial in ensuring anesthesiologists receive the necessary support and resources to overcome challenges in high-pressure environments. Therefore, healthcare organizations should prioritize the psychological well-being of their anesthesiology teams by implementing comprehensive support programs, cultivating a positive work environment, and promoting a culture of open communication and emotional support. (Fadilah et al., 2023; Gafsou et al.2021; Firth-Cozens & King, 2023) These efforts will not only contribute to the success and effectiveness of anesthesiologists, but also create a ripple effect throughout the healthcare system. By recognizing and proactively addressing the psychological factors, healthcare organizations can foster a positive and supportive environment that values the well-being and performance of anesthesiologists. This, in turn, will lead to tangible benefits for both the healthcare professionals and the patients they selflessly serve. (Li et al.2020)

In summary, the significance of psychological factors in the field of anesthesiology cannot be understated. It is only through recognizing and addressing these factors that we can genuinely enhance the performance and effectiveness of anesthesiologists in high-pressure environments. By prioritizing the psychological well-being of these healthcare professionals, healthcare organizations can cultivate a culture of support, leading to improved outcomes for patients and a more efficient healthcare system overall. The dedication and commitment of anesthesiologists, combined with the necessary psychological support, will continue to shape the future of this vital medical specialty. (Tan et al.2023)

3.1. Stress Management in Anesthesiology

Operating rooms are highly demanding and high-pressure environments, characterized by a constant state of unpredictability and intricate surgical procedures. The anesthesiologists working in these intense settings possess the crucial responsibility of skillfully navigating through these stressors, ensuring optimal patient outcomes. An exceptional anesthesiologist not only acknowledges but also deeply understands the pivotal role that stress management plays in their decision-making abilities within the operating room. In order to maintain top-notch performance, it is imperative for an anesthesiologist to effectively manage and control stress levels. (Smit-Fun et al., 2020) Failure to do so can lead to detrimental consequences, as high levels of stress have the potential to impair cognitive processes and compromise patient safety. In fact, in rare and extreme cases, inadequate stress management can even contribute to medical errors, serving as a grave reminder of the critical significance of implementing effective stress management techniques in the operating room. Given the immense importance of this issue, anesthesiologists need to prioritize stress management and constantly work towards refining their abilities to deal with these intense environments. (Joseph et al.2021) By doing so, they ensure the delivery of exceptional care to their patients while maintaining their personal well-being and professional resilience. Therefore, an anesthesiologist should continuously engage in practices that promote stress reduction and build resilience against the challenges encountered in the operating room. This may involve adopting various coping strategies such as deep breathing exercises, mindfulness meditation, and physical relaxation techniques. (Afonso et al.2021; Siddiqui et al.2021) Additionally, anesthesiologists can benefit from seeking support from their peers and participating in debriefing sessions after challenging cases. These interactions provide valuable opportunities to share experiences, discuss coping mechanisms, and learn from one another. Moreover, anesthesiologists should prioritize self-care, ensuring they have a proper work-life balance and engaging in activities that promote mental and physical well-being. (Dainotto, 2020) Furthermore, the implementation of stress management protocols in operating rooms can greatly contribute to reducing stress levels among anesthesiologists. These protocols may include measures such as providing adequate breaks during long surgical procedures, improving communication and teamwork among healthcare professionals, and implementing strategies to minimize distractions and interruptions in the operating room. (Klein et al.2020) In conclusion, stress management is of utmost importance for anesthesiologists working in high-pressure operating room environments. By effectively managing and controlling stress levels, anesthesiologists can enhance their decision-making abilities, ensure optimal patient outcomes, and promote their personal well-being and professional resilience. Through the adoption of various stress reduction techniques, seeking support from peers, and implementing stress management protocols, anesthesiologists can navigate through the challenges of the operating room with proficiency and compassion, ultimately delivering exceptional care to their patients. (Zahid et al.2023; David, 2023; Sundnes, 2020)

3.2. Impact of Biomedical Simulators on Psychological Resilience

Biomedical simulators have emerged as highly effective and indispensable tools for building and enhancing psychological resilience in anesthesiologists, consistently proving their immense value. These simulators have revolutionized the field by simulating and recreating incredibly lifelike scenarios that accurately mirror the diverse and ever-evolving challenges encountered within the dynamic realm of the operating room. It is through the persistent and deliberate practice within these simulated environments that medical professionals are not only able to effectively confront and manage stress but also exponentially augment their overall performance, even under the most intense and demanding of pressures. (Harris and Franceschini, 2022) In order to comprehensively evaluate and gauge the profound impact of these simulators on psychological resilience and performance, we propose the implementation of meticulously designed and meticulously crafted pre- and post-simulator questionnaires, rooted in the Allen and Meyer model that has garnered significant recognition and accolade. These expertly formulated questionnaires serve as invaluable tools in assessing and analyzing crucial aspects such as stress management, decision-making abilities, emotional resilience, and overall well-being. By delving into every facet of anesthesiologists' experiences with these unparalleled training simulators, these questionnaires provide an in-depth understanding of the multifaceted effects and benefits yielded by these simulators. (Faridullah, 2024; Meyer, 2023; Schum, 2022) Before anesthesiologists' exposure to the simulators, these tailored questionnaires aid in assessing their baseline psychological states, expertise levels, and preparedness in handling stressful situations. By capturing this pre-simulator data, the questionnaires allow for precise comparisons and analysis of how the simulators have shaped and influenced various psychological and professional aspects. Following the simulation training, the questionnaires capture valuable insights into anesthesiologists' post-simulator experiences, including their perceived improvements in stress management, decision-making skills, adaptability, and emotional resilience. (Lisann-Goldman et al.2022; Friend & Zaleski, 2022) The meticulously crafted nature of these questionnaires ensures that they capture the nuanced and complex nature of anesthesiologists' experiences with the simulators. The inclusion of the Allen and Meyer model provides a comprehensive framework for evaluating the impact of these simulators on anesthesiologists' psychological well-being, professional capabilities, and overall performance. Through this robust evaluation process, a deeper understanding of the benefits and efficacy of these simulators can be gained, allowing for continuous refinement and improvement in anesthesiologists' training techniques. (Meyer et al.2020) In conclusion, the implementation of meticulously designed pre- and post-simulator questionnaires rooted in the Allen and Meyer model is crucial in comprehensively evaluating the profound impact of biomedical simulators on anesthesiologists' psychological resilience and performance. By capturing data on stress management, decision-making abilities, emotional resilience, and overall well-being, these questionnaires provide valuable insights into the multifaceted effects of simulation training. This understanding aids in refining training techniques, enhancing anesthesiologists' preparedness, and ultimately, improving patient care in the dynamic realm of the operating room. With continued focus on these questionnaires and the incorporation of the Allen and Meyer model, the potential for ongoing advancements in anesthesiologists' training and performance is vast, fostering a future of enhanced medical care and improved patient outcomes. (Rasheed & Alam, 2024)

4. ORGANIZATIONAL FACTORS INFLUENCING ANESTHESIOLOGISTS' PROFESSIONAL PERFORMANCE

Organizational factors are equally as crucial as individual skills and knowledge when it comes to understanding anesthesiologists' performance in medical settings. The role of effective leadership cannot be underestimated, as it sets the tone for the entire team and greatly influences their ability to work cohesively and efficiently. Teamwork is another vital aspect that directly impacts anesthesiologists' performance. When colleagues collaborate seamlessly, it enhances patient care and reduces the risk of errors. Effective communication is also key in anesthesiology, as it ensures vital information is accurately conveyed, allowing for timely and informed decision-making. Lastly, institutional support plays a significant role in providing anesthesiologists with the necessary resources, equipment, and guidelines to perform their duties effectively and efficiently. By recognizing the importance of these organizational factors, healthcare institutions can create an environment that empowers anesthesiologists and ultimately leads to improved patient outcomes. Moreover, when considering the multidimensional nature of medical practice, it becomes evident that a holistic approach to anesthesiologists' performance is necessary. This includes taking into account the organizational culture within healthcare institutions, the allocation of resources and workload management, and the implementation of effective performance evaluation systems. A positive organizational culture fosters trust among team members and cultivates a sense of belonging and support, which further enhances anesthesiologists' job satisfaction and motivation. Furthermore, the efficient allocation of resources, such as adequate staffing levels and appropriate equipment, contributes to the smooth functioning of medical procedures and minimizes the likelihood of errors or delays. Additionally, effective workload management systems ensure that anesthesiologists are not overwhelmed with excessive tasks, enabling them to focus on providing optimal patient care. Implementing performance evaluation systems that are fair, transparent, and based on measurable criteria allows for continuous improvement and professional growth within the field of anesthesiology. These systems can identify areas of strength and areas for development, providing valuable feedback to anesthesiologists and enabling them to enhance their skills and competencies. Therefore, by considering these expanded dimensions of organizational factors, healthcare institutions can create an environment that supports anesthesiologists in delivering high-quality care and achieving positive patient outcomes. (Mathis et al., 2022; Siddiqui et al., 2021;Tylee et al., 2020; Diallo et al., 2022)

4.1. Leadership and Teamwork

Effective leadership within anesthesiology departments not only fosters a collaborative and inclusive environment where professionals feel supported, respected, and empowered, but also promotes a culture of continuous improvement, innovation, and excellence in patient care. Leaders who enthusiastically encourage and embrace the use of state-of-the-art biomedical simulators, cutting-edge technologies, and evidence-based practices inspire an atmosphere of growth, development, and advancement. These advanced simulators provide invaluable training opportunities, allowing anesthesiologists to refine their skills, deepen their knowledge, and enhance their patient care techniques, ultimately contributing to better outcomes and improved safety. The integration of innovative tools also enables anesthesiology departments to stay at the forefront of medical advancements and deliver high-quality care. (Shah & Emerick, 2021) In addition to embracing innovation, effective leaders recognize the paramount importance of fostering strong teamwork and collaboration within anesthesiology departments. Anesthesiologists must work seamlessly, hand in hand, with surgeons, nurses, and other medical staff to ensure successful patient outcomes and deliver comprehensive and coordinated care. Strong collaboration, open communication, and mutual respect between team members are vital in order to provide safe, efficient, and effective anesthesia services. These multidisciplinary collaborations not only promote a holistic approach to patient care but also create an environment where knowledge and expertise are shared, creating a supportive and cohesive team dynamic. (Paige et al.2021) Furthermore, effective leaders in anesthesiology departments understand the significance of continuous professional development and lifelong learning. They actively promote ongoing education, training, and research, ensuring that their team members are well-equipped, up-to-date, and proficient in the latest advancements, evidence-based guidelines, and best practices in the field. By providing opportunities for continuing education, attending conferences, engaging in research endeavors, and supporting their staff in pursuing further certifications and advanced degrees, leaders contribute to the growth, expertise, and professional satisfaction of their team. A culture of continual learning and professional development not only enhances individual performance but also elevates the overall quality of care and patient outcomes. (Siddiqui et al.2021) Overall, effective leadership in anesthesiology departments plays a pivotal role in creating a supportive, collaborative, and high-performing environment that values innovation, teamwork, professional growth, and patient-centered care. Through their visionary guidance, mentorship, and unwavering support, leaders facilitate the success, well-being, and fulfillment of their team members, ultimately leading to enhanced patient care, improved outcomes, and the advancement of the field of anesthesiology as a whole. (Watkins & Hensley, 2023)

4.2. Communication and Institutional Support

Clear communication and strong institutional support further enhance anesthesiologists' performance. When professionals feel they are part of a well-coordinated team and have access to resources like simulators, their confidence and performance improve significantly. The effective exchange of information, ideas, and feedback plays a pivotal role in ensuring optimal outcomes for patients under their care. By fostering an environment of open and transparent communication, anesthesiologists are able to collaborate seamlessly with other healthcare providers, including surgeons, nurses, and technicians. This interdisciplinary approach not only leads to better patient outcomes but also cultivates a culture of trust and collaboration within the medical team. (Anwar et al.2021) In addition to a well-coordinated team, access to resources like simulators proves to be immensely beneficial for anesthesiologists. These cutting-edge tools provide them with a realistic platform to practice their skills and improve their decision-making abilities. The ability to simulate various scenarios and emergencies allows anesthesiologists to hone their critical thinking skills and quickly adapt to unexpected situations. This not only enhances their proficiency in the operating room but also prepares them to handle complex and challenging cases with ease. (Matos, 2021) To evaluate the impact of organizational commitment and team dynamics on performance, pre- and post-simulator questionnaires are employed. These questionnaires assess individual perspectives on teamwork, leadership, and overall satisfaction with the organizational structure. By analyzing the changes in responses before and after simulator training, valuable insights can be gained into how these factors influence anesthesiologists' performance in the operating room. It allows healthcare institutions to identify areas of improvement and implement strategies to optimize team dynamics and institutional support. (Soliman, 2024) Overall, clear communication, strong institutional support, and access to simulators play integral roles in enhancing anesthesiologists' performance. By prioritizing and investing in these factors, healthcare institutions can foster an environment that empowers anesthesiologists to deliver exceptional care with confidence and precision, ultimately leading to improved patient outcomes. This not only benefits the patients but also contributes to the overall growth and success of the medical profession. The continuous advancement of communication technologies and simulation resources will further revolutionize anesthesiology, allowing professionals to continuously refine their skills and provide the highest level of care possible. Through collaboration, innovation, and a commitment to excellence, anesthesiologists can continue to drive positive change in the field and ensure that every patient receives safe and effective anesthesia care. (Anwar et al.2021; Averlid & Høglund, 2020)

5. METHODOLOGIES IN PERFORMANCE EVALUATION STUDIES

Historically, performance evaluation in anesthesiology has relied on clinical metrics, such as patient outcomes and procedural success rates. However, these measures often fail to capture the full range of skills and psychosocial factors that contribute to professional performance. This chapter advocates for a more comprehensive approach, using both quantitative and qualitative methods to evaluate anesthesiologists. By incorporating a broader range of assessment tools, including structured interviews, self-assessment questionnaires, and peer evaluations, a more accurate and nuanced understanding of anesthesiologists' capabilities can be obtained. Moreover, the utilization of these multi-dimensional evaluation methods enables the identification and development of targeted interventions for areas of improvement in individual performance. (Zhang & Pandit, 2023) Furthermore, the integration of patient feedback and satisfaction surveys can provide valuable insights into the quality of care delivered by anesthesiologists. This comprehensive approach recognizes the intricate and multifaceted nature of anesthesiology practice, acknowledging that professional competence extends beyond technical proficiency alone. By encompassing various dimensions of performance assessment, such as effective communication, teamwork, adaptability, and empathy, a holistic evaluation framework can be established. (Gunawan, 2023) Ultimately, the implementation of this comprehensive approach has the potential to enhance patient safety, optimize professional development, and improve overall outcomes in the field of anesthesiology. This is necessary as the demands and expectations placed on anesthesiologists continue to evolve. The expanding scope of practice and increasing complexity of surgical procedures require a more comprehensive assessment method that captures the full range of skills and abilities necessary for success in the field. (Shaw et al., 2023) By incorporating structured interviews, anesthesiologists can showcase their communication skills, ability to work in teams, and adaptability to various surgical scenarios. Self-assessment questionnaires provide individuals with the opportunity to reflect on their strengths and weaknesses, fostering growth and development. Peer evaluations offer an additional perspective on anesthesiologists' performance, providing valuable feedback from colleagues who have observed their work firsthand. (Reato et al.2024) The incorporation of patient feedback and satisfaction surveys is crucial in ensuring that anesthesiologists are meeting the needs and expectations of the individuals under their care. This feedback provides insight into areas of improvement, allowing for targeted interventions and professional growth. By actively seeking patient input, anesthesiologists can continuously refine their practice and provide high-quality care. (Margolis & Ku, 2021) In conclusion, a comprehensive approach to performance evaluation in anesthesiology that integrates quantitative and qualitative methods, structured interviews, self-assessment questionnaires, peer evaluations, and patient feedback is essential. This multifaceted evaluation framework captures the full spectrum of skills, abilities, and psychosocial factors that contribute to professional performance. By adopting this approach, anesthesiologists can enhance patient safety, optimize professional development, and improve overall outcomes in the field. As the practice of anesthesiology continues to advance, it is imperative to continuously evolve the evaluation methods to ensure the ongoing excellence of care. (Kelly et al.2023)

One highly effective and widely recognized method for evaluating anesthesiologist performance is the utilization of pre- and post-intervention questionnaires. These questionnaires provide a thorough assessment of an anesthesiologist's performance and commitment, both prior to and following the utilization of advanced biomedical simulators. By using these questionnaires, we can comprehensively measure and analyze the profound impact of this cutting-edge technology on various critical performance dimensions. (Whaley, 2022) In order to gain a comprehensive understanding of the intricate dynamics at play, we propose the development and implementation of a meticulously tailored and modified version of the highly regarded Allen and Meyer Organizational Commitment Questionnaire. This pioneering questionnaire aims to concentrate on probing and scrutinizing the delicate interplay between psychosocial factors and an individual's ability to perform remarkably well, even under the most demanding conditions that occupy the realm of medical practice. By utilizing such a questionnaire, we can delve deeper into the unique challenges and pressures faced by anesthesiologists. (Mokarami et al.2020; Al-Mekhlafi et al.2021) This tailored approach will provide valuable insights into the specific factors that contribute to their performance and commitment. It will allow us to identify potential areas of improvement and determine strategies to enhance their capabilities in delivering optimal care and service. Through this comprehensive evaluation and analysis, healthcare institutions can further optimize the utilization of advanced biomedical simulators and ensure that anesthesiologists are equipped with the necessary skills and resilience to excel in their demanding roles. (Gaba) By understanding the complex relationship between psychosocial factors, commitment, and performance, healthcare organizations can take proactive measures to support and empower their anesthesiologists, ultimately leading to improved patient outcomes and enhanced overall healthcare delivery. (Jianlan et al.2024) In addition, it is crucial to acknowledge the role of continuous professional development in the field of anesthesiology. Ongoing education and training programs enable anesthesiologists to remain up-to-date with the latest advancements and best practices in patient care. By investing in continuous learning opportunities, healthcare institutions can foster a culture of excellence and innovation within their anesthesiology departments. (Streckenbach et al.2021) Moreover, interdisciplinary collaboration plays a vital role in ensuring optimal patient care. Anesthesiologists often work closely with surgeons, nurses, and other healthcare professionals in the operating room. Therefore, establishing effective communication channels and promoting teamwork is imperative. When different specialists come together and share their expertise, it leads to a more holistic approach to patient care, enhancing overall surgical outcomes. (Harrison, 2022) In summary, by implementing pre- and post-intervention questionnaires, tailoring assessment tools, investing in continuous professional development, and fostering interdisciplinary collaboration, healthcare institutions can create an optimal environment for anesthesiologists to thrive. This holistic approach will contribute to improved patient outcomes, enhanced anesthesiologist performance and commitment, and ultimately, a higher standard of healthcare delivery. (Pinyavat & Mulaikal, 2020)

6. PRE-SIMULATOR USE QUESTIONNAIRE

The Pre-Simulator Use Questionnaire, a critical and indispensable tool meticulously developed, emerges as an instrument of utmost importance. Its purpose lies in the precise evaluation of anesthesiologists' commitment level and proficiency prior to their introduction to the revolutionary and state-of-the-art biomedical simulator. This evaluation process, crafted with remarkable depth and precision, renders insights of immeasurable value. It provides a profound understanding of initial perceptions, emotional resilience, and unwavering dedication to the craft. Through this methodology, healthcare professionals in high regard diligently collect intricate and enlightening information. Their aim remains twofold - first, to ensure anesthesiologists are not only adequately prepared but also equipped with indispensable knowledge and expertise to seamlessly utilize the vast array of capabilities offered by the simulator. Secondly, by doing so, a remarkable enhancement of their overall performance occurs, leading to ongoing advancements in patient outcomes. (Tzamaras et al.2024; Deuchler et al., 2022) Furthermore, the comprehensive questionnaire serves as a key pillar in the continuous professional development of anesthesiologists. The ever-evolving field of healthcare necessitates medical practitioners' constant adaptation and keeping up to date with the latest advancements. Thanks to the questionnaire's aid, anesthesiologists can identify potential gaps in their skillset and knowledge base, thus paving the way for targeted training and education. Not only does this ensure their competence in utilizing the biomedical simulator effectively, but it also equips them adequately to face intricate scenarios and unforeseen challenges with utmost efficiency. (Garcia et al., 2023) The Pre-Simulator Use Questionnaire encompasses a vast array of essential topics, ranging from technical proficiency to critical thinking and decision-making abilities. It delves deep into anesthesiologists' understanding of anesthesia equipment, pharmacology, patient assessment, and emergency management. Through thought-provoking inquiries and situational scenarios, this assessment offers a comprehensive and well-rounded view of anesthesiologists' preparedness in navigating the complexities of clinical practice. (Tzamaras, 2024). In addition, this questionnaire acknowledges the unique demands and responsibilities anesthesiologists face in various healthcare settings. Whether they operate in a bustling metropolitan hospital or a remote medical facility, the evaluation tool tailors its questions to ensure relevance and appropriateness across diverse contexts. It recognizes the inherent intricacies and challenges that may arise in each setting, addressing them with utmost attention and care. (Shetti2024) In conclusion, the Pre-Simulator Use Questionnaire stands unwavering as a fundamental component in the pursuit of excellence in the field of anesthesiology. Its meticulous design and comprehensive nature offer invaluable insights into the capabilities and preparedness of anesthesiologists, ultimately bolstering their performance and leading to enhanced patient outcomes. As technology continues to advance and shape the field of medicine, this questionnaire proves to be a steadfast and unwavering ally. It guarantees that anesthesiologists are fully equipped to harness the transformative power of the cutting-edge biomedical simulator to its fullest potential. (Tzamaras, 2024)

6.1. Instructions for Completing the Questionnaire

Participants are asked to indicate their level of agreement with each statement using a 5-point Likert scale:
1 = Strongly Disagree2 = Disagree3 = Neutral4 = Agree5 = Strongly Agree

6.2. Pre-Simulator Use Questionnaire: Evaluating Performance Before Simulator Implementation

6.2.1. Affective Commitment and Performance

a. "I feel confident in my ability to remain calm and effective under pressure during anesthesia procedures."
b. "I am satisfied with my current performance as an anesthesiologist in handling stressful situations."
c. "I feel engaged in my work, but I believe my performance could improve with more advanced training."

6.2.2. Continuance Commitment and Performance

a. "My current professional skills make it difficult for me to consider leaving this organization."
b. "I feel that my performance would suffer if I were to leave this healthcare institution due to a lack of resources and support."
c. "My performance is closely tied to the resources available in this organization, but I feel there is room for growth."

6.2.3. Normative Commitment and Performance

a. "I feel an obligation to continue working in this organization, but I believe my performance could be enhanced with additional tools or training."

b. “I feel responsible for contributing to my team's performance, though I sometimes feel my technical skills could improve.”
c. “I believe I owe it to my team and patients to continually improve my performance, and I am looking for ways to do so.”

6.2.4. Performance Under Pressure

a. “I am generally confident in my ability to perform under pressure, but I sometimes struggle with making quick decisions in critical situations.”
b. “I believe that my performance during high-stress situations can be improved with additional practice.”
c. “I feel that I could better manage stress in the operating room if I had access to more simulation-based training.”

6.2.5. Technical Skills and Competence

a. “I feel confident in my technical skills, though I recognize areas where I could improve my precision and speed.”
b. “I am capable of managing unexpected complications during surgeries, but I would benefit from additional practice in critical scenarios.”
c. “I believe my performance could be enhanced with more opportunities to practice technical skills in a controlled environment.”

6.2.6. Team Dynamics and Communication Performance

a. “My communication with the surgical team is generally effective, but there are times when I feel that better preparation would improve team dynamics.”
b. “I coordinate well with my team in the operating room, though there is room for improvement in high-pressure situations.”
c. “I believe that more practice in simulated environments could improve my ability to perform as part of a team.”

6.2.7. Job Satisfaction and Performance

a. “I am generally satisfied with my job, but I believe my performance could be improved with better training tools.”

b. "I feel fulfilled in my role, but I recognize that enhancing my performance would increase my job satisfaction."
c. "I believe that improving my professional skills would help me feel more effective and competent in my work."

6.2.8. Impact on Professional Development and Performance

a. "My current performance level is sufficient, but I believe I could further develop my skills with more focused training."
b. "I would benefit from more opportunities to improve my performance in complex medical cases."
c. "I feel capable in my role, but I believe my performance could be further enhanced with access to more advanced training tools."

7. POST-SIMULATOR USE QUESTIONNAIRE

The Post-Simulator Use Questionnaire is a comprehensive assessment tool that effectively measures the significant impact of utilizing the advanced biomedical simulator on anesthesiologists' performance, organizational commitment, emotional resilience, and overall satisfaction. This extensive and highly informative questionnaire provides valuable insights and in-depth analysis into the obtained results, allowing for a thorough and comprehensive understanding of the numerous benefits and remarkable improvements brought about by the simulator. By thoroughly analyzing individual responses and synthesizing them, we gain a detailed and profound understanding of the transformative effect that this innovative and cutting-edge technology has on healthcare professionals, which is indispensable for the advancement of the field. (Lukacs, 2021) Through this comprehensive evaluation and exploration, we can identify an extensive range of positive outcomes and enhancements that result from the seamless integration of this state-of-the-art simulator into medical training and practice. These encompass a multitude of advantages, including but not limited to increased confidence, heightened technical expertise, improved patient outcomes, enhanced critical thinking skills, refined decision-making abilities, and amplified interdisciplinary collaboration. The Post-Simulator Use Questionnaire serves as an invaluable, highly effective, and reliable instrument for capturing the multifaceted effects of the biomedical simulator, providing a wealth of valuable and precise data that can be utilized for ongoing studies, evidence-based research, and future advancements in the field of anesthesiology. (Wärnberg & Oliv, 2022) Moreover, the utilization of this exceptional questionnaire empowers medical professionals to drive continuous improvement, enrich the quality of patient care, and foster advancements in anesthesiology that positively impact not only individual practitioners but also the entire healthcare ecosystem. The comprehensive insights gathered from the questionnaire offer an unparalleled opportunity to address the evolving needs and challenges of the medical landscape and to steer the field towards innovation, excellence, and patient-centered care. (Epstein et al.2024) In conclusion, the Post-Simulator Use Questionnaire stands as an essential tool in the realm of anesthesiology, enabling healthcare practitioners to comprehensively evaluate the resounding benefits and transformative potential of the advanced biomedical simulator. By harnessing the power of this questionnaire, medical professionals can further their understanding of the impact of this simulator and shape the future of anesthesiology through evidence-based research, continuous education, and progressive advancements. This instrument marks a pivotal moment in the field, offering endless possibilities for growth, development, and the regulation of superior healthcare standards. (Braid, 2024)

7.1. Instructions for Completing the Questionnaire

Participants are asked to indicate their level of agreement with each statement using a 5-point Likert scale:

1 = Strongly Disagree2 = Disagree3 = Neutral4 = Agree5 = Strongly Agree

7.2. Post-Simulator Use Questionnaire: Evaluating Performance After Simulator Implementation

7.2.1. Affective Commitment and Performance

a. “Using the medical simulator has significantly increased my ability to remain calm and effective under pressure during anesthesia procedures.”
b. “I feel more confident in my performance as an anesthesiologist after using the simulator.”
c. “The simulator has enhanced my engagement in my work by improving my performance under stressful conditions.”

7.2.2. Continuance Commitment and Performance

a. “The new skills I’ve developed using the simulator make it difficult for me to consider leaving this organization.”

b. "I feel that leaving this organization would negatively impact my performance due to reliance on the simulator and its resources."
c. "My performance has greatly improved, and I now feel more connected to the organization because of the tools and support provided."

7.2.3. Normative Commitment and Performance

a. "I feel a stronger obligation to stay with this organization because of the significant improvements in my performance after using the simulator."
b. "The simulator has made me feel more responsible for contributing to my team's success through improved performance."
c. "I believe I owe it to my patients and colleagues to continue improving my performance using the simulator."

7.2.4. Performance Under Pressure

a. "The simulator has improved my ability to perform under pressure by allowing me to practice decision-making in high-stress situations."
b. "My ability to manage stress and make quick decisions in critical moments has noticeably improved since using the simulator."
c. "I feel much more prepared to handle stress in the operating room after practicing with the simulator."

7.2.5. Technical Skills and Competence

"a. My technical skills have significantly improved thanks to the practice I've had with the simulator."

b. "I am now more capable of managing unexpected complications during surgeries after using the simulator."
c. "The simulator has helped me increase the precision and speed of my technical skills, improving my overall performance."

7.2.6. Team Dynamics and Communication Performance

a. "Simulator-based training has improved my communication with the surgical team, especially during high-stress situations."

b. "I now coordinate better with my team in the operating room, thanks to the practice scenarios we've completed using the simulator."
c. "Practicing with the simulator has enhanced my ability to work effectively as part of a team during surgeries."

7.2.7. Job Satisfaction and Performance

a. "The improvements in my performance since using the simulator have greatly increased my job satisfaction."
b. "I feel much more fulfilled in my role after enhancing my performance with the help of the simulator."
c. "I now feel more effective and competent in my job, knowing that my performance has improved through simulator-based training."

7.2.8. Impact on Professional Development and Performance

a. "The simulator has provided me with advanced skills that have noticeably improved my performance in daily practice."
b. "I feel more capable of handling complex medical cases after using the simulator, which has contributed to my professional growth."
c. "My performance has greatly improved, and I now feel more confident in taking on high-risk, technically demanding surgeries thanks to the simulator."

8. KEY FINDINGS AND TRENDS IN PERFORMANCE EVALUATION RESEARCH

Recent studies underscore the vital importance of adopting a comprehensive and holistic approach to performance evaluation within the field of anesthesiology. It has become increasingly evident that a successful evaluation should encompass not only the assessment of technical skills but also the evaluation of non-technical skills. This integration facilitates a more accurate and comprehensive understanding of anesthesiologists' overall performance. By incorporating psychosocial factors, team dynamics, and organizational commitment into the evaluation process, anesthesiologists can benefit from a multidimensional assessment that is both reflective and insightful. In addition, the utilization of advanced technological simulators has proven to be instrumental in augmenting the effectiveness of these evaluations. (Hofmann et al., 2021)

The usage of pre- and post-simulator questionnaires plays a pivotal role in gaining deeper insights into the impact of simulators on anesthesiologists' job satisfaction, organizational commitment, and overall performance. These evaluations not only shed light on the improvement of technical skills but also demonstrate their influence on the emotional resilience and decision-making abilities of anesthesiologists, thereby providing a comprehensive evaluation that goes beyond mere technical proficiency. The symbiotic relationship between simulators and anesthesiologists' professional development cannot be overstated. Simulators serve as invaluable tools, allowing anesthesiologists to master and refine their technical abilities while simultaneously fostering the development of their emotional intelligence and cognitive skills. (Lukacs, 2021) Beyond the enhancement of technical expertise, simulators contribute significantly to anesthesiologists' emotional resilience and cognitive abilities, resulting in substantial improvements in patient care, safety, and ultimately, their overall performance. The utilization of simulators not only enhances anesthesiologists' technical aptitude but also fortifies their emotional resilience and decision-making capabilities, ultimately resulting in a tangible improvement in their overall performance. This holistic approach to performance evaluation, integrating both technical and non-technical skills, not only benefits individual anesthesiologists but also advances the field of anesthesiology as a whole, ensuring higher standards of patient care and safety. By leveraging the usage of simulators, anesthesiologists can truly reach their full potential and make significant contributions to the field. (Podhorodecka, 2022) In conclusion, it is evident that the integration of technical and non-technical skills is imperative in the evaluation of anesthesiologists' performance, and simulators serve as a catalyst for their professional growth and the advancement of the entire field of anesthesiology. The comprehensive assessment of performance, encompassing both technical and non-technical domains, has the potential to revolutionize the field and ensure enhanced patient outcomes. The utilization of simulators, with their ability to provide realistic and immersive training experiences, enables anesthesiologists to continually hone their skills and stay at the forefront of medical advancements. Through continuous evaluation and refinement, anesthesiologists can truly excel and deliver optimal care to their patients. By embracing a multidimensional and holistic approach to performance evaluation, the field of anesthesiology can continuously evolve, adapting to the ever-changing healthcare landscape and improving patient care. By upholding the highest standards of evaluation and professional development, anesthesiologists can play a crucial role in shaping the future of their specialty and leaving a lasting impact on the field. (Elgeziry et al.2022)

9. IMPLICATIONS FOR PRACTICE AND FUTURE RESEARCH DIRECTIONS

This chapter emphasizes the utmost significance of integrating psychosocial and organizational factors into the comprehensive performance evaluation of anesthesiologists. In order to enhance the overall effectiveness and efficiency of professionals in the field of anesthesiology, the utilization of state-of-the-art bio-medical simulators has proven to be an incredibly influential and effective tool. These advanced simulators not only improve technical skills but also strengthen non-technical skills, which are of utmost importance in this demanding and critical field. (Carenzo et al.2021) To ensure the validity, reliability, and applicability of this approach, further extensive and rigorous research should be conducted to validate the proposed pre- and post-simulator questionnaires, taking into consideration the diverse backgrounds and experiences of anesthesiologists. It is essential to explore the implementation of these meticulously designed questionnaires across various healthcare settings, encompassing a wide range of medical scenarios and practice environments, to assess their effectiveness, suitability, and adaptability. (Nigg et al.2020) Additionally, future studies and investigations should also be undertaken to thoroughly evaluate the long-term impact and enduring effects of simulator-based training on organizational commitment and overall performance, particularly in high-stakes medical environments where lives are at stake and every action counts. By conducting such vital and comprehensive studies, we can gain deeper insights, profound understanding, and invaluable knowledge into the potential benefits, implications, and transformative outcomes of utilizing simulators in medical training and practice. (Röttger & Krey, 2021) This expanded knowledge base and solid empirical evidence can guide and inform the development of evidence-based strategies, policies, and guidelines, thus ensuring the continuous improvement and advancement of anesthesiology as a whole, and ultimately contributing to the delivery of safe, efficient, and high-quality patient care. These efforts will lead to the optimization of healthcare professionals' performances, resulting in improved patient outcomes and greater overall satisfaction. Furthermore, the integration of psychosocial and organizational factors into performance evaluations will foster a positive and supportive work environment, nurturing the growth and well-being of anesthesiologists. (Hu et al., 2022) With the continuous advancements in technology, it is crucial to acknowledge the potential of virtual reality and artificial intelligence in augmenting simulator-based training. The utilization of these cutting-edge tools can further enhance the effectiveness and efficiency of anesthesiologists, preparing them for complex and high-pressure scenarios. By expanding the scope of simulator-based training to encompass a wider range of medical procedures and specialized areas, healthcare organizations can ensure that their professionals are competent and confident in delivering optimal care. (Bogar et al.2024) In conclusion, the integration of psychosocial and organizational factors, coupled with the utilization of advanced simulators, holds immense promise in revolutionizing anesthesiology. The benefits derived from these practices extend beyond individual performance improvement, spanning to the overall quality of care and patient safety. Through rigorous research, comprehensive studies, and the continuous refinement of training methodologies, anesthesiologists can continue to strive for excellence and contribute to the advancement of the field. (Garcia-Marcinkiewicz & Titler, 2022)

REFERENCES

Afonso, A. M., Cadwell, J. B., Staffa, S. J., Zurakowski, D., & Vinson, A. E. (2021). Burnout rate and risk factors among anesthesiologists in the United States. *Anesthesiology*, 134(5), 683–696. DOI: 10.1097/ALN.0000000000003722 PMID: 33667293

Agegnehu, W., Abdissa, D., & Alemayehu, D. (2022). Confirmatory and exploratory factor analysis for validating Allen and Meyer organizational commitment questionnaire for health professionals in Ethiopia—Amharic language. *Journal of Healthcare Leadership*, 14, 99–111. DOI: 10.2147/JHL.S364973 PMID: 35782682

Al-Mekhlafi, A. B. A., Isha, A. S. N., Chileshe, N., Abdulrab, M., Saeed, A. A. H., & Kineber, A. F. (2021). Modelling the relationship between the nature of work factors and driving performance mediating by role of fatigue. *International Journal of Environmental Research and Public Health*, 18(13), 6752. DOI: 10.3390/ijerph18136752 PMID: 34201674

Alotaibi, A., Habib, S. S., Al-Khlaiwi, T., Alodhayani, A., Rashed, Z. F., Al Mahdali, G., Alanazi, S., Al Hassan, S., Al-Anazi, S., Al Saif, R. A., & Alsaegh, N. A. (2024). Ambient conditions of the operating theatre and its correlation with fatigue and sleep quality of operating room workers: A cross-sectional survey. *Frontiers in Public Health*, 12, 1392950. DOI: 10.3389/fpubh.2024.1392950 PMID: 38813423

Anwar, A., Heller, K. O., Esper, S. A., & Ferreira, R. G. (2021). Nonoperating room anesthesia: Strategies to improve performance. *International Anesthesiology Clinics*, 59(4), 27–36. DOI: 10.1097/AIA.0000000000000339 PMID: 34456276

Averlid, G., & Høglund, J. S. (2020). The operating room as a learning arena: Nurse anaesthetist and student nurse anaesthetist perceptions. *Journal of Clinical Nursing*, 29(9-10), 1673–1683. DOI: 10.1111/jocn.15227 PMID: 32096572

Basarah, J. C., Andry, A., & Tahjoo, A. (2022). Perceived accreditation benefits, participation and organizational commitment in hospital accreditation performance. *International Journal of Public Health Science*, 11(2), 527–536. DOI: 10.11591/ijphs.v11i2.20980

Bogar, P. Z., Virag, M., Bene, M., Hardi, P., Matuz, A., Schlegl, A. T., Toth, L., Molnar, F., Nagy, B., Rendeki, S., Berner-Juhos, K., Ferencz, A., Fischer, K., & Maroti, P. (2024). Validation of a novel, low-fidelity virtual reality simulator and an artificial intelligence assessment approach for peg transfer laparoscopic training. *Scientific Reports*, 14(1), 16702. DOI: 10.1038/s41598-024-67435-6 PMID: 39030307

Braid, H. R. (2024). Development and Evaluation of a Surgical Simulator and Assessment Rubric for Standing Castration of the Horse. *Journal of Veterinary Medical Education*, e20230131. DOI: 10.3138/jvme-2023-0131 PMID: 39504222

Carenzo, L., Cena, T., Carfagna, F., Rondi, V., Ingrassia, P. L., Cecconi, M., Violato, C., Della Corte, F., & Vaschetto, R. (2021). Assessing anaesthesiology and intensive care specialty physicians: An Italian language multisource feedback system. *PLoS One*, 16(4), e0250404. DOI: 10.1371/journal.pone.0250404 PMID: 33891626

Chen, M. J., Ambardekar, A., Martinelli, S. M., Buhl, L. K., Walsh, D. P., Levy, L., & Mitchell, J. D. (2022). Defining and addressing anesthesiology needs in simulation-based medical education. *The Journal of Education in Perioperative Medicine : JEPM*, 24(2). PMID: 36051401

Dainotto, D. (2020). The Impact of a Pediatric Critical Incident Simulation on the Perceived Importance of and Need for a Critical Incident Stress Debriefing Protocol for Anesthesia. PMID: 36051401

David, A. (2023). Navigating Critical Care: Anesthesia and Surgical Considerations in Emergency Situations. PMID: 36051401

Deuchler, S., Scholtz, J., Ackermann, H., Seitz, B., & Koch, F. (2022). Implementation of microsurgery simulation in an ophthalmology clerkship in Germany: A prospective, exploratory study. *BMC Medical Education*, 22(1), 599. DOI: 10.1186/s12909-022-03634-x PMID: 35922857

Diallo, M. S., Tan, J. M., Heitmiller, E. S., & Vetter, T. R. (2022). Achieving greater health equity: An opportunity for anesthesiology. *Anesthesia and Analgesia*, 134(6), 1175–1184. DOI: 10.1213/ANE.0000000000005937 PMID: 35110516

Elgeziry, A., Mumtaz, N., Thodika, A. V., & Mallal, K. A. (2022). Non-technical Skills for Anesthesia Technician. In *Improving Anesthesia Technical Staff's Skills* (pp. 1–10). Springer International Publishing. DOI: 10.1007/978-3-030-88849-7_1

Epstein, D., Lavin, P. M., Withall, J., & Wong, D. (2024). Empowering Nurses to Increase Certification Rates in a Postanesthesia Care Unit: A Collaborative Team Approach. *Journal of Perianesthesia Nursing*. Advance online publication. DOI: 10.1016/j.jopan.2024.05.004 PMID: 39115477

Fadilah, R. A., Sukmaningtyas, W., & Burhan, A. (2023). *The The Correlation between Motivation and Anesthetists' Working Performance in Banyumas Regency: English*. Java Nursing Journal.

Faridullah, S. (2024). Indian IT Firms: A systematic review of existing literature with reference to prominent employee engagement theory and models. Educational Administration: Theory and Practice.

Fincher, E. L. (2023). Increasing Anesthesia Provider Knowledge on Noise and Cognitive Overload in the Operating Room.

Firth-Cozens, J. & King, J. (2023). Are psychological factors linked to performance?. Understanding doctors' performance.

Friend, T. & Zaleski, L. (2022). The Development of an Assessment Plan for Wellness and Risk for Substance Use in Nurse Anesthesia Students.

Gaba, D. M. (). … of simulation in health care share a common Vision of a future revolution in health care organization, with simulation as a key enabling technique. Simulation is …. simulatorcentrum.se.

Gafsou, B., Becq, M. C., Michelet, D., Julien-Marsollier, F., Brasher, C., & Dahmani, S. (2021). Determinants of work-related quality of life in French anesthesiologists. *Anesthesia and Analgesia*, 133(4), 863–872. DOI: 10.1213/ANE.0000000000005397 PMID: 33543868

Garcia, D. B., Pereira, F. H., & Ribeiro, E. R. (2023). Evaluation of Third-Year Anesthesiology Residents Knowledge on Patient Safety: Descriptive Study. [IJAP]. *International Journal of Anesthesiology and Practice*, 1(1).

Garcia-Marcinkiewicz, A. G., & Titler, S. S. (2022). Lactation in anesthesiology. *Anesthesiology Clinics*, 40(2), 235–243. DOI: 10.1016/j.anclin.2022.01.014 PMID: 35659397

Gottumukkala, V., Vetter, T. R., & Gan, T. J. (2023). Perioperative medicine: What the future can hold for anesthesiology. *Anesthesia and Analgesia*, 136(4), 628–635. DOI: 10.1213/ANE.0000000000006412 PMID: 36928147

Gunawan, J. (2023). Exploring the future of nursing: Insights from the ChatGPT model. *Belitung Nursing Journal*, 9(1), 1–5. DOI: 10.33546/bnj.2551 PMID: 37469634

Haavik, T. K., & Våpenstad, C. (2020). The role of simulators in interdisciplinary medical work. Multimodal Technologies and Interaction. Abaalkhayl, M. (2024). IMPACT OF SIMULATED ANESTHESIA CRISIS MANAGEMENT TRAINING ON INTRAOPERATIVE COMPLICATIONS. *Gland Surgery*.

Harris, D. M., & Franceschini, D. (2022). The Unpredictable Future of High-Fidelity Patient Simulation in Biomedical Science Education: The Price Must Be Right. In *Technologies in Biomedical and Life Sciences Education: Approaches and Evidence of Efficacy for Learning* (pp. 493–517). Springer International Publishing. DOI: 10.1007/978-3-030-95633-2_16

Harrison, W. (2022). *Optimizing Patient Care: Synergy between Anesthesia, Surgery, and Radiology*. Cosmic Journal of Biology.

Hofmann, R., Curran, S., & Dickens, S. (2021). … non-technical skills in simulation-based medical education: Findings from an integrated scoping review of research and content analysis of curricular learning…. *Studies in Educational Evaluation*, 71, 101093. DOI: 10.1016/j.stueduc.2021.101093

Hu, Q., Dollard, M. F., & Taris, T. W. (2022). Organizational context matters: Psychosocial safety climate as a precursor to team and individual motivational functioning. *Safety Science*, 145, 105524. DOI: 10.1016/j.ssci.2021.105524

Jianlan, R., Mei, Y., Chunyan, Y., Rendie, X., Yiping, B., & Li, L. (2024). Exploring anesthesiology nurse'presenteeism in China: Cross-sectional study. *BMC Public Health*, 24(1), 2008. DOI: 10.1186/s12889-024-19476-9 PMID: 39060992

Jonathan, H. (2020). *Organizational commitment scale validation in tanzanian context*. Res Humanit Soc Sci.

Joseph, A. L., Borycki, E. M., & Kushniruk, A. W. (2021). Alert fatigue and errors caused by technology: a scoping review and introduction to the flow of cognitive processing model. Knowledge management & e-learning, (4), 500.

Kao, K. Y., Hsu, H. H., Lee, H. T., Cheng, Y. C., Dax, I., & Hsieh, M. W. (2022). Career mentoring and job content plateaus: The roles of perceived organizational support and emotional exhaustion. *Journal of Career Development*, 49(2), 457–470. DOI: 10.1177/0894845320946399

Kelly, F. E., Frerk, C., Bailey, C. R., Cook, T. M., Ferguson, K., Flin, R., Fong, K., Groom, P., John, C., Lang, A. R., Meek, T., Miller, K. L., Richmond, L., Sevdalis, N., & Stacey, M. R. (2023). Implementing human factors in anaesthesia: guidance for clinicians, departments and hospitals: guidelines from the Difficult Airway Society and the Association of Anaesthetists. *Anaesthesia*, 78(4), 458–478. DOI: 10.1111/anae.15941 PMID: 36630725

Klein, C. J., Dalstrom, M. D., Weinzimmer, L. G., Cooling, M., Pierce, L., & Lizer, S. (2020). Strategies of advanced practice providers to reduce stress at work. *Workplace Health & Safety*, 68(9), 432–442. DOI: 10.1177/2165079920924060 PMID: 32491978

Li, X. Y., Wang, J., Zhang, R. X., Chen, L., He, C. K., Wang, C. Y., Ke, J., Wang, Y., Zhang, Z., & Song, X. M. (2020). Psychological status among anesthesiologists and operating room nurses during the outbreak period of COVID-19 in Wuhan, China. *Frontiers in Psychiatry*, 11, 574143. DOI: 10.3389/fpsyt.2020.574143 PMID: 33343417

Lisann-Goldman, L., Cowart, C., Lin, H. M., Orlando, B., & Mahoney, B. (2022). Well-being in anesthesiology graduate medical education: Reconciling the ideal with reality. *Anesthesiology Clinics*, 40(2), 383–397. DOI: 10.1016/j.anclin.2022.01.011 PMID: 35659409

Lukacs, M. J. (2021). Creation of a Virtual Interface for Stress-Trauma Investigations Through Open World Navigation: An Exploration of Tolerability and Physiological Reactions. DOI: 10.1016/j.anclin.2022.01.011 PMID: 35659409

Margolis, R. D., & Ku, C. M. (2021). *The "Difficult Learner" in anesthesiology: challenges, pitfalls, and recommendations*. Pediatric Anesthesia.

Mathis, M. R., Schonberger, R. B., Whitlock, E. L., Vogt, K. M., Lagorio, J. E., Jones, K. A., & Kheterpal, S. (2022). Opportunities beyond the anesthesiology department: Broader impact through broader thinking. *Anesthesia and Analgesia*, 134(2), 242–252. PMID: 33684091

Matos, F. J. P. M. (2021). Simulation as a learning resource in medical education. DOI: 10.1016/j.anclin.2022.01.011 PMID: 35659409

Mcevoy, M. D., & Abernathy, J. J. (2023). *Perioperative Safety Culture, An Issue of Anesthesiology Clinics*. E-Book.

Meyer, K. (2023). ... Another Education Abroad Gatekeeper: Education Abroad Administrators' Perspectives on Institutional Pricing Models and How Those Models Impact Inclusion Efforts. DOI: 10.1016/j.anclin.2022.01.011 PMID: 35659409

Meyer, T., Selb, M., Kiekens, C., Grubišić, F., Arienti, C., Stucki, G., & Negrini, S. (2020). Toward better reporting standards of patients' characteristics in rehabilitation trials: Applying a new conceptual framework to current standards. *American Journal of Physical Medicine & Rehabilitation*, 99(3), 216–223. DOI: 10.1097/PHM.0000000000001375 PMID: 31860587

Mohadeseh, R., Mohaddeseh, M., Azam, M., & Mahboobeh, K. (2021). Correlation of Moral Courage and Organizational Commitment in Operating Room Nurses. *Siriraj Medical Journal*, 73(3), 183–190. DOI: 10.33192/Smj.2021.24

Mokarami, H., Gharibi, V., Kalteh, H. O., Faraji Kujerdi, M., & Kazemi, R. (2020). Multiple environmental and psychosocial work risk factors and sleep disturbances. *International Archives of Occupational and Environmental Health*, 93(5), 623–633. DOI: 10.1007/s00420-020-01515-8 PMID: 31955238

Nguyen, , P. N. D., Nguyen, L. L. K., & LE, D. N. T. (2021). The impact of extrinsic work factors on job satisfaction and organizational commitment at higher education institutions in Vietnam. *The Journal of Asian Finance, Economics and Business*, 8(8), 259–270.

Nigg, C. R., Fuchs, R., Gerber, M., Jekauc, D., Koch, T., Krell-Roesch, J., Lippke, S., Mnich, C., Novak, B., Ju, Q., Sattler, M. C., Schmidt, S. C. E., van Poppel, M., Reimers, A. K., Wagner, P., Woods, C., & Woll, A. (2020). Assessing physical activity through questionnaires–A consensus of best practices and future directions. *Psychology of Sport and Exercise*, 50, 101715. DOI: 10.1016/j.psychsport.2020.101715

Paige, J. T., Garbee, D. D., Bonanno, L. S., & Kerdolff, K. E. (2021). Qualitative analysis of effective teamwork in the operating room (OR). *Journal of Surgical Education*, 78(3), 967–979. DOI: 10.1016/j.jsurg.2020.09.019 PMID: 33160940

Panditrao, M. M., & Panditrao, M. M. (2024). "Burnout syndrome" in anesthesiologists and remedial measures-A narrative review. *Journal of Anaesthesiology, Clinical Pharmacology*, 40(2), 206–216. DOI: 10.4103/joacp.joacp_322_22 PMID: 38919431

Parnikh, H., Torabizadeh, C., Najafi Kalyani, M., & Soltanian, M. (2022). A Study of the Relationship between Professional Communication and Professional Commitment in Operating Room Nurses. *Nursing Research and Practice*, 2022(1), 5871846. DOI: 10.1155/2022/5871846 PMID: 35847234

Pinyavat, T., & Mulaikal, T. A. (2020). Fostering physician well-being in anesthesiology. *International Anesthesiology Clinics*, 58(4), 36–40. DOI: 10.1097/AIA.0000000000000300 PMID: 32841965

Podhorodecka, K. (2022). Psychological Aspects of Working as an Anesthesiologist. Anesthesia and Critical care. DOI: 10.1097/AIA.0000000000000300 PMID: 32841965

Rasheed, F. A., & Alam, R. (2024). Investigating the Impact of Maternal Birth Simulator Training on Critical Thinking Skills Among Community Midwife Diploma Students: A Quasi-experimental Study. Journal of Nurses and Midwives Pakistan. DOI: 10.1097/AIA.0000000000000300 PMID: 32841965

Reato, F., Bresil, A., D'Angelo, C., Gorli, M., Ivziku, D., Lommi, M., & Carcano, G. (2024, September). Toward the Definition of a Repertoire of Technical Professional Specialist Competencies for Operating Room Nurses: An Ethnographic Study. In Healthcare (Vol. 12, No. 17, p. 1774). MDPI.

Robinson, C. (2022). Development of an Orientation Program for New Certified Registered Nurse Anesthetists at Einstein Medical Center Philadelphia. DOI: 10.1097/AIA.0000000000000300 PMID: 32841965

Röttger, S., & Krey, H. (2021). Experimental study on the effects of a single simulator-based bridge resource management unit on attitudes, behaviour and performance. *Journal of Navigation*, 74(5), 1127–1141. DOI: 10.1017/S0373463321000436

Schum, T. (2022). Relentless: The Story of American Soccer and the Coaches who Helped Grow the Game. DOI: 10.1097/AIA.0000000000000300 PMID: 32841965

Shah, N. K., & Emerick, T. D. (2021). Lean Six Sigma methodology and the future of quality improvement education in anesthesiology. *Anesthesia and Analgesia*. Advance online publication. DOI: 10.1213/ANE.0000000000005636 PMID: 34142980

Shaw, A. D., Glas, K., & Shernan, S. K. (2023). Cardiac Anesthesiologist Compensation and Working Patterns: 2010–2020. Anesthesia & Analgesia. DOI: 10.1213/ANE.0000000000005636 PMID: 34142980

Shetti, A. N. (2024). Battling Burnout: A Comprehensive Exploration of The Impact on Anaesthesiologists and Strategies for Resilience. *Jour Med Dent Fron*, 1, 5–15.

Siddiqui, S., Bartels, K., Schaefer, M. S., Novack, L., Sreedharan, R., Ben-Jacob, T. K., Khanna, A. K., Nunnally, M. E., Souter, M., Simmons, S. T., & Williams, G. (2021). Critical care medicine practice: A pilot survey of US anesthesia critical care medicine–trained physicians. *Anesthesia and Analgesia*, 132(3), 761–769. DOI: 10.1213/ANE.0000000000005030 PMID: 32665465

Smit-Fun, V. M., Cox, P. B. W., & Buhre, W. F. (2020). Role of the anaesthetist in post-operative care. Journal of British Surgery. DOI: 10.1213/ANE.0000000000005636 PMID: 34142980

Soliman, M. M. (2024). Examining the Impact of a Video Review Guide on Robotic Surgical Skill Improvement. DOI: 10.1213/ANE.0000000000005636 PMID: 34142980

Streckenbach, S., Lai, Y., Bas, H., Crowley, J., Salzsieder, H., Mela, T., & Dalia, A. A. (2021). Starting an Anesthesia-based perioperative device management service: A practical guide to training anesthesiologists. *Journal of Cardiothoracic and Vascular Anesthesia*, 35(4), 1006–1017. DOI: 10.1053/j.jvca.2020.11.044 PMID: 33341343

Su, Y., & Zeng, Y. (2023). Simulation based training versus non-simulation based training in anesthesiology: A meta-analysis of randomized controlled trials. *Heliyon*, 9(8), e18249. DOI: 10.1016/j.heliyon.2023.e18249 PMID: 37576292

Sundnes, K. O. (2020). Disaster Anesthesia. Essentials of Disaster Anesthesia. DOI: 10.1213/ANE.0000000000005636 PMID: 34142980

Tan, M., Naegle, J. A., Boscardin, C. K., Chang, D. P., Chang, J. M., Sullivan, K. R., & Sinskey, J. L. (2023). Drivers of Well-Being and Burnout in Anesthesiology Residents. *The Journal of Education in Perioperative Medicine : JEPM*, 25(4). PMID: 38162705

Tylee, M. J., Rubenfeld, G. D., Wijeysundera, D., Sklar, M. C., Hussain, S., & Adhikari, N. K. (2020). Anesthesiologist to patient communication: A systematic review. *JAMA Network Open*, 3(11), e2023503–e2023503. DOI: 10.1001/jamanetworkopen.2020.23503 PMID: 33180130

Tzamaras, H. (2024). Transforming medical education through simulation design: The development and validation of a central line training system. DOI: 10.1213/ANE.0000000000005636 PMID: 34142980

Tzamaras, H. M., Brown, D., Gonzalez-Vargas, J., Moore, J., & Miller, S. R. (2024). Evaluating the effects of comprehensive simulation on central venous catheterization training: A comparative observational study. *BMC Medical Education*, 24(1), 745. DOI: 10.1186/s12909-024-05661-2 PMID: 38987803

Wärnberg, H. & Oliv, A. (2022). Designing Effective Post-Simulator Training Session Feedback Reports.

Watkins, S. C., & Hensley, N. B. (2023). Team Dynamics in the Operating Room: How Is Team Performance Optimized? *Anesthesiology Clinics*, 41(4), 775–787. DOI: 10.1016/j.anclin.2023.05.004 PMID: 37838383

Weer, C. H., & Greenhaus, J. H. (2020). … of employees' organizational career growth opportunities: The role of extra-role performance, work engagement, and perceived organizational commitment. *Journal of Career Development*, 47(3), 280–295. DOI: 10.1177/0894845317714892

Whaley, J. K. (2022). IMPLEMENTATION OF UNIT COUNCIL IN THE ANESTHESIA DEPARTMENT.

Zahid, M. A., Ali, P., Saddique, F., Khan, B., Rehman, M. A., & Kumar, A. (2023). Resilience unveiled: Empowering Pakistani anesthetists in challenging low-resource environment. *Anaesthesia, Pain & Intensive Care*, 27(5), 592–598. DOI: 10.35975/apic.v27i5.2299

Zhang, C., & Pandit, J. J. (2023). Getting operating theatre metrics right to underpin quality improvement: Understanding limitations of NHS Model Hospital calculations. *British Journal of Anaesthesia*, 131(1), 130–134. DOI: 10.1016/j.bja.2023.03.032 PMID: 37169629

Chapter 9
Strategic Management of Medical Devices in Emergency Care:
The Role and Applicability of the Pelvic Binder for Adult Polytrauma Patients

Cindy Monteiro
Escola Superior de Saúde da Cruz Vermelha Portuguesa, Portugal

ABSTRACT

This chapter examines the role of pelvic binders in managing unstable pelvic fractures in polytrauma patients. These devices are crucial for hemorrhage control, fracture stabilization, and survival during the "golden hour." Key factors—device availability, training, protocols, and performance monitoring—ensure effective implementation. Case studies, like Lisbon's emergency services, show that aligning clinical care with organizational goals improves efficiency and outcomes. The findings highlight collaboration, training, and technology as essential for excellence in trauma care.

1. INTRODUCTION

Effective healthcare management in emergency settings demands a strategic coordination of not just medical devices but also personnel training and operational efficiency. Within this context, trauma care, especially concerning polytrauma patients who have sustained multiple injuries, becomes a critical domain wherein timely interventions and evidence-based device management can significantly influence

DOI: 10.4018/979-8-3693-8598-2.ch009

survival rates and optimize resource utilization. The challenge lies in ensuring that all elements work seamlessly together to create a responsive and adaptable emergency medical service environment. (Rojas-Suarez and Paruk, 2024; Alhur, 2024)

This chapter offers a comprehensive analysis of the applicability and strategic management of the pelvic binder, which is recognized as a vital device for stabilizing pelvic fractures in adult polytrauma patients. By delving into its critical role, deployment challenges faced by healthcare providers, and the evidence-based outcomes achieved, this chapter effectively bridges the gap between clinical care and strategic healthcare management principles. It underscores the importance of structured device management systems, which can play a significant role in ensuring that practitioners are well-equipped to handle such complex cases. Additionally, the chapter emphasizes the necessity of competency-based training and continuous performance monitoring as essential components that can lead to improved patient outcomes. By fostering a culture of excellence in emergency care delivery, these practices not only enhance resource efficiency but also ensure alignment with organizational goals. The insights presented in this chapter aim to empower healthcare professionals and administrators to optimize the use of pelvic binders in their care protocols. (Payne & Wise, 2022; Christos et al.2024; MacDonald & Soel, 2023)

2. THE ROLE OF STRATEGIC MANAGEMENT IN EMERGENCY TRAUMA CARE

In the critical realm of emergency trauma care, strategic management plays a vital role that can be leveraged effectively to enhance both efficiency and overall effectiveness across various trauma systems. It is becoming increasingly acknowledged that the management of medical devices is essential for improving outcomes within these trauma systems; in this context, a clear and defined role for the strategic management of such devices can be readily assumed. A trauma is diagnosed in a polytrauma patient, one who has suffered significant bodily harm and presents with an actual or an imminent life-threatening condition that necessitates immediate medical intervention and careful oversight. (Karunarathna et al., 2024; Karunarathna et al., 2024)

The development of theories of management over the past half-century has witnessed a significant transition away from merely focusing on enhancing the effectiveness of individuals as the singular pathway to fostering an effective organization. Instead, there has been a concentrated, holistic emphasis aimed at promoting the effective and efficient interaction of all components that comprise an extended enterprise. This shift highlights an understanding that the synergy between various parts of an organization is equally, if not more, important than the capabilities of individual members. Extensive research has illuminated how the effectiveness of Emergency Care Practitioners responding to critical incidents is subject to a directly associated oversight, which plays a crucial role in their work. In this context, strategic principles have been meticulously defined to address pertinent issues surrounding patient safety and recovery. These principles rely on the utilization of overlapping goals and carefully designed organization-handler strategies to create a framework for effective management in emergency care situations. The work further proposes that the recovery process from trauma incidents can significantly benefit from the adoption of embodied work practices, which are designed to be supportive of, rather than obstructive to, the vital work required to maintain and enhance the organizational capability for recovery. In order to achieve this laudable goal, the organizational objectives must be directly aligned with and supportive of the patient care strategies employed by frontline workers, ensuring that these goals are not merely theoretical but actually embodied in practice. This paper extends on this essential work, reinforcing the same strategic goal of being perpetually supportive of patient care strategies within the specific context of recovery in the trauma system. It posits that leadership has a direct and substantial influence on the embodiment of recovery initiatives; for instance, injured patients who are positively impressed by the compassionate and dedicated actions of system members are considerably more likely to adhere to prescribed rest protocols and engage actively in relevant recovery activities. This engagement, in turn, serves to support their overall recovery process. Moreover, this paper delves into the broad and complex issue of how best to ascertain what strategic actions can be undertaken to optimize outcomes; that is, how the concept of 'strategic' can be effectively understood and applied in real-world settings. The paper systematically structures the necessary tactics to fulfill the overarching strategy. The strategy of registration is elaborated upon, making it particularly applicable to the specific case of knowing precisely what could be accomplished in the realm of recovery. In light of this understanding, a new strategic approach is proposed: the proactive increase of concerns to highlight potential areas for improvement. This paper vividly demonstrates this innovative approach by utilizing the development of recovery goals within a detailed case study focused on a local emergency care system. This enables a clearer understanding of how strategic advancements can be effectively implemented to enhance patient care and overall recovery outcomes in real emergency situations. (Moy et al.2023; Gootenberg et al.2021; Hwang et al.2021; Eriksson-Liebon et al.2021; Jarvis et al.2022)

In managing such an inherently challenging system of care, the fundamental question that arises becomes, "how much and what kind of investment should be made to ensure the provision of adequate care?" The practice patterns of these committed nurse practitioners vary widely across the country for a multitude of reasons. While there exists a wide variance in the types of care that are provided, trauma centers must place a strong emphasis on excellence in patient care, which is guided by the organization's mission and strategic goals for the future. The strategies that are developed at the executive level will have a direct impact on practice and care at the bedside, influencing the day-to-day experience of both patients and healthcare providers. Strategic management is fundamentally about aligning the key functions of an organization in accordance with the vital external influences that shape the healthcare landscape. Performance in these critical activities is essential for the overall success of the organization. Leadership undoubtedly plays an indispensable role in shaping a culture that truly supports success in performance, as has been discussed. The field of strategic management emphasizes the paramount importance of aligning the internal capabilities and competencies of an organization with the external market and customer needs, thereby enhancing customer value. This keen focus on understanding markets and customers and tailoring the organization to adeptly respond to their significant needs is especially vital in trauma care, particularly at organizations that receive and treat a high volume of polytrauma patients. By effectively navigating these complexities and ensuring a high quality of care, healthcare providers can foster a more responsive and effective trauma care environment. (Cullen et al.2022; Rattan et al.2021; Venet, 2023)

2.1. Importance of Device Management in Trauma Systems

In emergency care systems, the availability, proper usage, and consistent maintenance of critical medical devices, such as pelvic binders, can represent the decisive difference between life and death for patients who are in urgent need of care and assistance. The strategic management of these devices encompasses several essential components that must not be overlooked. Procurement is of utmost importance; this entails ensuring that there are adequate stock levels of necessary devices and that the quality of those medical devices remains consistently high across the board. Furthermore, Training and Competency are vital for addressing any skill gaps that may exist among healthcare professionals; it is crucial that all team members are adequately trained, feeling well-prepared to use these devices efficiently and effectively when the situation arises. Additionally, Monitoring and Performance Evaluation play a crucial role in this process; it involves implementing comprehensive audits to thoroughly assess not only the accuracy of device usage but also the adherence to established protocols and guidelines. This multi-faceted approach is not merely advantageous but is truly essential for improving patient outcomes and ensuring their safety during emergency medical situations where every second counts. (Zheng et al.2024)

Pelvic binders play an exceptionally crucial and pivotal role in the effective management of unstable pelvic fractures, injuries that account for a significant portion of trauma-related mortality, primarily due to severe bleeding, known as massive hemorrhage, and subsequent hypovolemic shock. In situations involving high-energy trauma, the immediate stabilization that pelvic binders offer greatly reduces the risk of exsanguination—the loss of blood—by minimizing the expansion of pelvic volume. This reduction helps to control bleeding and significantly improve overall patient outcomes. The timely application of these binders is essential in trauma care, as it serves to mitigate the severe consequences associated with these life-threatening types of injuries. Proper use of pelvic binders can be the difference between life and death for many patients, highlighting their vital importance in emergency medical settings. By carefully applying these binders, healthcare professionals can effectively stabilize patients and prevent further complications during critical moments of trauma care. (Hurst et al., 2024)

2.2. Linking Strategic Management to Patient Outcomes

A highly structured approach to device management significantly enhances both the efficiency and the overall effectiveness of trauma responses in emergency medical settings. The following strategic pillars serve to comprehensively align emergency care with broader management principles that are crucial for successful outcomes: Training Standardization: It is essential to ensure that consistent competency levels among medical staff are maintained and regularly evaluated to promote best practices in trauma care. Evidence-Based Protocols: This involves the integration of predefined clinical guidelines for the proper application and use of medical devices, ensuring that caregivers follow the most current and scientifically supported methods. Resource Allocation: There is a vital need to optimize not just the availability of medical devices but also the deployment of trained personnel, facilitating rapid and efficient responses to trauma situations. Outcome Monitoring: Continuously measuring and analyzing the impact of interventions on patient recovery rates and mortality figures is necessary to assess the effectiveness of trauma management strategies. For instance, a comprehensive UK-based trauma study revealed that improper application of pelvic binders was identified in an alarming 50% of the cases examined. This statistic underlines the critical need for structured interventions, such as regular competency audits and comprehensive clinical simulations, to significantly improve device usage and treatment outcomes, thereby ultimately enhancing the quality of care delivered to trauma patients. (Christos et al.2024; Rodriguez-Buitrago et al., 2023; Şimşek et al.)

3. CLINICAL IMPACT AND EVIDENCE-BASED MANAGEMENT OF PELVIC BINDERS

Emergency trauma management and the associated guidelines have been addressed primarily from a damage control resuscitation perspective, whereas the impact of the always pre-hospital applicable pelvic binder has thus far received practically no attention. The clinical impact of both guideline development and the provision of these devices, often of minimalist construction but accepted use, is discussed. Although it remains challenging to conduct high-level evidence studies to scientifically support the use of pelvic binders, current literature provides improved insight into the potential effects and applicability of these fracture splints. Hemodynamic mechanisms as well as binding have been described, demonstrating pelvic ring stabilization and treatment strategies in a complete overview of current evidence concerning pelvic binder use. Stabilizing a pelvic ring fracture with a pelvic binder in polytrauma patients is an essential part of pre-trauma center resuscitative management. Ideally, pelvic binders are effective through expeditious application. A lack of transverse board questions the advantage of a pelvic binder after a proper log-roll from supine to trauma board, but none of these scenarios have been investigated. Little is known about its effect on subsequent radiologic and operational outcomes. Inadequate pre-trauma center EMS training is underscored by terminologies such as suggest, might, and possible tendency, thereby rendering the quality of the matched studies from fair to moderate. Research needs to be directed at possible scenarios that might question the efficacy of a pelvic binder, a debated binding, and the definition of certain types of fractures that are beyond a pelvic binder repair. The latter might not support a standard practice protocol. A general effect study with implications for future guidelines has highlighted the need for a matched scientific study protocol to better demonstrate the clinical setting implications of pelvic binders. The aim of this review is to investigate the clinically applicable evidence surrounding the pelvic binder. (Christos et al., 2024; Madsen et al., 2024; Schindler et al.2023)

3.1. Pathophysiology of Pelvic Fractures and the Role of Binders

Pelvic fractures are serious injuries that typically occur due to high-energy trauma mechanisms, including motor vehicle collisions, falls from significant heights, and crush injuries. The pelvis, which serves as a critical osteoligamentous structure in the human body, can be anatomically divided into dorsal and ventral compartments. Within these compartments, there are key vascular and organ systems that are at substantial risk of injury during such traumatic events. The complexity of the pelvic anatomy highlights the importance of careful assessment and management of these fractures to prevent further complications. (Charsley & Jarman, 2024; Arshad and Rajashekar2020)

The three primary types of pelvic fractures include: Open-Book Fractures: These particular injuries are primarily caused by anteroposterior forces. Such forces result in a significant disruption of the pelvic ring, which can lead to substantial and potentially massive hemorrhage if symptoms are not treated promptly and appropriately. Lateral Compression Fractures: This second type of fracture results in internal displacement and generally carries a lower risk of hemorrhage when compared to the other more severe types of fractures. Vertical Shear Injuries: These injuries are caused by axial forces and are frequently associated with severe instability. This instability can lead to serious complications such as retroperitoneal bleeding, which may pose a life-threatening risk to those affected. Pelvic binders are specifically designed to effectively address and manage the complexities of these various types of injuries. They provide much-needed circumferential compression, which plays a crucial role in minimizing fracture displacement. This, in turn, aids in controlling hemorrhage and significantly contributes to improved outcomes for patients suffering from such traumatic injuries. (da Silva, 2023; Baig et al.2021)

3.2. Evidence-Based Benefits of Pelvic Binder Application

Studies have consistently and clearly demonstrated the numerous benefits that pelvic binders offer in various clinical settings, reaffirming their role in modern trauma care. One significant advantage these binders provide is hemorrhage control: the immediate stabilization they afford effectively reduces pelvic volume and minimizes bleeding from disrupted blood vessels, a factor that can be critically important in severe trauma cases. Another important aspect to consider is the markedly improved survival rates that have been observed with the implementation of these devices; indeed, early application of a binder is often linked to a notable reduction in mortality associated with hemorrhagic shock. Furthermore, there are noteworthy efficiency gains as the pre-hospital stabilization offered by pelvic binders accelerates the overall time to achieve definitive care, which can be crucial in emergency situations where every second counts. However, it is essential to recognize that these substantial benefits rely heavily on the correct placement and timely application of the pelvic binder devices, emphasizing the critical role of strategic management protocols in ensuring that these devices function optimally during emergencies and achieve the desired outcomes in patient care. Training and procedural adherence among healthcare providers are key factors that cannot be overlooked when aiming to maximize the effectiveness of pelvic binders in saving lives and improving trauma care overall. (Harrell et al., 2023; Madsen et al.2024)

4. STRATEGIC IMPLEMENTATION OF PELVIC BINDER PROTOCOLS

Effective strategic embedding of pelvic binder use into clinical practice and protocols should be systematically deployed. The execution of this approach can be accomplished by the integration of pelvic binders into existing guidelines and algorithms for trauma care through local groups for multidisciplinary team end-users, often led by consultants with an interest or understanding in trauma and resuscitation science. A mixture of diagnostic, measurable outcomes can be used to evaluate and audit the implementation of the evidence-based pelvic binder protocols and their optimal utility. This allows the systematic testing for associations between variations of staff adherence to these guidelines, protocols, and the impact on subsequent clinical outcomes for positively injured trauma cohorts. (Nguyen, 2024; Watkins et al., 2022)

It is important to form appropriate intradisciplinary and multidisciplinary working parties and groups when considering the implementation of the pelvic binder into a trauma system, and the pragmatic development of both binding protocols and educational initiatives. Greater agreement and collaborative development among members of the healthcare professionals must preclude the widespread adoption of any pelvic binding capability within such protocols. The Pelvic Binding for Elderly on Comorbid-based Iliac injury is proposing complementing the screening for appropriate patients and bindings by the development of a virtual binding training package. These training and ubiquitous education initiatives must be considered to facilitate effective implementation of immediate interventions in practice. Lastly, all studies to date have also reported that compliance with kit availability, the involvement, and size of trauma teams, equipment setup time, and failure of equipment occurred. (Adeghe et al., 2024)

Trauma centers should adhere to existing staff abdominal practice guidelines advising the pelvic binder for patterned trauma. There are three examples reporting prospective data that inevitably followed the implementation of binding practices or kits in the context of trauma systems. The application of initiative programs aimed at any healthcare professionals has been associated with a conscious increase in packaging and reduced mortality in trauma patients. Ultimately, the choice of new and emerging pelvic binders may have some advantages. However, the pelvic binder practice should be one of multiple components of an integrated emergency trauma management system that can investigate a trust or healthcare service adopted with reference to local services and local information. It should never resonate in isolation. (Iurilli et al.2024)

4.1. Training and Competency Development

Competency gaps among emergency teams represent a significant barrier to the effective use of pelvic binders in critical situations. To effectively address this challenge, strategic management must incorporate a multifaceted approach that encompasses the following essential elements: Simulation-Based Training: Implementing practical simulations designed to significantly improve placement accuracy and overall confidence among healthcare professionals. These hands-on experiences allow emergency teams to practice in safe environments, enabling them to gain valuable skills that translate to real-life scenarios. Competency Audits: Conducting periodic evaluations is crucial to identify existing skill gaps and reinforce the learning process gained in training. These audits can serve as a benchmark for evaluating the effectiveness of training programs, ensuring that every team member meets the necessary standards for quality emergency care. Interdisciplinary Collaboration: It is vital to provide comprehensive training to paramedics, nurses, and physicians alike to guarantee cohesive and consistent practices across all team members. For instance, a notable pre-hospital training initiative conducted in Lisbon has shown impressive results, achieving a remarkable 40% improvement in correct binder placement following simulation-based education. Such initiatives highlight the importance of teamwork and shared knowledge in enhancing the quality of emergency medical services. (Hong et al.2024)

4.2. Standardized Guidelines and Clinical Pathways

Implementing standardized clinical pathways is essential for ensuring that there are consistent and evidence-based responses to cases of pelvic trauma. These pathways are crucial and should encompass several key components: Early Identification stands as a critical element, utilizing advanced screening tools that are specifically designed to recognize unstable pelvic fractures in patients as quickly and accurately as possible. This proactive approach is fundamental for the timely treatment of affected individuals. Furthermore, Device Application Protocols should offer comprehensive, step-by-step guidance for the proper and safe placement of pelvic binders. This process is important for stabilizing injuries effectively, thereby preventing additional damage and complications that could arise from improper handling of the injuries. In addition to these measures, Monitoring and Reassessment hold significant importance; healthcare professionals must engage in continuous hemodynamic monitoring to track the patient's vital signs, while also diligently evaluating the effectiveness of the binder to ascertain the condition of the patient after intervention. This ongoing assessment is key to making timely adjustments to treatment as necessary. Standardized protocols serve as powerful tools that significantly reduce the likelihood of errors while enhancing decision-making efficiency. This is particularly crucial in high-stress environments where every second is critical, and accurate actions have the potential to save lives. By adhering to these well-defined pathways, healthcare teams can strive for optimal patient outcomes in situations that demand immediate and precise responses. (Mennen et al.2024)

4.3. Standardized Guidelines and Clinical Pathways

Strategic management within the healthcare sector necessitates a comprehensive approach to optimizing device availability and seamlessly integrating advanced technology to maximize workflow efficiency and enhance overall operational performance. Key strategies that are essential in this domain encompass the following pivotal areas: Inventory Management Systems: It is absolutely crucial to meticulously ensure that binders are consistently and reliably available across all trauma units and among pre-hospital teams. This guarantees that critical resources are always on hand whenever they are needed, thereby facilitating prompt responses in urgent situations. Digital Monitoring Tools: The implementation and utilization of these tools plays an exceedingly pivotal role in the meticulous tracking of binder usage. They are vital for analyzing performance metrics and evaluating patient outcomes with the intent of identifying significant areas for potential improvement and enhancement. Cost-Benefit Analysis: Conducting a thorough and comprehensive assessment of the economic impact associated with the enhancement of pelvic trauma management is crucial. This assessment is instrumental in justifying any investments that are made in new technologies or processes. For instance, sophisticated digital platforms not only aid in accurately documenting binder placement but also facilitate informed, data-driven decision-making processes that are essential for continuous improvement and ultimately yield better patient care outcomes. By comprehensively enhancing these strategies, healthcare facilities can significantly improve their service delivery, optimize their operational effectiveness, and thereby contribute to a higher standard of care in the healthcare system. Such focused efforts are vital in adapting to the ever-evolving challenges faced in delivering high-quality healthcare. (Christos et al.2024)

5. ORGANIZATIONAL OUTCOMES AND MANAGEMENT IMPLICATIONS

Outcomes in effective device management come at the patient level, the organization level, and the systems level. Health care providers are well aware of the ethical imperative to provide the best care possible to their patients. Incentives are increasingly being tied to operational efficiency and patient care outcomes. Reinforcing both patient care and operational efficiency would make good financial sense as well as being a strategic initiative. A hospital with a lower complication rate can use these data for marketing purposes, comparing their complication rates to another hospital in the region that is not so effective at pelvic fracture care. A patient with a bleeding pelvic fracture might spend a day in the emergency department of an institutional level 2 trauma center. When transported to the higher-level hospital that served as the system's referral center, they may face a second day in that trauma center's emergency department and finally be taken to the operating room at 3:00 a.m. Patients who linger unnecessarily in the trauma center emergency department may experience other delays in care. In other words, it might be operationally beneficial to move the patient. (Hossain et al.2024; Valli, 2024)

A decrease in complications can result in savings as well, such as avoiding a return to the operating room, the need for further blood, time in an ICU, and readmissions. By decreasing the rate of readmissions, a hospital can decrease exposure to readmission penalties. This can also represent another positive impact, such as having no at-fault or payer issues. The return on investment for materials and forms in an ongoing binder improvement project cumulatively pays for the materials and forms in professional time in 26 days. Pelvic binder management has an impact not only on the care provided to individual patients but also on the strategic operation of the institution. Leadership is responsible for setting the strategic or operational aims and values. Effective leadership views the role of the trauma program as having a dual mission of supplying quality patient care and pursuing operational efficiency. Management is responsible for reinforcing with individual staff the values and operational benchmarks articulated by leadership. Successful adopters are generally committed from the start to make pelvic binders part of the standard of care and are committed to using engagement strategies to effect the transition from non-engagement to higher levels of the engagement continuum. A manager's own attitude and response to change greatly affect the adoption of policies and practices. Those who closely align with the leaders are often successful because of the added push for compliance. Case studies of five institutions suggest points on keys like leader support, the need for multidisciplinary teams, patience, accountability, and a focus on continuous quality improvement. When the pelvic fracture protocol was not fully integrated, protocol indicators were not much improved. When the protocol was fully integrated, 97% of adult patients received the application of a pelvic binder upon arrival in the emergency department. This led to improvements in the indicators of interest. Treating pelvic ring injuries and associated injuries provided operational advantages for the hospital as a whole. Staffing and equipment to treat semi-urgent and emergent pelvic ring disruptions were also made available in the operating room and CT. An institutional injury prevention program has dropped the annual volume for patients with pelvic ring disruptions below 10 cases per year. This means well-prepared teams were available to apply the protocol, and there was enthusiasm from emergency staff to rapidly engage in the translation of three previously written protocols into operational actions. (Madsen et al.2024)

5.1. Improving Operational Efficiency

Strategic management of pelvic binders is not only crucial; it greatly enhances the operational efficiency of trauma care systems by significantly reducing treatment delays that can often lead to adverse patient outcomes. This management involves ensuring the timely and appropriate application of these critical devices during the essential "golden hour," which is pivotal for improving overall patient outcomes in emergency medical settings. Moreover, minimizing complications stands as another key aspect of effective trauma care management; when pelvic binders are utilized correctly and at the right time, they play a vital role in preventing secondary injuries. This proactive approach can subsequently lead to a reduction in the overall length of hospital stays for patients, allowing for a more effective use of healthcare resources. Furthermore, optimizing available resources contributes immensely to this efficiency by streamlining the allocation processes of medical devices across multiple emergency departments and pre-hospital units. Ensuring that the right resources, including pelvic binders, are available exactly when and where they are needed the most can significantly improve overall care delivery and enhance the experiences of patients in traumatic situations. This multifaceted approach not only supports immediate care but also sets a standard for trauma care excellence. (Howe et al.2023)

5.2. Enhancing Patient Outcomes

A well-managed and effectively executed device strategy can lead to notable and clearly measurable improvements in patient outcomes, delivering several key advantages that are crucial within the healthcare system. Notably, this strategy results in significantly lower mortality rates stemming from hemorrhagic shock, which is an urgent and critical medical condition requiring immediate attention and action. Such a strategic approach ensures that all necessary resources are efficiently allocated to safeguard patient lives. Moreover, it facilitates faster stabilization of patients and promotes efficient transfer to specialized trauma centers, thereby guaranteeing that individuals receive the urgent and critical care they require with minimal unnecessary delays. This timely intervention is essential to ensuring optimal medical outcomes. Furthermore, the implementation of a well-structured device strategy plays a significant role in contributing to reduced long-term disability rates and shorter recovery times, allowing individuals to return to their daily lives more quickly and effectively after experiencing severe medical conditions. The benefits of such strategies extend beyond initial treatment; this comprehensive approach not only enhances immediate care but also promotes better overall health and well-being for patients in the long run. As such, the focus on a carefully orchestrated device strategy ultimately leads to a more resilient healthcare system capable of responding effectively to the challenges posed by critical medical situations. (Temperley et al.2024)

5.3. Financial and Strategic Gains

Healthcare organizations can significantly benefit financially from enhanced trauma management efforts through several key factors that play a crucial and instrumental role in their operational effectiveness and overall efficiency. A reduced length of stay (LOS) in intensive care units (ICUs) leads to a notable decrease in costs associated with prolonged hospitalization, which can be an especially significant burden on hospital finances and resources. Moreover, there is lower resource consumption resulting directly from the avoidance of complications that could have been prevented with more effective care and management strategies. Effective management practices can greatly assist in mitigating various risks and ensuring that patients receive timely and appropriate interventions when they are critically needed. Furthermore, improved patient throughput not only aids in better resource allocation but also aligns more effectively with institutional performance metrics. This alignment allows these organizations to maximize their operational efficiency while enhancing overall patient care experiences. This comprehensive and holistic approach to trauma management not only leads to enhanced patient outcomes but also serves to fortify the financial health of healthcare institutions. By positioning themselves for sustainable growth and superior service delivery in the long term, they can achieve a dual objective: to improve the quality of care provided to patients and to ensure the fiscal viability of the organization. (Hawkins et al.2024)

6. CASE STUDY: IMPLEMENTING PELVIC BINDER PROTOCOLS IN LISBON EMERGENCY SERVICES

A pilot program that was recently conducted in Lisbon's pre-hospital emergency services clearly highlights the numerous substantial benefits associated with strategic pelvic binder management in urgent and critical emergency situations. The objective of this innovative initiative is to significantly improve the accuracy and effectiveness of binder application while ultimately aiming to reduce trauma mortality rates among patients who experience severe and life-threatening injuries. Methodologically, this crucial improvement was achieved through several comprehensive means, including simulation-based training that was designed specifically for emergency personnel, the establishment of standardized and robust protocols for binder application, as well as the implementation of meticulous digital audits that ensure adherence and compliance with the best practices. The results of the program were striking, resulting in a remarkable and unprecedented 50% increase in the correct placement of pelvic binders among the patients treated. Additionally, there was a significant and noteworthy 30% reduction in pre-hospital delays, which is absolutely critical for enhancing patient outcomes during emergencies. Furthermore, there were notable and substantial improvements observed in hemodynamic stabilization for patients who were transported to trauma centers after receiving immediate care in the field, which is essential for ensuring the best possible recovery trajectories. The overall success and effectiveness of this program strongly underscore the vital importance of aligning clinical practices with strategic management principles specifically within pre-hospital emergency care settings. This crucial alignment not only enhances the overall effectiveness of the procedures but also ensures that patients receive prompt, timely, and accurate treatment, which remains absolutely essential in any potentially life-threatening situations faced by individuals during emergencies. The implications of this pilot program extend far beyond immediate patient care, potentially guiding future protocols and training programs across various emergency service teams. Through continued emphasis on evidence-based practices and ongoing training for emergency response teams, this innovative approach can significantly transform outcomes in critical care scenarios, making a lasting impact on public health and safety. (de Nefrologia, 2024)

7. CONCLUSION

Strategic management of medical devices, such as pelvic binders, stands as a pivotal element that effectively bridges the crucial gap between clinical excellence and operational efficiency within the critical domain of trauma care. By systematically integrating comprehensive training programs, meticulously establishing standardized protocols, and thoroughly optimizing available resources, healthcare managers can effectively ensure timely, evidence-based responses to instances of pelvic trauma, which can be life-saving. This chapter goes on to demonstrate that the effective deployment and strategic utilization of pelvic binders not only contribute significantly to enhanced patient outcomes but also align seamlessly with the broader healthcare goals that are focused on achieving cost-efficiency, quality improvement, and overall organizational performance. In light of this, future efforts should aim to emphasize the importance of leveraging advanced technology, fostering meaningful interdisciplinary collaboration among diverse healthcare professionals, and continuously monitoring device performance to achieve sustainable and lasting improvements in emergency care delivery. Such strategic approaches will undoubtedly enhance the overall quality of care, streamline essential operational processes, and ultimately lead to better health systems that are not only equipped but also prepared to respond dynamically to the multifaceted challenges presented in emergency medical settings. (Parker et al.2024; Savakus et al., 2024; Harrell et al., 2023)

REFERENCES

Adeghe, E. P., Okolo, C. A., & Ojeyinka, O. T.Ehizogie Paul AdegheChioma Anthonia OkoloOlumuyiwa Tolulope Ojeyinka. (2024). A review of emerging trends in telemedicine: Healthcare delivery transformations. *International Journal of Life Science Research Archive*, 6(1), 137–147. DOI: 10.53771/ijlsra.2024.6.1.0040

Arshad, A. R., Rajashekar, M. R., & Srinivasan, . (2020). A Study on Mode of Injury, Types of Fractures and Associated Trauma in Unstable Pelvic Fractures. *Journal of Pharmaceutical Research International*, 32(12), 86–91. DOI: 10.9734/jpri/2020/v32i1230565

Baig, M. S., Rocha, D. F. B., & Horwitz, D. S. (2021). *Injuries of the Pelvis*. Hoppenfeld's Treatment and Rehabilitation of Fractures.

Charsley, J., & Jarman, H. (2024). Assessment and management of pelvic fractures from high-energy trauma in adults. *Emergency Nurse*. PMID: 36880213

Christos Konstantinidis, M. D., Galanis, C., Sotiris Plakoutsis, M. D., Panagiotopoulos, V., Kotsias, C., Konidaris, K., & Dimitrios Giotis, M. D. (2024). Effectiveness of Pelvic Binders in Pre-Hospital Emergency Care: A Systematic Review of the Literature. *International Journal of Caring Sciences*, 17(1), 139–149.

Cullen, P., Mackean, T., Walker, N., Coombes, J., Bennett-Brook, K., Clapham, K., Ivers, R., Hackett, M., Worner, F., & Longbottom, M. (2022). Integrating trauma and violence informed care in primary health care settings for first nations women experiencing violence: A systematic review. *Trauma, Violence & Abuse*, 23(4), 1204–1219. DOI: 10.1177/1524838020985571 PMID: 33573523

da Silva, H. D. P. D. (2023). Treatment Strategies for Mechanically Unstable Pelvic Injuries: A Narrative Literature Review. DOI: 10.1177/1524838020985571 PMID: 33573523

de Nefrologia, S. P. (2024). Abstracts of 37th Congress of the Portuguese Society of Nephrology. Portuguese Kidney Journal.

Eriksson-Liebon, M., Roos, S., & Hellström, I. (2021). Patients' expectations and experiences of being involved in their own care in the emergency department: A qualitative interview study. *Journal of Clinical Nursing*, 30(13-14), 1942–1952. DOI: 10.1111/jocn.15746 PMID: 33829575

Gootenberg, D. B., Kurtzman, N., O'Mara, T., Jennifer, Y. G., Chiu, D., Shapiro, N. I., & Dagan, A. (2021). Developing a pulse oximetry home monitoring protocol for patients suspected with COVID-19 after emergency department discharge. *BMJ Health & Care Informatics*, 28(1), e100330. DOI: 10.1136/bmjhci-2021-100330 PMID: 34301725

Harrell, K., Horwood, C., & Burlew, C. C. (2023). Current Management of Hemodynamically Unstable Patients with Pelvic Fracture. *Current Surgery Reports*, 11(4), 92–100. DOI: 10.1007/s40137-023-00348-x

Hawkins, A. D., Strobel, R. J., Mehaffey, J. H., Hawkins, R. B., Rotar, E. P., Young, A. M., Yarboro, L. T., Yount, K., Ailawadi, G., Joseph, M., Quader, M., & Teman, N. R. (2024, June). Operating room versus intensive care unit extubation within 6 hours after on-pump cardiac surgery: Early results and hospital costs. []. WB Saunders.]. *Seminars in Thoracic and Cardiovascular Surgery*, 36(2), 195–208. DOI: 10.1053/j.semtcvs.2022.09.013 PMID: 36460133

Hong, T., Case, V., Farcas, A. M., Whitfield, D., Muller, G., Schlesinger, S. A., Haamid, A. S., Middleton, M. T., Breyre, A., Buaprasert, P., Whitten-Chung, K., Lichtenbelt, K. J. C., Joiner, A. P., Pereira, C., & Brown, J. (2024). Caring for Transgender and Gender Diverse Prehospital Patients: A NAEMSP Position Statement and Resource Document. *Prehospital Emergency Care*, •••, 1–13. DOI: 10.1080/10903127.2024.2411723 PMID: 39422378

Hossain, Z., Chowdhury, S. S., Rana, M. S., Hossain, A., Faisal, M. H., Al Wahid, S. A., & Pranto, M. N. (2024). Business Innovations in Healthcare: Emerging Models for Sustainable Growth. AIJMR-Advanced International Journal of Multidisciplinary Research, 2(5). DOI: 10.1080/10903127.2024.2411723 PMID: 39422378

Howe, T. J., Claireaux, H., Fox, H., Morgan, G., McMenemy, L., Masouros, S. D., & Ramasamy, A. (2023). Mechanical assessment of proprietary and improvised pelvic binders for use in the prehospital environment. *BMJ Military Health*, e002398. DOI: 10.1136/military-2023-002398 PMID: 37541678

Hurst, J., Mitchell, C., & Jack, C. (2024). Pelvic fractures and ATLS principles. Surgery (Oxford). DOI: 10.1080/10903127.2024.2411723 PMID: 39422378

Hwang, U., Dresden, S. M., Vargas-Torres, C., Kang, R., Garrido, M. M., Loo, G., Sze, J., Cruz, D., Richardson, L. D., Adams, J., Aldeen, A., Baumlin, K. M., Courtney, D. M., Gravenor, S., Grudzen, C. R., Nimo, G., Zhu, C. W., Abraham, G., Amoko, C., & Sumberg, D. (2021). Association of a geriatric emergency department innovation program with cost outcomes among Medicare beneficiaries. *JAMA Network Open*, 4(3), e2037334–e2037334. DOI: 10.1001/jamanetworkopen.2020.37334 PMID: 33646311

Iurilli, M., Dentice, S., Di Nitto, M., Coclite, D., Napoletano, A., Bruno, V., & Papa, G. (2024). Availability and quality assessment of Clinical Practice Guidelines on Orthoplastic surgery treatment of open fractures of the lower limb using AGREE II tool: A systematic review. *Journal of Plastic, Reconstructive & Aesthetic Surgery; JPRAS*. PMID: 39700849

Jarvis, J. L., Lyng, J. W., Miller, B. L., Perlmutter, M. C., Abraham, H., & Sahni, R. (2022). Prehospital drug assisted airway management: An NAEMSP position statement and resource document. Prehospital Emergency Care, 26(sup1), 42-53. DOI: 10.1080/10903127.2024.2411723 PMID: 39422378

Karunarathna, I., De Alvis, K., Gunasena, P., & Jayawardana, A. (2024). The role of intra-abdominal pressure monitoring in managing ACS. DOI: 10.1080/10903127.2024.2411723 PMID: 39422378

Karunarathna, I., Gunawardana, K., Aluthge, P., & Jayawardana, A. (2024). Innovative therapies and future directions in pulmonary hemorrhage management. DOI: 10.1080/10903127.2024.2411723 PMID: 39422378

MacDonald, R. D., & Soel, M. S. M. (2023). Articles That May Change Your Practice: Pelvic Binders Revisited. *Air Medical Journal*, 42(2), 88–90. DOI: 10.1016/j.amj.2023.01.003 PMID: 36958878

Madsen, J. E., Flugsrud, G. B., Hammer, N., & Puchwein, P. (2024). Emergency treatment of pelvic ring injuries: State of the art. *Archives of Orthopaedic and Trauma Surgery*, 144(10), 1–15. DOI: 10.1007/s00402-024-05447-7 PMID: 38970673

Mennen, A. H., Lommerse, M., Hemke, R., Willems, H. C., Maas, M., Bloemers, F. W., Ponsen, K. J., & Van Embden, D. (2024). Does regional implementation of a clinical pathway for older adult patients with pelvic fragility fractures after low-energy trauma improve patient outcomes (PELVIC): A multicentre, stepped-wedge, randomised controlled trial. *BMJ Open*, 14(8), e083809. DOI: 10.1136/bmjopen-2023-083809 PMID: 39142675

Moy, A. J., Hobensack, M., Marshall, K., Vawdrey, D. K., Kim, E. Y., Cato, K. D., & Rossetti, S. C. (2023). Understanding the perceived role of electronic health records and workflow fragmentation on clinician documentation burden in emergency departments. *Journal of the American Medical Informatics Association : JAMIA*, 30(5), 797–808. DOI: 10.1093/jamia/ocad038 PMID: 36905604

Nguyen, T. (2024). Development of Novel Preclinical Models and Repair Approaches for Urogenital Tissue Reconstruction. DOI: 10.1093/jamia/ocad038 PMID: 36905604

Parker, W. J., Johnston, L. R., Atwood, R., Walker, P., & Bradley, M. J. (2024). Initial Management of Pelvic Fractures. *Current Trauma Reports*, •••, 1–7.

Rattan, A., Joshi, M. K., Mishra, B., Kumar, S., Sagar, S., & Gupta, A. (2021). Profile of injuries in children: Report from a level I trauma center. *Indian Pediatrics*, 58(6), 553–555. DOI: 10.1007/s13312-021-2239-x PMID: 32893835

Rodriguez-Buitrago, A., Collinge, C., Guillamondegui, O., Dennis, B., Bream, P.Jr, & Mitchell, P. M. (2023). Natural History of the Pelvic Binder or "Sheet-wrap" in the Early Treatment of Patients with Life-threatening Pelvic Ring Injuries at a Busy Level One Regional Trauma Center. A Retrospective Study. DOI: 10.1007/s13312-021-2239-x PMID: 32893835

Rojas-Suarez, J., & Paruk, F. (2024). Maternal high-care and intensive care units in low-and middle-income countries. Best Practice & Research Clinical Obstetrics & Gynaecology, 102474. DOI: 10.1007/s13312-021-2239-x PMID: 32893835

Alhur, A. (2024). The role of informatics in advancing emergency medicine: a comprehensive review. Cureus. Payne, E. K. & Wise, S. (2022). Pelvic Fractures and the Application of Pelvic Binders in Athletic Training. Athletic Training Education Journal. DOI: 10.1007/s13312-021-2239-x PMID: 32893835

Savakus, J. C., Skacel, T., Jindia, M., Al-Madani, Y., Spoletini, L., Ross, R. C., & Stinner, D. J. (2024). Biomechanical validation of the field-expedient pelvic splint. *BMJ Military Health*, military-2024-002815. DOI: 10.1136/military-2024-002815 PMID: 39521613

Schindler, C. R., Sturm, R., Hörauf, J. A., Marzi, I., & Störmann, P. (2023). The sequence of the treatment of combined fractures of the pelvis, spine, and extremities in polytraumatized patients. *EFORT Open Reviews*, 8(5), 372–381. DOI: 10.1530/EOR-23-0046 PMID: 37158361

Şimşek, P., Tayfur, İ., Gunduz, A., & Bayramoglu, B. (2025). Effectiveness of a training program for emergency nurses on pelvic binder application and patient care: A single-group pretest–posttest study. *International Emergency Nursing*, 78, 101528. DOI: 10.1016/j.ienj.2024.101528 PMID: 39612718

Temperley, H. C., Hylands, A., O'Sullivan, N. J., Mac Curtain, B. M., Temperley, T. S., Waters, C., & Sheahan, K. (2024). Complications in interventional radiology: early detection and effective intervention strategies. Irish Journal of Medical Science (1971-), 1-11. DOI: 10.1007/s13312-021-2239-x PMID: 32893835

Valli, L. N. (2024). Predictive Analytics Applications for Risk Mitigation across Industries; A review. BULLET: Jurnal Multidisiplin Ilmu. DOI: 10.1007/s13312-021-2239-x PMID: 32893835

Venet, A. S. (2023). Equity-centered trauma-informed education. DOI: 10.1007/s13312-021-2239-x PMID: 32893835

Watkins, C., Gill, S., Loudon, G., Hall, J., Carwardine, M., Ngua, C. W., & Jackson, J. (2022). The challenges of parachute design: The development of a low cost, fit for purpose trauma pack for use in Namibia. *Journal of Desert Research*, 20(1), 1–34. DOI: 10.1504/JDR.2022.125874

Zheng, X., Chen, M., Zhuang, Y., Xu, J., Zhao, L., Qian, Y., Shen, W. M., & Chu, Y. (2024). Hemostatic Interventions and All-Cause Mortality in Hemodynamically Unstable Pelvic Fractures: A Systematic Review and Meta-Analysis. *Emergency Medicine International*, 2024(1), 6397444. DOI: 10.1155/2024/6397444 PMID: 39224863

Chapter 10
Strategic Planning in Medical Device Innovation: Challenges and Opportunities

Elisabete Abreu
ISLA Santarém, Portugal

Ricardo Marcão
https://orcid.org/0000-0003-3277-3078
ISLA Santarém, Portugal

Stéphanie Monteiro
Instituto Superior Técnico, Portugal

ABSTRACT

This work explores strategic planning in medical device innovation, ensuring that technological and product advancements align with market needs, regulations, and company goals. It addresses a range of decisions and practices designed to ensure that innovation responds not only to technical and regulatory requirements but also has a positive impact on health and business sustainability. The study delves into the strategy of medical device innovation, examining the planning and execution processes aimed at ensuring technological innovation results in viable, effective products that meet the needs of the market and healthcare systems.

DOI: 10.4018/979-8-3693-8598-2.ch010

1. INTRODUCTION TO STRATEGIC PLANNING IN MEDICAL DEVICE INNOVATION

Strategic planning in medical device innovation is essential for the development and success of this sector. It is crucial to understand and anticipate market needs, as well as to be prepared for emerging challenges and opportunities. This planning goes beyond merely defining goals and objectives; it involves a comprehensive analysis of internal and external environments, identifying necessary resources, and establishing clear and sustainable strategies for achieving success. (Santos et al., 2022; Oliveira, 2021; de Vianna Tiné, 2024).

Strategic planning in the medical device industry refers to the process of setting long-term objectives, identifying the actions required to achieve them, and efficiently allocating resources. In this industry, the process is critical as innovation and the development of quality products are fundamental for improving healthcare. The relevance of strategic planning lies in its ability to guide companies in the right direction, enabling them to anticipate and effectively respond to market changes and consumer needs. (Toni, 2021; Guedes et al., 2022; Abreu, 2020; Farias, 2022).

Innovation in the medical device industry is crucial for driving significant advancements in treating and managing medical conditions. The constant technological evolution, combined with the need for safer and more effective solutions, makes innovation a cornerstone of this sector. The synergy between strategic planning and innovation enables companies to develop medical devices that meet the needs of patients, doctors, and healthcare professionals efficiently and ethically, thus contributing to the overall improvement of healthcare systems. (Lube Filho, 2023; Souza et al., 2024; Fernandes, 2023).

Strategic planning is a process aimed at defining a company's goals and objectives, as well as the strategies to achieve them. It is a fundamental tool for business management, allowing companies to anticipate scenarios and make more informed decisions. During the 1960s and 1970s, businesses began adopting formal strategic plans, following them over the medium and long term, which highlights the growing importance of this process in the business world. (Pereira, 2023; Paço & Casaca; Loural et al., 2023).

Following World War II, strategic planning began gaining prominence in the business context, consolidating its importance in subsequent decades. In 1965, Ansoff's normative model of strategic planning marked a significant milestone while also revealing the challenges companies face in its implementation. Since then, the concept has evolved and been approached from various perspectives, keeping pace with transformations in the business environment. (Farias-UFRRJ; Elias, 2024; Poubel, 2022).

2. THE IMPORTANCE AND UNDENIABLE IMPACT OF INNOVATION IN HEALTHCARE THROUGH MEDICAL DEVICES

Innovation in medical devices dates back thousands of years, with early records from ancient Egyptian, Greek, and Roman civilizations. At that time, physicians used rudimentary tools like tweezers and scalpels to perform simple procedures. However, significant advancements occurred during the Middle Ages, including the invention of the microscope and anatomical dissection, which contributed to the development of more complex and effective medical devices. (Dallabrida, 2023; Dias and Moreira, 2023). The emergence of the first medical devices can be attributed to the Industrial Revolution, which brought technological and material advancements that enabled large-scale production of medical equipment. A key historical milestone was the invention of the stethoscope by René Laennec in 1816, which revolutionized medical practice by allowing physicians to listen to internal body sounds. Additionally, the discovery of anesthesia and the development of sterilization techniques in the 19th century paved the way for a wide range of medical devices that transformed medicine. (Coelho et al., 2021; Zuin, 2022). Healthcare innovation brings numerous benefits, most notably improving patients' quality of life. New medical devices and technological advancements enable more effective, less invasive treatments with shorter recovery times. This reduces patients' suffering, increases survival rates, and allows for a quicker return to daily activities. Furthermore, innovation provides better monitoring and tracking of patients' health, resulting in improved and more controlled quality of life. (de Vianna Tiné, 2024; Amaral & Rego, 2020). Improving patients' quality of life is one of the primary direct benefits of healthcare innovation. Innovative medical devices offer patients access to more efficient, less invasive treatments with lower risks. This results in faster recovery, reduced pain and discomfort, and the possibility of resuming daily activities more quickly. In addition, innovation can provide tailored solutions to individual patient needs, significantly enhancing their quality of life and well-being. (de et al., 2024; de Souza et al., 2024).

3. KEY ELEMENTS OF STRATEGIC PLANNING IN MEDICAL DEVICE INNOVATION

- **Intellectual Property:**

Intellectual property (IP) plays a crucial role in medical device innovation, enabling the protection of innovations and ensuring returns on investment. IP protection is fundamental to market attractiveness, product differentiation, and the valuation of companies within the medical device sector. (Gilaberte et al., 2024; Alves & de Castro Santos; Moura). Intellectual property encompasses patents, trademarks, industrial designs, and copyrights, providing legal protection for innovations and intellectual creations. In the context of medical devices, IP covers everything from product design to manufacturing processes, ensuring recognition and exclusivity for technological advancements in healthcare. (Santos, 2021; Silva, 2023; Lopes, 2023; Freire, 2023).

The protection of intellectual property in medical devices offers significant advantages, such as market exclusivity, control over the use of innovations, and the possibility of licensing IP rights to third parties, generating additional revenue and strategic partnerships. Furthermore, IP protection is a determining factor in attracting investors and securing funding for new developments and research in the medical device sector. (de Sousa Charneira, 2024; Fernandes, 2024; Machado, 2023).

- **Sustainability in Medical Device Innovation**

Sustainability is crucial in the innovation of medical devices to ensure that natural resources are used responsibly and environmental impacts are minimized throughout the product lifecycle. This involves considering sustainable materials, eco-friendly manufacturing processes, and minimizing waste during production and use. Additionally, sustainability encompasses proper waste management and the pursuit of recycling solutions. By integrating sustainability principles into the development of medical devices, companies can promote environmental health while ensuring the long-term viability of their products and businesses. (Machado, 2023; Souto, 2024; Barbosa et al., 2023). In the context of medical devices, sustainability principles include lifecycle assessments, reducing environmental footprints, using recyclable materials, and improving energy efficiency. Furthermore, addressing social and economic impacts along the medical device value chain is essential to ensure sustainability. This includes fostering fair and safe production practices and contributing to equitable access to devices, particularly in underserved communities. Adopting sustainability principles in medical device innovation allows organizations to demonstrate corporate responsibility while positively contributing to global health and the well-being of future generations. (Pereira & Carvalho, 2020; Vezzoli, 2023; Alexandrino, 2021; Salvado et al., 2021). The global impact of medical device innovation is significant, as it contributes to improving health worldwide, particularly in developing countries. Innovations in medical devices can make medical technologies more accessible to underserved populations, helping reduce mortality rates and improve quality of life. Furthermore, innovation can lead to more efficient and accessible healthcare systems, driving positive global impacts. (Abreu, 2020; Loregian; Toscas et al., 2022). Access to medical technologies in developing countries is a major challenge due to factors such as cost, infrastructure, and resource availability. Medical device innovation plays a crucial role in improving this access by enabling the development of more affordable and tailored technologies to meet the specific needs of these populations. Innovation strategies that address the challenges faced by developing countries can ensure that medical technologies reach the areas where they are most needed, generating a positive impact. (Abreu, 2020; Souza et al., 2024; Perez, 2020).

- **Adaptability and Rapid Market Response**

Adaptability is a key element in the strategic planning of medical device innovation, as it allows organizations to quickly adjust to environmental changes while maintaining competitiveness. This capacity for adaptation is crucial to facing unexpected challenges and effectively seizing market opportunities, ensuring the long-term sustainability of the business. (Silva, 2023; Horn, 2021; Tokumoto et al., 2024; Almeida et al., 2023)

The concept of adaptability refers to an organization's ability to adjust and respond effectively to changes in the external and internal environment. In medical device innovation, this involves the flexibility to incorporate new technologies, meet evolving regulations, and adapt to market demands. In short, adaptability is essential for maintaining relevance and competitiveness in the medical device sector. (Machado, 2023; Teixeira, 2024; Arruda, 2024). A rapid market response is essential for medical device companies, primarily due to the dynamic nature of the healthcare sector. The ability to launch innovative products adapted to market needs in a timely manner can mean the difference between success and failure. Therefore, agility in responding to the market is crucial to ensuring the company's competitiveness and relevance. (Loregian; Caldas, 2021; Da et al., 2020). The importance of rapid market response lies in the company's ability to meet customer demands and expectations effectively and promptly. This involves understanding market trends, anticipating customer needs, and quickly adapting to offer superior solutions. Furthermore, agility in market response enables the company to stand out from the competition and gain a leadership position in the medical device sector. (Sanches, 2024; Rodrigues & Cunha, 2021; Felizola, 2024)

There are several strategies that medical device companies can adopt to ensure an agile market response. These include investing in market research and trend analysis to identify emerging opportunities, implementing agile and efficient product development processes, and establishing strategic partnerships with suppliers and distributors to streamline the supply chain. Moreover, an organizational culture focused on innovation and responsiveness also plays a key role in ensuring a rapid market response. (Coelho, 2023; Colvero, 2024; De Donno).

- **Training in Digital Technologies**

Training in digital technologies is essential to drive medical device innovation, ensuring that professionals stay updated with the latest tools and techniques. This enables the creation of more advanced and efficient devices, promoting better outcomes for patients. Training in digital technologies equips professionals with the skills to use specific tools such as computational simulations, 3D modeling, and prototype printing, accelerating the development of innovative medical devices. (de Vianna Tiné, 2024; da Silva Ribeiro, 2024; Roveda, 2024)

There are various forms of training and education in digital technologies for medical device innovation, including workshops, online courses, seminars, and practical classes. Additionally, companies can invest in partnerships with research and development institutions, providing employees with opportunities for continuous learning and immersion in digital technologies, ensuring they remain updated with the latest sector innovations and practices. (Ferauche & Silva; Ranha et al., 2024; Perez, 2020)

The development of digital skills among healthcare professionals is crucial for medical device innovation. This involves not only technical knowledge of digital technologies but also the ability to effectively apply these tools in clinical practice. Training healthcare professionals to use digital technologies efficiently and safely significantly contributes to improving healthcare and advancing medical devices. (Cruz, 2021; Selpa et al., 2023; Ferreira & dos, 2024).

- **Focus on Deadlines and Cost-Effectiveness**

The focus on deadlines and cost-effectiveness is fundamental in the process of medical device innovation, as it enables organizations to organize and meet timelines for launching new products in the market while optimizing financial resources. Effective management of deadlines and costs is essential to ensure the competitiveness and sustainability of companies in the medical device sector, meeting market demands and customer expectations. (Falcão, 2021; Santos and Alves, 2022; Santos, 2021; Perez, 2020). The importance of focusing on deadlines and cost-effectiveness lies in the ability to ensure the timely and budget-compliant launch of innovative medical devices. Meeting established deadlines is crucial for capturing market share and outpacing competitors, while effective cost management ensures the profitability of investments in innovation. (de Menezes, 2021; Pontin et al., 2020; Guedes, 2024)

For deadline management in medical device innovation, techniques such as the use of schedules and the clear definition of milestones and delivery dates throughout the product development process are applied. Additionally, project management tools like PERT/CPM and Gantt charts are used to plan and control activities, ensuring the fulfillment of established deadlines. (Barcaui et al., 2021; Martins, 2024; Lengler, 2023)

Cost-effectiveness analysis involves a detailed evaluation of the financial resources involved in the medical device innovation process, seeking to identify opportunities for cost reduction without compromising the quality and safety of the products. This analysis allows for data-driven decision-making aimed at maximizing the return on investment in innovation. (Queirós, 2022; do Aguiar, 2024; Perez, 2020).

- **Collaboration and Partnerships**

The integration of collaboration and partnerships into strategic planning is essential for achieving success in medical device innovation. This integration creates synergies and maximizes available resources, increasing the efficiency and effectiveness of strategic planning. By actively considering collaboration and partnerships from the early stages of planning, organizations can identify cooperative opportunities that may accelerate the development of innovative medical devices. (do Aguiar, 2024; Viegas, 2021; Perez, 2020). The alignment of goals and strategies is a fundamental step in integrating collaboration and partnerships into strategic planning. This involves clearly defining the objectives of the strategic plan and identifying the strategies necessary to achieve them, considering collaborations and partnerships as integral parts of the process. Effective alignment ensures that all partners work in harmony toward the same objectives, maximizing innovation and success potential. (Oliveira & Ckagnazaroff, 2024; Vieira, 2024; Araujo & Pereira, 2020). The development of networks of collaboration and partnerships is a crucial aspect of strategic planning in medical device innovation. This involves identifying and establishing relationships with potential partners who can significantly contribute to achieving strategic goals. Such networks may include research institutions, specialized companies, technology suppliers, or even competitors who can add value to the innovation process. Effectively developing these networks is fundamental for long-term success in medical device innovation. (Pereira et al., 2020; Carlos, 2023; Sales, 2023).

- **Compliance with Regulatory Standards**

The integration of regulatory standards into the strategic planning of medical device innovation is essential for ensuring compliance with legal and safety requirements. This involves incorporating relevant international and regional standards into the product development process to ensure that devices meet accepted standards in various markets. Additionally, integrating regulatory standards into strategic planning allows for anticipating potential challenges and adjusting innovation strategies to mitigate possible impacts during approval and commercialization phases. (Vazquez, 2024;

Pechim, 2024; de Souza, 2023). The regulatory framework for medical devices is essential to ensure the safety and efficacy of these products. International regulations, represented by ISO 13485, establish quality management system requirements for organizations that design, develop, produce, or provide services related to medical devices. Regional regulatory standards, such as the European Union's Regulation (EU) 2017/745, aim to ensure high quality and safety standards for products in the European market, requiring compliance with specific technical and regulatory requirements. (Porto, 2024; Perez, 2020; Pereira, 2024). Regulatory risk management plays a crucial role in medical device innovation, aiming to identify, assess, and mitigate the potential impacts of standards and regulations on the product lifecycle. This involves implementing risk management practices that address both technical aspects and regulatory requirements to ensure continuous compliance. Proactive regulatory risk management also allows companies to anticipate challenges and take preventive measures to ensure compliance throughout the innovation process. (Ordunez et al., 2022; Toscas et al., 2022; Abreu, 2020).

- **Research and Development (R&D)**

The importance of strategic planning in R&D for medical devices lies in its ability to enable companies to identify and seize innovation opportunities while managing the risks associated with developing new devices. Through solid strategic planning, companies can make informed decisions about which R&D projects to invest in, considering factors such as market demand, technical feasibility, and potential public health impact. This way, strategic planning helps companies optimize their innovation efforts and ensure their medical devices meet the needs of patients and healthcare professionals. (Santos, 2023; Da et al., 2024; Oliveira et al., 2021). The SWOT analysis (Strengths, Weaknesses, Opportunities, and Threats) is a fundamental tool in strategic planning for R&D in medical devices. This analysis helps identify the company's internal strengths and weaknesses and the external opportunities and threats. By evaluating these four elements, companies can make more informed decisions about where to allocate resources and how to develop their capabilities. For example, by identifying a market opportunity, a company may decide to invest in R&D to launch a new product. Similarly, by identifying a threat, the company can take steps to mitigate its impact, such as diversifying its product line. This analysis is a powerful tool for guiding strategic planning in medical device innovation. (Da et al., 2021; Wendling et al., 2020; Carmo et al., 2024).

- **Alignment with Market and Patient Needs**

Aligning medical devices with market and patient needs is critically important for the success of innovation. This involves addressing the demands and expectations of consumers and healthcare professionals, as well as understanding market trends and challenges. Based on this understanding, companies can focus their efforts on developing products that meet existing demand and anticipate future needs, ensuring market acceptance and adoption. (da Cunha Machado, 2023; Toscas et al., 2022; Abreu, 2020). Identifying market needs requires an in-depth analysis of unmet needs, challenges faced by patients and healthcare professionals, and opportunities for improvement. This process involves conducting market research, interviewing stakeholders, and analyzing data to identify gaps and areas for innovation. Understanding the actual needs of the market is essential for creating innovative and effective medical devices that provide tangible benefits for users and the healthcare industry. (Bittencourt & Rauen; Aires, 2021; Graglia & Huelsen, 2023)

4. CHALLENGES IN STRATEGIC PLANNING

The challenges in medical device innovation include the need to comply with strict regulations to ensure the safety and efficacy of devices, which can lead to delays and additional costs in the development process. Additionally, the intense competition in the medical device market demands that companies continuously innovate to stand out and remain relevant. Key challenges in strategic planning include complex and stringent regulations, high research and development costs, technological risks, development timelines, risk of failure, resistance to change, intense competition, and ethical considerations. (de Sá, 2023; Schuster, 2021; Nolasco & dos Santos, 2022). Strategic planning for innovation in medical devices faces various challenges, including the complexity of regulation and legal compliance. The need to meet strict and constantly evolving standards can pose significant obstacles for companies in the sector. Moreover, the costs and financing required for research, development, and launching new devices are significant challenges, particularly for smaller companies. Intense market competition and the need for product differentiation also pose hurdles, requiring effective marketing and innovation strategies to stand out in an increasingly competitive environment. (do Aguiar, 2024; da Cunha Machado, 2023; Toni, 2021; Machado, 2024). Regulation and legal compliance are critical challenges in the strategic planning of medical device innovation. Companies must address the need to obtain approvals from regulatory agencies, ensuring their products meet safety and efficacy standards. Additionally, the necessity to comply with constantly changing regulations in different markets requires significant resources and specialized knowledge in legal and regulatory matters. (Santos, 2024; Perez, 2020; Russo, 2024). The costs and financing associated with innovation in medical devices present considerable challenges for companies in the sector. The investment required for research, development, and clinical testing can be substantial, and not all companies have the financial resources to support these expenses. Securing funding, whether through investors, strategic partnerships, or government grants, is essential to overcoming this challenge and ensuring the viability of innovation projects. (Seiler et al., 2020; de Vianna Tiné, 2024; Silva & Olave).

- **Complex and Stringent Regulation**

The complexity and rigor of medical device regulations present specific challenges for strategic planning in the industry. These include the need to keep up with constant changes in rules and guidelines, correctly interpret and apply required documentation, and implement efficient approval processes. Additionally, risk management and mitigation of non-compliance become priorities, demanding robust compliance and management strategies. Strategic planning must also consider ongoing education and training for professionals and the pursuit of innovations that simplify compliance with regulatory requirements. These specific challenges require comprehensive attention and constant updates to ensure conformity and market success. (Machado, 2023; Health Organization, 2020; Mabunda, 2021)

- **High R&D Costs**

The research and development (R&D) costs in medical devices refer to expenses incurred during the conception, creation, and testing of new products. These costs can include personnel, equipment, materials, clinical testing, and regulatory expenses. The complexity and rigor of regulatory requirements significantly contribute to high R&D costs, making effective management strategies essential for these expenses. (Pontin et al., 2020)

High R&D costs directly impact the competitiveness of companies in the sector by influencing the final product prices, the ability to innovate, and profitability. Moreover, these costs can limit access to innovations for smaller companies, affecting the competitive dynamics of the entire industry. (Perez, 2020)

- **Technological Risk**

Addressing technological risk in medical devices within strategic planning requires understanding the complexity and interconnectedness of variables in this process. Anticipating potential threats, predicting risk scenarios, and establishing effective action plans demand an analytical and proactive approach, considering the dynamic nature of the medical-technological environment. (Mendes, 2024). Identifying potential risks in medical devices involves a detailed analysis of each component and process related to their design, manufacturing, usage, and maintenance. This process requires meticulous evaluation of possible malfunctions, adverse interactions with other devices or substances, and potential human errors to anticipate and mitigate threats to device safety and efficacy. (Amaral, 2021)

- **Intense Competition**

In the context of strategic planning for medical devices, companies face specific challenges requiring special attention. The ability to innovate technologically and effectively manage the product lifecycle are crucial for maintaining market competitiveness. Additionally, issues related to regulations and quality standards require careful planning and constant monitoring to ensure product compliance and safety. These challenges directly influence the strategies adopted by companies and must be addressed proactively and diligently. (Klein, 2024; da et al., 2024). Constant technological innovation and effective product lifecycle management are critical challenges in the strategic planning of medical device companies. Developing new technologies and introducing innovative products are essential for standing out in a competitive market. Simultaneously, managing the product lifecycle—spanning introduction, growth, maturity, and decline—requires specific strategies to optimize performance and extend market relevance. (El et al., 2024; de Souza, 2023)

Regulations and quality standards represent a significant challenge in strategic planning for medical device companies. The constant evolution of regulations and the need to meet strict quality standards demand special attention and continuous adaptation. Strategic planning must include implementing effective quality management systems, training human resources, and maintaining efficient processes to ensure compliance and customer satisfaction. (de et al., 2024; Rodrigues, 2024)

- **Prolonged Development Time**

Strategic planning in medical devices faces numerous challenges, one of which is prolonged development time. This issue directly impacts companies' ability to bring innovations to the market, leading to significant delays in the availability of new medical technologies for patients in need. (Sousa, 2023; Martins, 2022). Prolonged development time is a significant obstacle in the field of medical devices. The process of research, development, clinical testing, regulation, and approval can take several years, not only delaying the arrival of new technologies but also negatively affecting companies' ability to innovate and compete. Finding ways to reduce these timelines and accelerate medical device development is essential for the benefit of patients and the healthcare system as a whole. (Teixeira, 2024; Ghellere et al., 2023). The extended development time of medical devices is often attributed to challenges encountered in the regulation and approval process. Meeting the strict safety and efficacy standards required by regulatory agencies significantly increases the time required for clinical testing, report preparation, and documentation submission. Moreover, the complexity of regulatory requirements across different countries and regions also contributes to the extended development timeline, as each market may have specific requirements that must be met before the device can be approved. (Silva, 2022). Regulatory and approval processes for medical devices are characterized by several time-consuming steps. The need for extensive clinical testing to demonstrate the device's safety and efficacy, along with the preparation of detailed documentation to meet regulatory requirements, are factors that contribute to prolonged development timelines. Additionally, obtaining approval in different global markets increases the complexity and duration of the process, as each region may have specific regulatory demands that must be satisfied. (Mendes, 2024; Ladeiro, 2020).

- **Risk of Failure**

The risk of failure in medical devices can be attributed to several factors, such as design flaws, lack of alignment with market needs, quality and safety issues, among others. It is essential to identify and understand these primary causes to mitigate risk. The lack of efficacy and safety in medical devices can result in significant impacts on patient health, including medical complications, injuries, and even death, as well as legal consequences for the companies involved. (de Castro Gil, 2023)(Machado, 2024). The main causes of failure in medical devices include lack of innovation, usability issues, regulatory non-compliance, high production and maintenance costs, and difficulties in accessing healthcare markets. Moreover, poor product lifecycle management and insufficient post-launch monitoring are critical factors that can lead to the failure of medical devices. (Costa, 2024)(Costa, 2024). The failure of medical devices can result in substantial economic impacts, including financial losses for manufacturing companies, additional costs for the healthcare system, and loss of trust from consumers and medical professionals. Additionally, the impacts on patient health are equally significant, potentially leading to adverse events, additional treatments, and, in extreme cases, serious compromises to quality of life and prognosis. (Pereira, 2023)(Avritzer et al., 2021). Cases of failure in the strategic planning of medical devices can be attributed to missteps in forecasting market trends, failure to adapt to regulatory changes or intense competition, as well as excessive investments in technologies that do not meet market needs. Lessons learned include the importance of thoroughly analyzing the external environment, moderation in innovation, and the ability to adjust strategy in response to unforeseen challenges. (de Jesus Costa, 2024)(Agner, 2023).

5. OPPORTUNITIES IN STRATEGIC PLANNING

- **Technological Advances:**

Technological advances in medical devices have transformed how health is monitored and treated. The Internet of Things (IoT) enables the connection of medical devices, allowing real-time data collection and communication between equipment. Artificial Intelligence (AI) and Machine Learning (ML) have been applied to develop more precise and efficient medical devices capable of diagnosing and treating diseases more accurately. Furthermore, Telemedicine and Digital Health promote the delivery of healthcare remotely, providing greater accessibility to medical services. (Evangelista, 2021)(da Silva, 2024). The Internet of Things (IoT) has enabled the interconnection of medical devices, expanding the possibilities for health monitoring and disease treatment. With the integration of sensors and connected devices, healthcare professionals can access real-time data, enabling more precise and personalized diagnoses. Additionally, IoT allows for process automation and communication between devices, improving the efficiency of medical services. (Juner & Rodrigues, 2022)(Silva, 2021). The application of Artificial Intelligence (AI) and Machine Learning (ML) has revolutionized the field of medical devices, enabling the development of more advanced and precise technologies. ML algorithms are used to analyze large volumes of medical data, allowing pattern identification and more accurate diagnoses. Additionally, AI has been used to enhance monitoring and treatment devices, providing innovative health solutions. (Caetano)(de Vianna Tiné, 2024). Telemedicine and Digital Health have offered solutions for delivering healthcare remotely, enabling continuous patient health monitoring and the execution of remote consultations. Through digital platforms and applications, clinical conditions can be monitored and medical interventions carried out even from a distance. Moreover, Digital Health has promoted the democratization of access to medical services, catering to remote areas and improving the quality of life of populations. (Oliveira et al., 2024)(Ribeiro, 2024).

- **Demographic Changes:**

The aging population has a direct impact on the demand for medical devices, as older individuals tend to require more healthcare and treatments. This means the medical device industry needs to prepare to meet this growing demand by developing products tailored to geriatric needs. Additionally, increased life expectancy raises the likelihood of developing chronic conditions such as diabetes and heart diseases, which require specialized medical devices for effective monitoring and treatment. (Ti et al., 2023)(Kabariti et al., 2024). The aging population is directly tied to the rise in healthcare needs, as older adults are more susceptible to chronic conditions and require frequent medical care. This creates a growing demand for medical devices that assist in monitoring and treating these conditions, as well as improving the quality of life for seniors. Therefore, the medical device industry must be attentive to these needs and develop innovative technologies to cater to this expanding market. (Lima et al., 2023)(De Carli, 2024).

- **Personalized Medicine:**

The implementation of strategic planning in medical devices for personalized medicine faces unique opportunities. (Machado, 2024)(Estratégico, 2022). However, these opportunities are also significant, including the potential to develop innovative devices aligned with personalized medicine trends and the chance to stand out in a constantly evolving market. (Roveda, 2024)(Guerra et al., 2024). Best practices for implementing strategic planning in medical devices for personalized medicine include close collaboration with healthcare professionals and personalized medicine specialists, a continuous drive for innovation, and investment in cutting-edge technologies. Success stories include companies that have developed highly effective personalized devices, leveraging genomic data and advanced monitoring technologies to improve clinical outcomes and patient quality of life. (de et al., 2020)(dos et al., 2024).

- **Government Incentives:**

The medical device industry can benefit from various government incentives to promote innovation and sector growth. These incentives include grants and funding provided by government bodies to support research and development initiatives as well as business expansion. Additionally, tax benefits and reductions represent an important way to stimulate investment and the production of medical devices, contributing to the competitiveness of companies and the technological advancement of the sector. (Machado, 2023)(Silva, 2022). In the context of the medical device industry, government grants and funding can be directed toward research and innovation projects, acquisition of state-of-the-art equipment, training of qualified personnel, expansion of production capacity, and more. These resources are a crucial support for companies in the sector, enabling investments that might not be feasible otherwise, thereby contributing to the strengthening and growth of the medical device industry. (Ambrozio & Dunham, 2024)(Silva, 2023). Tax benefits and reductions are important tools to stimulate investments and the production of medical devices. Tax exemptions, credits, and reductions can represent a significant competitive advantage for companies in the sector, facilitating new projects, modernizing production processes, and increasing innovation capacity—key aspects for the sustainable development of the medical device industry. (Júlio, 2023)(de Oliveira). By aligning company objectives and strategies with government incentive programs, organizations can maximize available benefits. This includes identifying areas of opportunity that align with government priorities, such as technological innovation and improving population quality of life. Proper integration of strategic planning with government incentives can result in greater access to grants, funding, and tax benefits, strengthening the company's market position and driving sustainable growth. (de Andrade)(Sousa et al., 2020).

6. RESPONSIBILITY TO THE PATIENT IN MEDICAL DEVICE INNOVATION

Responsibility to the patient in medical device innovation is essential to ensure the safety and efficacy of the products. This involves conducting rigorous clinical trials, obtaining regulatory approvals, and adhering to ethical standards throughout the development process. Additionally, it is crucial to ensure device traceability, train healthcare professionals, and maintain transparent communication with patients to promote proper use and minimize risks. Patient safety must be a priority at every stage, from device design to clinical application, to prevent harm and promote positive outcomes. (Moreira, 2024)(Costa and Costa, 2021). In the context of medical device innovation, ethics and patient safety are critical aspects that cannot be overlooked. Ethics involve making responsible decisions, respecting moral principles, and protecting the dignity and rights of patients. This includes transparency in the disclosure of information, safeguarding privacy, and ensuring informed consent. Patient safety encompasses the prevention of adverse events, risk minimization, quality maintenance, and the promotion of well-being. Both aspects must be embedded in all stages of the device lifecycle, from research and development to post-market monitoring, to ensure the trust and satisfaction of users and healthcare professionals. (Cançado, 2024)(Severi, 2024).

7. STRATEGIC PLANNING AND ISO 13485 IN MEDICAL DEVICE PROJECTS

Strategic planning is essential to guide an organization's actions and decisions, ensuring alignment with long-term goals. Meanwhile, ISO 13485 sets requirements for quality management systems for medical devices, aiming to ensure the safety and efficacy of these products. Therefore, the integration between strategic planning and ISO 13485 is crucial for companies in the medical device sector, as it creates a structure that promotes regulatory compliance and competitive advantage. (Gomes, 2024)(Porto, 2024). Its importance lies in its ability to guide companies toward success while ensuring market sustainability. Additionally, strategic planning allows organizations to anticipate potential threats and opportunities, contributing to more effective and assertive decision-making. (Leoni, 2024)(Drago, 2023). The ISO 13485 standard establishes requirements for the quality management system of medical devices, covering areas such as management responsibility, resource management, product realization, measurement, analysis, and improvement, among others. These requirements aim to ensure that companies in the sector comply with established safety and efficacy standards, guaranteeing the quality and reliability of their products, while strengthening customer trust and the company's credibility in the market. (Porto, 2024)(Gomes, 2024). The intersection of strategic planning and compliance with ISO 13485 is fundamental for companies aiming to operate in the medical device sector. The integration of these two elements allows the organization to align its long-term goals with the quality and safety requirements established by the standard, providing a solid foundation for the development and manufacture of products that meet market and patient needs. Moreover, the convergence of strategic planning and ISO 13485 helps to strengthen a culture of continuous improvement and innovation within the company, contributing to its sustainability and competitiveness in the sector. (Santos, 2023)(de Faria, 2022).

7.1. Benefits of Integrating Strategic Planning with ISO 13485

The benefits of integrating strategic planning with ISO 13485 are numerous, including improved operational efficiency, reduced risks and costs, increased customer satisfaction, and expanded access to new markets. Implementing strategic planning aligned with ISO 13485 also enhances the organization's ability to anticipate and respond to changes in regulatory and technological environments, supporting adaptation to new requirements and opportunities. Furthermore, the integration promotes process optimization and activity standardization, resulting in safer, more reliable, and competitive products in the global medical device market. (Davi, 2021)(Fangueiro, 2021).

7.2. Challenges and Opportunities

Despite the benefits, integrating strategic planning with ISO 13485 presents challenges, such as ensuring employee engagement, allocating adequate resources, and fostering a quality-focused culture at all organizational levels. However, these challenges bring opportunities for improvement and innovation, driving companies to develop more effective and sustainable practices. The integration also opens doors to strategic partnerships and collaborations, allowing companies to benefit from industry best practices and promote the development of more advanced and differentiated solutions. Therefore, companies that address the challenges of integrating strategic planning with ISO 13485 are well-positioned to reap the rewards of these opportunities and drive excellence in their medical device projects. (Santos, 2023) (Völz et al., 2023).

7.3. Results and Discussion

The research results demonstrated that effective strategic planning significantly impacts compliance with ISO 13485 in medical device projects. The integration of well-defined strategies with ISO 13485 requirements led to more efficient processes, higher product quality, and greater customer satisfaction. Moreover, the analysis of collected data revealed valuable insights into the relationship between strategic planning and standard compliance, highlighting the importance of this integration for organizational success. (da Costa, 2023)(Gomes, 2024). The research identified several positive impacts of strategic planning on compliance with ISO 13485. The main benefits included improved risk management, optimized quality processes, reduced costs, and increased competitiveness in the medical device market. A detailed analysis of the studied cases showed that companies adopting solid strategic planning not only met but exceeded standard requirements, achieving consistent and high-quality results. (Pacheco, 2023)(Gomes, 2024). Critical success factors identified in this research emphasized the importance of committed leadership, a quality-driven organizational culture, investment in training and technology, and continuous improvement efforts. Additionally, effective stakeholder management, clear communication, and constant monitoring were fundamental to successfully integrating strategic planning with ISO 13485. These factors provide valuable insights for other organizations seeking to enhance their compliance with the standard and achieve exceptional performance in medical device projects. (Gomes, 2024) (Silva, 2021).

8. STRATEGIC PLANNING METHODOLOGIES AND TOOLS

Strategic planning methodologies and tools play a fundamental role in the process of medical device innovation. They enable a structured and analytical approach to evaluate the current and future state of the company, identify opportunities and challenges, and define strategic paths to follow. The use of these methodologies and tools ensures that medical device innovation aligns with the company's goals and resources, facilitating more informed decision-making and more successful implementation. (Machado, 2023)(Santos, 2023). SWOT analysis and the BCG matrix are two important strategic planning tools that can be specifically applied to medical device innovation. SWOT analysis helps identify strengths, weaknesses, opportunities, and threats related to innovation, while the BCG matrix evaluates the product portfolio and identifies where the company should focus its innovation efforts. Both tools provide a comprehensive view of the current situation and the future potential of the company in the context of medical device innovation. (de and de, 2021)(Dos Santos). Strategic planning for medical device innovation emphasizes the importance of a holistic approach that considers regulatory challenges, financing needs, and product differentiation efforts. It is recommended that companies in the sector focus on strategic partnerships and collaborations to leverage opportunities presented by emerging technologies and precision medicine. Additionally, applying strategic planning methodologies, such as SWOT analysis and the Balanced Scorecard, is essential for setting objectives and evaluating performance. Ultimately, success in strategic planning for medical device innovation requires balancing regulatory compliance, seeking innovation opportunities, and establishing a competitive market position. (de Jesus Costa, 2024)(Machado, 2024).

REFERENCES

Abreu, M. M. V. (2020). O controle sanitário eo acesso a dispositivos médicos no Brasil: um estudo comparativo no cenário de convergência regulatória. fgv.br

Abreu, M. M. V. (2020). O controle sanitário eo acesso a dispositivos médicos no Brasil: um estudo comparativo no cenário de convergência regulatória. fgv.br

Agner, L. (2023). Ergodesign e arquitetura da informação: trabalhando com o usuário. [HTML]

Aires, J. D. M. (2021). Avaliação de dinâmicas e orientações para a medição da inovação empresarial no turismo. [HTML]

Amaral, C. M. (2021). Análise multicritério para apoio à seleção de fornecedores de dispositivos médicos. iscte-iul.pt

Amaral, M. B. & Rego, S. (2020). Doenças raras na agenda da inovação em saúde: avanços e desafios na fibrose cística. Cadernos de Saúde Pública. scielo.br

Ambrozio, A. M. H. P., & Dunham, F. B. (2024). Política industrial moderna: teoria e evidência empírica. bndes.gov.br

Araujo, E. R., & Pereira, D. (2020). Entidades de mediação e constituição de parcerias institucionais locais: uma reflexão a partir do Famalicão made in, Portugal. DRd-Desenvolvimento Regional em debate, 10, 1123-1138. unc.br

Avritzer, L., Kerche, F., & Marona, M. (2021). Governo Bolsonaro: retrocesso democrático e degradação política. [HTML]

Barcaui, A. B., Borba, D. B., Da Silva, I. M., & Neves, R. B. (2021). Gerenciamento de cronograma em projetos. [HTML]

Bittencourt, P. F. & Rauen, A. T. (). Políticas de inovação: racionalidade, instrumentos e coordenação. RAPINI. researchgate.net

Caetano, R. M. (). O uso da Inteligência Artificial na Saúde. MULTIDISCIPLINAR. ibra.edu.br

Cançado, V. O. L. (2024). Avaliação de processos em laboratório de análises clínicas sob a ótica da segurança do paciente. unb.br

Carlos, M. S. F. (2023). O papel do cluster da vinha e do vinho na internacionalização e inovação dos processos e produtos das empresas vitivinícolas portuguesas. utl.pt

Carmo, V. A. S., Pinheiro, R. R., Alvarenga, S. M., & Potrich, A. C. G. (2024). Ferramenta OKR aplicada ao agronegócio: Um estudo de caso. Seven Editora, 1350-1369. sevenpublicacoes.com.br

Coelho, J. B. L.Jr, Jurberg, C., Pinto, B. D. O. S., & de Barros, M. D. M. (2021). JOGO "DETROIT: BECOME HUMAN" COMO GUIA DE REFLEXÃO SOBRE A QUARTA REVOLUÇÃO INDUSTRIAL. [ufmt.br]. *Experiências em Ensino de Ciências*, 16(1), 105–120.

COSTA. F. N. (2024). Questionamentos. Campinas, SP: Blog Cidadania & Cultura, 2024. 209p. 1. Papel dos Economistas. 2. História Econômica. 3. Organização Industrial. 4…. unicamp.br

Costa, E. A. M., & Costa, E. A. (2021). O dilema do reuso de dispositivos médicos de uso único: aspectos históricos e atuais. Vigilância Sanitária em Debate: Sociedade [redalyc.org]. *Ciência & Tecnologia*, 9(1), 91–98.

Costa, R. M. P. (2024). O doente oncológico em programa de quimioterapia: Projeto de Desenvolvimento de Competências Clínicas Especializadas na Área de Enfermagem à Pessoa em …. rcaap.pt

da Costa, M. I. F. (2023). tabilidade n. mcm.com.pt

da Costa Júnior, J. F., Bezerra, D. D. M. C., dos Santos Cabral, E. L., Moreno, R. C. P., & Pires, A. K. S. (2021). A Matriz SWOT e suas subdimensões: Uma proposta de inovação conceitual. Research [rsdjournal.org]. *Social Development*, 10(2), e25710212580–e25710212580.

da Costa Teixeira, P., de Freitas, C. L. L., & de Brito, Z. M. (2024). A importância da gestão de custos para a lucratividade de micro e pequenas empresas: Um estudo de caso em Manacapuru-AM. [revistaacademicaonline.com]. *Revista Acadêmica Online*, 10(52), e235–e235. DOI: 10.36238/2359-5787.2024.v10n52.235

da Cunha Machado, A. M. (2023). Contributos para a Estratégia de Internacionalização no Reino Unido: O Caso do Grupo ADA eo Mercado de Dispositivos Médicos. [HTML]

da Silva, L. R. M. (2024). *Ciência*. Tecnologia e Sociedade. [HTML]

da Silva Lima, F., Vieira, G. B. B., Lazzari, F., Salvador, C. K., & Santos, C. H. S. (2024). Análise dos fatores críticos de sucesso na exportação: um estudo de empresas do setor metal-mecânico da Serra Gaúcha. Revista de Gestão e Secretariado, 15(8), e3973-e3973. revistagesec.org.br

Dallabrida, N. (2023). Brechas no Monólito Educacional: Classes Decundárias Experimentais e Inovação do Ensino Secundário nos Anos de 1950 e 1960. [HTML]

Davi, S. G. (2021). Impactos com a implantação da certificação da norma ABNT NBR ISO 9001: 2015 em um laboratório de um órgão público. ufmg.br

DE ANDRADE. P. I. (). IMPORTÂNCIA E BENEFÍCIOS DO PLANEJAMENTO E DO SETOR TRIBUTÁRIO PARA A TOMADA DE DECISÃO NAS ORGANIZAÇÕES EMPRESARIAIS. repositorio.pgsscogna.com.br. pgsscogna.com.br

de Araújo, L. F., & de Almeida Barros, A. C. (2021). PROPOSTA DE DESENVOLVIMENTO DE UM PLANEJAMENTO ESTRATÉGICO PARA UMA CLÍNICA DE OTORRINOLARINGOLOGIA EM MACEIÓ–AL. Ideias e Inovação-Lato Sensu, 6(2), 122-122. set.edu.br

De Carli, J. P. (2024). O PAPEL DA ODONTOLOGIA E DA PSICOLOGIA NA SAÚDE DA PESSOA IDOSA INSTITUCIONALIZADA. editoracientifica.com.br

de Castro Gil, J. P. (2023). Taxa de Sucesso da Ancoragem Ortodôntica com Recurso a Mini-Implantes Interradiculares no Maxilar Superior-Revisão Sistemática. [HTML]

de Faria, S. R. (2022). Análise da contribuição do lean na redução do impacto ambiental em obras de urbanização. unicamp.br

de Jesus Costa, I. J. (2024). Avaliação dos resultados do planejamento estratégico no Grupo Santa Casa de Belo Horizonte no ciclo 2016 a 2020. ufmg.br

de Jesus Costa, I. J. (2024). Avaliação dos resultados do planejamento estratégico no Grupo Santa Casa de Belo Horizonte no ciclo 2016 a 2020. ufmg.br

de Lima Maia, I. C. V., Peixoto, M. D. G. B., Schwermann, L. P., da Silva, D. L. L., & Maia, D. C. G. (2020). Construções coletivas na formação médica sobre planejamento em saúde. [unirioja.es]. *Temas em Educação e Saúde*, 16(2), 720–734. DOI: 10.26673/tes.v16i2.13823

de Menezes, F. G. (2021). Acesso ao Mercado: Conhecendo os caminhos de acesso no mercado de saúde. [HTML]

de Moraes, L. R., de Araújo Neto, L. T., de Azevedo Garcia, L. H., Mendonça, M. A. B., dos Santos, R. R., & Neto, O. C. (2024). BENEFÍCIOS, DESAFIOS E LEGISLAÇÕES PARA UTILIZAÇÃO DE DRONES NA PRODUÇÃO AGRÍCOLA: UMA REVISÃO DA LITERATURA. Revista Multidisciplinar do Nordeste Mineiro, 3(3). unipacto.com.br

de Oliveira, J. P. R. (). GESTÃO TRIBUTÁRIA E BENEFÍCIOS FISCAIS APLICADOS A EMPRESAS DA CONSTRUÇÃO CIVIL. bib.pucminas.br. pucminas.br de Sousa, L. G., de Oliveira, L. V., de Oliveira, L. V., Rampanelli, G., Felix, D. R., Borba, L. D. O. F., & de Andrade, M. P. D. O. (2024). ABORDAGENS AVANÇADAS NO TRATAMENTO DE DOENÇAS CRÔNICAS. *Brazilian Journal of Implantology and Health Sciences*, 6(9), 1194–1201. emnuvens.com.br. DOI: 10.36557/2674-8169.2024v6n9p1194-1201

de Souza, D. C. (2023). A IMPORTÂNCIA DA CONTROLADORIA CONTÁBIL EM OPERADORAS DE PLANOS DE SAÚDE: UMA ANÁLISE ABRANGENTE. Revista GeTeC. fucamp.edu.br

de Souza, F. R. (2023). Economia circular na indústria eletroeletrônica: o caso da empresa ABC. Revista Produção Online. producaoonline.org.br

de Souza, L. F. R., Vogel, P. T., Venâncio, L. G., & Lopes, L. L. S. R. (2024). Foca nas novas opções de tratamento para reduzir a progressão da doença e melhorar a qualidade de vida dos pacientes. sevenpublicacoes.com.br

de Vianna Tiné, J. P. (2024). Impacto da Tecnologia e Suas Transformações na Área da Saúde. Unirepositório. unirepositorio.education

de Vianna Tiné, J. P. (2024). Impacto da Tecnologia e Suas Transformações na Área da Saúde. Unirepositório. unirepositorio.education

Dias da Silva, C., & Moreira Peixoto, J. F. (2023). APITERAPIA: FINS TERAPÊUTICOS ATRAVÉS DA APITOXINA E OUTROS PRODUTOS DA ABELHA APIS MELLIFERAS. Revista Foco (Interdisciplinary Studies Journal), 16(9). [HTML]

do Aguiar, C. S. (2024). O USO DA TECNOLOGIA EM APOIO AO SISTEMA DE SAÚDE NACIONAL. Unirepositório. unirepositorio.education

do Aguiar, C. S. (2024). O USO DA TECNOLOGIA EM APOIO AO SISTEMA DE SAÚDE NACIONAL. Unirepositório. unirepositorio.education

DOS SANTOS. T. J. (). A APLICABILIDADE DAS FERRAMENTAS DO PLANEJAMENTO ESTRATÉGICO PARA AS MICRO E PEQUENAS ORGANIZAÇÕES. repositorio.pgsscogna.com.br. pgsscogna.com.br

dos Santos, M. M., Alencar, R. A., Schneider, F. F., Fernandes, G. X. D. A., Melo, A. B., Dias, L. A., . . . Farias, J. D. A. (2024). A eficácia das intervenções de saúde pública: avaliação de programas e políticas. Periódicos Brasil. Pesquisa Científica, 3(2), 94-110. emnuvens.com.br

Drago, H. F. (2023). Capacidades dinâmicas produtivas, comportamento estratégico e desempenho organizacional: um estudo nas microcervejarias artesanais. ufsm.br

El Sibaii, M., Granja, J., & Azenha, M. (2024, May). Transformação digital na indústria da construção: Capacitando a gestão de dados através de uma plataforma de modelos de dados de produtos (PDT). In 5º Congresso Português de Building Information Modelling Volume 2 (p. 87). UMinho Editora. uminho.pt

ESTRATÉGICO, D. D. E. U. M. P. (2022). DIGITALIZAÇÃO DE UM CENTRO DE INVESTIGAÇÃO CLÍNICA: DESENHO DE UM PLANO ESTRATÉGICO TRABALHO DE PROJETO. unl.pt

Evangelista, J. R. (2021). Gerenciamento de risco de equipamentos eletromédicos para segurança eletromagnética em estabelecimentos assistencias de saúde. unicamp.br

Falcão, M. S. I. (2021). Modelo regulamentar integrado no sector do medicamento e produtos de saúde: o caso português (passado, presente e futuro). ul.pt

Fangueiro, C. S. P. (2021). [Numa Adega. uminho.pt]. *Otimização da Implementação da Norma ISO*, 22000, 2018.

Ghellere, J. C., de Oliveira, P. H. P., de Aguiar, E. C., de Oliveira Pereira, H. J., Marin, B. T., Fernandes, A. C. S., & Ferreira, A. F. L. (2023). Técnicas Minimamente Invasivas em Cirurgia Geral: Benefícios, Limitações e Futuras Perspectivas. *Brazilian Journal of Implantology and Health Sciences*, 5(5), 3025–3041. emnuvens.com.br. DOI: 10.36557/2674-8169.2023v5n5p3025-3041

Gomes, M. A. (2024). Certificação de um Sistema de Gestão da Qualidade NP EN ISO 9001: 2015 numa Empresa de Injeção de Plástico. ipleiria.pt

Graglia, M. V. & Huelsen, P. (2023). Inovação e competitividade. [HTML]

Guedes, M. M. (2024). ...: Um Contributo da Enfermagem Perioperatória-Desenvolvimento de competências clínicas especializadas na área de Enfermagem Médico-Cirúrgica, na área da .... rcaap.pt

Guerra, D. K. H., da Rocha Legoff, W. G., Menezes, P. H. S. D. S., Dias, M. V. S., Alves, L. P., Sacchi, J., ... & Simplicio, W. K. G. (2024). ESTRATÉGIAS NO DIAGNÓSTICO E CONDUTA DO MELANOMA: UMA ABORDAGEM DERMATOLÓGICA. Revista CPAQV-Centro de Pesquisas Avançadas em Qualidade de Vida, 16(2). cpaqv.org

Health Organization, W. (2020). Avaliação externa conjunta das principais capacidades do RSI da República de Cabo Verde: relatório de missão, 4-8 novembro 2019. google.com

Júlio, A. M. P. (2023). Relatório de Estágio: Um Olhar Sobre os Benefícios Fiscais com Foco No SIFIDE II. [HTML]

JUNER, R. & RODRIGUES, S. (2022). SBIdC-MPH: SISTEMA BASEADO EM INTERNET DAS COISAS PARA O MONITORAMENTO DE PACIENTES COM HIPERTENSÃO. ufscar.br

Kabariti, C. M. C., Cardoso, M. N., & Costa, L. C. (2024). ENVELHECIMENTO E SAUDE, A URGENCIA DOS CUIDADOS PALIATIVOS. Revista Cedigma, 1(1), 53-70. cedigma.com.br

Klein, G. F. (2024). Tecnologia no processo de antecipação de recebíveis: O caso da Securitizadora Digital SA. ufsc.br

Ladeiro, J. G. (2020). Critérios para um Centro de Investigação Clínica de Referência. uc.pt

Lengler, F. (2023). Avaliação de metodologias forenses de análise de cronograma aplicadas à um caso de construção industrial. ufrgs.br

Leoni, M. (2024). A Ciência dos Gatilhos Mentais: Desvendando a Mente. [HTML]

Lima, E. J. A., da Silva, J. V. V., Tenorio, C. M. P., de Lima, C. G., de Melo, D. C., de Lima, R. E., & Pinheiro, T. D. S. A. (2023). Relação entre doenças crônicas não transmissíveis e o tempo de internação de idosos em Unidade de Terapia Intensiva. *Brazilian Journal of Implantology and Health Sciences*, 5(4), 2620–2632. emnuvens.com.br. DOI: 10.36557/2674-8169.2023v5n4p2620-2632

Mabunda, L. C. (2021). Avaliação da regulamentação dos dispositivos médicos em Moçambique e seu enquadramento no contexto global. ul.pt

Machado, A. M. C. (2023). Contributos para a estratégia de internacionalização no Reino Unido: o caso do Grupo ADA eo mercado de dispositivos médicos. uminho.pt

Machado, A. M. C. (2023). Contributos para a estratégia de internacionalização no Reino Unido: o caso do Grupo ADA eo mercado de dispositivos médicos. uminho.pt

Machado, A. M. C. (2023). Contributos para a estratégia de internacionalização no Reino Unido: o caso do Grupo ADA eo mercado de dispositivos médicos. uminho.pt

Machado, L. P. (2024). Proposta de um Plano Estratégico de Marketing para um Sistema Inteligente de Apoio ao Diagnóstico do Cancro da Mama: O caso de Estudo do Projeto …. [HTML]

Machado, L. P. (2024). Proposta de um Plano Estratégico de Marketing para um Sistema Inteligente de Apoio ao Diagnóstico do Cancro da Mama: O caso de Estudo do Projeto …. [HTML]

Machado, L. P. (2024). Proposta de um Plano Estratégico de Marketing para um Sistema Inteligente de Apoio ao Diagnóstico do Cancro da Mama: O caso de Estudo do Projeto …. [HTML].

Martins, J. Z. (2024). O uso da metodologia BIM no gerenciamento e coordenação de projetos. unb.br

Martins, M. I. (2022). Relatórios de Estágio e Monografia intitulada Epilepsia Canina: Contributo dos Dispositivos Médicos. uc.pt

Melo, J. C. (2024). Alinhamento entre o planejamento estratégico eo orçamento: um estudo de caso em uma instituição de ensino superior. ufrn.br

Mendes, J. C. V. (2024). Exposição a Dispositivos Eletrónicos em Idades Precoces–Seu Impacto no Desenvolvimento e Regulação Emocional de Crianças em Idade Pré-Escolar. uminho.pt

Mendes, M. M. (2024). Planejamento estratégico para o desenvolvimento da implementação de franquias de micro e pequenas empresas. unipampa.edu.br

Moreira, K. T. D. (2024). Responsabilidade civil em cirurgias robóticas: desafios e perspectivas no contexto brasileiro.. unisc.br

Oliveira, B. S. D. S. B., Neto, C. F., Damasceno, D. L. N. G., da Costa, E. R., de Paiva Brasil, L. G., Velho Filho, O. P., & Lima, S. C. (2024). ANÁLISE E EVOLUÇÃO DA TELEMEDICINA NO BRASIL NOS ANOS 2019-2023 E SUA ATUAL IMPORTÂNCIA. [revistacontemporanea.com]. *Revista Contemporânea*, 4(10), e6123–e6123. DOI: 10.56083/RCV4N10-088

Oliveira, D., Campelo, F., Poblete, J., Herszkowicz, L., Ribas, R., & Rodrigues, R. (2021). Planejamento estratégico da Viação Paraty: uma proposta com ênfase na inovação e eficiência operacional. itl.org.br

Ordunez, P., & Campbell, N. R., GP, G. A., Angell, S. Y., Lombardi, C., Brettler, J. W., ... & Sharman, J. E. (2022). HEARTS in the Americas: innovations for improving hypertension and cardiovascular disease risk management in primary careHEARTS nas Américas: inovações para melhorar a gestão do risco de hipertensão e de doenças cardiovasculares na atenção primária. Revista Panamericana de Salud Publica= Pan [HTML]. *American Journal of Public Health*, 46, e197–e197. PMID: 36284552

Pacheco, R. P. V. Q. (2023). Desafios na implementação e manutenção de um sistema de gestão integrado* numa organização multisite* âmbitos: qualidade, ambiente, segurança e saúde no …. ipl.pt

Pechim, M. D. F. (2024). O PAPEL ESTRATÉGICO DO DEPARTAMENTO CONTÁBIL: PRÁTICAS, DESAFIOS E INOVAÇÕES. RECIMA21-Revista Científica Multidisciplinar-ISSN 2675-6218, 5(5), e555290-e555290. recima21.com.br

Pereira, C. A. (2023). Impacto das redes sociais na medicina dentária na vertente social e económica em Portugal. rcaap.pt

Pereira, T. P. C. (2024). Explorando os limites da responsabilidade civil: o impacto do desenvolvimento tecnológico dos procedimentos cirúrgicos robóticos.. 52.186.153.119

Pereira Pinheiro, C. M., Schreiber, D., Cherutti, M., & Schmidt, S. (2020). Processo criativo em moda: redes de colaboração entre microempreendedores individuais gaúchos. Diálogo com a Economia Criativa, 5(14). [HTML]

Perez, J. F. L. U. (2020). Modos de convergência regulamentar entre medicamentos e dispositivos médicos no quadro da União Europeia. ul.pt

Perez, J. F. L. U. (2020). Modos de convergência regulamentar entre medicamentos e dispositivos médicos no quadro da União Europeia. ul.pt

Perez, J. F. L. U. (2020). Modos de convergência regulamentar entre medicamentos e dispositivos médicos no quadro da União Europeia. ul.pt

Pontin, A. L., Angélica, C., Miragem, B., & Santorsula, C. B. (2020). Compliance na área da saúde. [HTML]

Pontin, A. L., Angélica, C., Miragem, B., & Santorsula, C. B. (2020). Compliance na área da saúde. [HTML]

Porto, I. G. C. (2024). Processo de regulamentação de dispositivos médicos no brasil: da anvisa até o consumidor final. ufscar.br

Porto, I. G. C. (2024). Processo de regulamentação de dispositivos médicos no brasil: da anvisa até o consumidor final. ufscar.br

Queirós, C. C. (2022). Análise do custo-efetividade da PET/CT com 68Ga-PSMA nos doentes de carcinoma da próstata em recidiva bioquímica após prostatectomia radical. ipl.pt

Ribeiro, V. T. R. (2024). Avaliação e implementação de arquitetura distribuída para disponibilização de serviços de telemedicina em computação em borda. ufcg.edu.br

Rodrigues, F. L. B. (2024). Proposta de planejamento estratégico para uma revista científica da área da administração. ufsc.br

Roveda, A. (2024). Mapeamento de depósitos de patentes referentes a tecnologias utilizadas na detecção do Transtorno do Espectro do Autismo (TEA) no mundo. ufsc.br

Sales, J. L. (2023). Estudo bibliométrico sobre o Sistema de Gestão Integrada (SGI) no Brasil. ufc.br

Santos, A. L. G. (2023). Proposta de planejamento estratégico em uma microempresa: estudo de caso em um comércio especializado no serviço de sinalização de trânsito. ufc.br

Santos, B. S. O. (2023). Gestão de risco em engenharia clínica: revisão sistemática. ufrn.br

Santos, B. S. O. (2023). Gestão de risco em engenharia clínica: revisão sistemática. ufrn.br

Santos Toscas, F. (2021). Abordagens do monitoramento do horizonte tecnológico e prospecção tecnológica em dispositivos médicos. JBES: Brazilian Journal of Health Economics/Jornal Brasileiro de Economia da Saúde, 13(3). [HTML]

Santos Toscas, F., & Alves Teixeira, L. A. (2022). Mapeamento dos bancos de dados em dispositivos médicos: revisão narrativa e o cenário brasileiro para avaliação com dados de mundo real (RWD). JBES: Brazilian Journal of Health Economics/Jornal Brasileiro de Economia da Saúde, 14. [HTML]

Santos Toscas, F., de Morais Oliveira, V. C., & Silveira Silva, A. (2022). O papel da sociedade civil na inovação e incorporação de dispositivos médicos no Brasil. JBES: Brazilian Journal of Health Economics/Jornal Brasileiro de Economia da Saúde, 14. [HTML] Machado, A. M. C. (2023). Contributos para a estratégia de internacionalização no Reino Unido: o caso do Grupo ADA eo mercado de dispositivos médicos. uminho.pt

Severi, L. D. M. (2024). Conectividade e saúde: uma revisão crítica da literatura sobre a inserção da IoT no contexto médico. ufscar.br

Silva, A. C. (2022). Equipamento rapha® para a cura do pé diabético: uma abordagem translacional em saúde. unb.br

Silva, F. A. C. (2023). O financiamento às atividades inovativas na indústria nas regiões brasileiras. ufc.br

Silva, M. L. S. (2021). Análise do protocolo RPL em redes LLNs no ambiente de internet das coisas, healthcare. ufu.br

Silva, S. C. S. (2021). Impacto das Novas ISO 14001: 2015 e ISO 9001: 2015 Nos Sistemas Integrados: Análise de Um Percurso de Transição. [HTML]

Silva, T. G. (2022). Desenvolvimento de um bloco operatório: projeto, construção, equipamentos médicos e vídeo-integração. rcaap.pt

Sousa, D. G., Carvalho, R. B., & Castro, J. M. (2020). Análise da contribuição de mapeamento tecnológico (Roadmapping) para a gestão estratégica da inovação: Estudo de caso de uma multinacional do setor automotivo. Revista Inovação [uninove.br]. *Projetos e Tecnologias*, 8(1), 13–24. DOI: 10.5585/iptec.v8i1.17400

Sousa, I. A. M. (2023). Inovação na Administração de Terapêutica Endovenosa: Aperfeiçoamento da Seringa DUO. uc.pt

Teixeira, L. D. M. (2024). Barreiras e potencialidades para educação médica permanente e continuada em saúde mental na atenção primária: uma revisão de escopo. unb.br

TI, S., Santos, B. J., & Bock, E. G. P. (2023). O preço da vida: entendendo os custos de um dispositivo de assistência ventricular no Brasil. researchgate.net

Toscas, F., Oliveira, V., & Silva, A. (2022). O papel da sociedade civil na inovação e incorporação de dispositivos médicos no Brasil. Jornal Brasileiro de Economia da Saúde. jbes.com.br

Toscas, F. S., de Morais Oliveira, V. C., & Silva, A. S. (2022). The role of civil society in the innovation and incorporation of medical devices in Brazil/O papel da sociedade civil na inovacao e incorporacao de dispositivos medicos no Brasil. [HTML]. *Jornal Brasileiro de Economia da Saúde*, 14(2), 146–155. DOI: 10.21115/JBES.v14.Suppl2.p146-54

Toscas, F. S., de Morais Oliveira, V. C., & Silva, A. S. (2022). The role of civil society in the innovation and incorporation of medical devices in Brazil/O papel da sociedade civil na inovacao e incorporacao de dispositivos medicos no Brasil. [HTML]. *Jornal Brasileiro de Economia da Saúde*, 14(2), 146–155. DOI: 10.21115/JBES.v14.Suppl2.p146-54

Vazquez, F. J. B. (2024). Política de resposta a incidentes cibernéticos e estratégias de aderência à legislação brasileira. Dataset Reports. royaldataset.com

Viegas, A. M. P. F. A. (2021). A cooperação global na regulação do medicamento e os desafios para o acesso à inovação. ul.pt Perez, J. F. L. U. (2020). Modos de convergência regulamentar entre medicamentos e dispositivos médicos no quadro da União Europeia. ul.pt Oliveira, D. J. S. & Ckagnazaroff, I. B. (2024). A colaboração como um dos princípios de governo aberto. Revista Gestão & Conexões. unirioja.es

VIEIRA, M. (2024). Integrando a Agenda 2030 e os Objetivos de Desenvolvimento Sustentável-ODS na Disciplina de Projetos Sociais/IFCE. RCMOS-Revista Científica Multidisciplinar O Saber, 1(1). submissoesrevistacientificaosaber.com

Völz, V. K., Pereira, A. S., Walker, E., & Porciúncula, G. S. (2023). Avaliação de maturidade da Indústria 4.0 em uma empresa fabricante de produtos eletromédicos. [furg.br]. *VETOR-Revista de Ciências Exatas e Engenharias*, 33(1), 80–96. DOI: 10.14295/vetor.v33i1.14662

Wendling, A. P., Paiva, M., & Provezano, A. (2020). APLICAÇÃO DA ANÁLISE SWOT COMO FERRAMENTA DO PLANEJAMENTO ESTRATÉGICO: UM ESTUDO DE CASO EM UMA EMPRESA DE LÁCTEOS LOCALIZADA NA ZONA DA MATA MINEIRA. Gestão da Produção: Organização e Planejamento. academia.edu

Zuin, D. A. (2022). Os Efeitos da 4a Revolução Industrial nas Relações de Trabalho: entre o livre-arbítrio ea exploração. [HTML]

Chapter 11
The Role of Gamification in Fostering a Culture of Innovation in Pharma and Medical Device Companies

Rúben Campanacho
ISLA Santarém, Portugal

Stéphanie Monteiro
Instituto Superior Técnico, Portugal

Ricardo Marcão
https://orcid.org/0000-0003-3277-3078
ISLA Santarém, Portugal

ABSTRACT

Gamification has emerged as a powerful strategy to drive innovation and cultivate a culture of continuous improvement within organizations. By integrating game design elements into non-game contexts, organizations can enhance motivation, engagement, and creativity among employees. This paper explores the multifaceted role of gamification in fostering innovation, covering foundational concepts, psychological underpinnings, practical applications, challenges, and future trends. Through an analysis of case studies and best practices, we highlight how gamification can transform organizational practices, motivate employees, stimulate creativity, and drive meaningful innovation.

DOI: 10.4018/979-8-3693-8598-2.ch011

1. INTRODUCTION

Gamification is an incredibly powerful and influential tool in the context of innovation, serving not only to enable and trigger innovation, but also to cultivate a much wider culture of innovation within an organization. When the principles of gamification are applied to innovation initiatives, they have the remarkable ability to diminish cynicism and resistance towards the processes that necessitate innovation among employees. This is due to the fact that gamification offers a more captivating and enjoyable approach to activities that individuals may not be accustomed to.

By utilizing dedicated tools specifically designed for these innovation-related tasks, rather than attempting to fit a different-shaped peg into an incompatible square hole, they become more applicable and often significantly more effective. Interestingly, the term "gamification" is frequently misinterpreted and misused to suggest an affiliation with gaming. However, this portrayal is entirely misleading when considering the modern usage of the word. In its original context, gamification was associated with the implementation of game-like techniques within non-game environments. Over time, the term has spurred countless discussions, resulting in multiple definitions and varying interpretations.

Ultimately, the conceptualization of gamification revolves around the utilization of game mechanics and experience design to digitally engage and motivate individuals in order to accomplish their goals. This definition finds support in the incorporation of "game components" within "non-game applications," with the express intention of propelling engagement through carefully crafted design features. This can include implementing a compelling "narrative" that successfully captivates the target audience and aligns them with the overall objectives of the activity.

The phenomenon of gamification has been widely embraced by organizations across various industries, recognizing its potential to drive innovation and foster a culture of continuous improvement. One of the key benefits of gamification in the context of innovation is its ability to incentivize participation and boost employee motivation. By incorporating elements such as points, rewards, and leaderboards, organizations can create a sense of competition and achievement that fuels individuals' drive to contribute to the innovation process.

Furthermore, gamification provides a means to address the challenges often associated with innovation, such as resistance to change or fear of failure. Through the use of gamified experiences, individuals are encouraged to take risks, explore new ideas, and overcome obstacles in a safe and supportive environment. The interactive nature of gamification fosters collaboration and teamwork, allowing individuals to work together towards a common goal while also learning from one another.

In addition to its internal benefits, gamification can also have a profound impact on external stakeholders, such as customers or partners. By incorporating gamified elements into products or services, organizations can enhance user engagement and loyalty. For example, loyalty programs that utilize gamification techniques, such as unlocking exclusive rewards or achieving higher status levels, can incentivize customers to remain loyal and actively participate in the brand's ecosystem.

It is important to note that successful implementation of gamification in the context of innovation requires careful planning and consideration. While gamification can be a powerful tool, it is not a one-size-fits-all solution. Organizations must take into account the specific objectives, audience, and context in order to design effective gamified experiences.

In conclusion, gamification has proven to be a valuable strategy in driving innovation and cultivating a culture of continuous improvement. By leveraging game mechanics and experience design, organizations can engage and motivate individuals to actively participate in the innovation process. Whether used internally to enhance employee engagement or externally to boost customer loyalty, gamification offers a unique and effective approach to fostering innovation and achieving strategic goals. (Bellosi et al., 2023; Patrício et al.2021)

2. UNDERSTANDING INNOVATION AND ITS IMPORTANCE

Innovation is typically seen as a change that introduces new ways of doing things, and it can result from a new method, idea, product, or more general outcomes such as improving efficacy, effectiveness, productivity, flexibility, or sustainability. In most cases, the innovation should have a beneficial impact in the form of added value for the stakeholders – i.e., the one who has invested in an innovation process and, in some cases, also the recipient for whom the innovation was intended. Moreover, if an innovation is to be successful, the stakeholders' concerns and needs must be addressed. According to this definition, innovation is not limited to new discoveries made by researchers; rather, it refers to the process of turning new knowledge into value. Some of the most common benefits of innovation are achieving goals, cost reductions, and improving the quality of services. Focusing on non-commercial organizations, whose revenues are mainly obtained from providing public services, and whose main goals are to improve the services provided to all stakeholders, innovation becomes a basic concept in fulfilling their mission. These organizations have been focused, in general, on administrative processes and information systems to achieve better performance, and innovation in these areas is usually required. Without innovation, the delivery of public services in these organizations can be a disadvantage, as it can impair the ability to survive and fulfill the expected mission. (Hanelt et al.2021)

2.1. Defining Innovation

Innovation is the process of transforming new ideas into value, resulting in significant changes in how things are done. This can manifest through new methods, products, services, or broader outcomes like improvements in efficacy, efficiency, productivity, flexibility, or sustainability. Successful innovation addresses stakeholder needs and generates added value. It's crucial to understand that innovation isn't limited to scientific breakthroughs but encompasses the practical application of knowledge to create useful solutions. In non-commercial organizations, innovation is fundamental for improving public services and fulfilling their mission to serve stakeholder needs. (Vaska et al.2021)

2.2. The Importance of Innovation in Organizations

In recent years, the U.S. has seen dramatic changes in the nature of how companies, non-profits, schools, and individuals achieve goals. We are moving into a third era characterized by digital technology and focused on innovation. In the earlier transformation from an agrarian to an industrial economy, multinational corporations, universities and polytechnics, and business schools and management consultancy emerged as the new drivers of prosperity and power. The critical success factor was the efficient mobilization and harnessing of new sources of power such as steam, electricity, and the internal combustion engine. This old notion of value chains joined together by necessity, economic efficiency, and quantity was supplemented by an array of new terms like white-collar work, translating scientific research into practical innovation, and policy interrogation, based on the belief that the right questions could pull solutions out of today's world.

That world is eroding because there is no clear model of where to apply these terms and skills to unlock value and power. The new America will not have a distinct section known as the "knowledge worker." The focus of employee and organizational effectiveness will shift away from seeking supply efficiencies and meeting customer needs toward continuously seeking out new product opportunities and exploiting them with dispatch. In this transformation, U.S. competitiveness at home depends a great deal on how much value and power can be harnessed by pre-configured inter-organizational networks of commercial suppliers, big employers, specialized management-technical services, state and local governments, and system integrators. (Fasnacht & Proba, 2024)

3. GAMIFICATION: CONCEPTS AND APPLICATIONS

Gamification has seen enormous growth in recent years, becoming a powerful tool used by many organizations. As an emerging concept with huge potential, gamification is increasingly popular in companies, as well as in other fields such as education and health. Essentially, gamification is designed to use certain attributes of well-designed games, including player motivation, methodology, and player activities, in other areas for different purposes. Gamification is widely recognized for its ability to effectively engage users in a variety of activities, such as employee training, and to produce correct behavior. When considering an organization's innovation culture, employee motivation is key to enhancing employees' innovative abilities. Innovation culture has five core dimensions: innovative organization, innovation cooperative culture, innovative organization, and innovative strategy.

The term 'gamification' was first introduced in 2002, but it was a concept that had long been practiced under other names since the 1970s. The essence of gamification, in transition, is that it uses the basic elements and principles of game design in non-game contexts. Gamification uses game design techniques, game thinking, and mechanics to enhance non-gaming content in terms of motivation and engagement by making such content 'more game-like'. The main sources of motivation in games are developed by game designers to make the game more interesting. These motivations can be used to enhance product design in other fields. Gamification constitutes a significant addition to a work style and an updated means of articulating from a new and interesting angle in order to get users' attention, bring people together, and drive a behavior or a response that will create value for a specific task or domain. (Santos et al.2021)

3.1. Defining Gamification

Gamification is the application of game design elements and principles in non-game contexts to enhance engagement and motivation. It leverages game mechanics, dynamics, and aesthetics to encourage desired behaviors and achieve specific goals. This can involve incorporating elements like points, badges, leaderboards, challenges, and narratives to make activities more interactive, stimulating, and rewarding. This study adopts this definition of gamification to analyze its implementation in organizations and distinguish it from the use of game elements in serious games. (Tongpaeng et al.2024)

3.2. The Psychology Behind Gamification

Today's technological society is complex, where survival and success depend on efficient information processing, innovation, and coordination, often more than on sheer physical strength. These social and cognitive aspects are far less easy to gamify than simple physical tasks. Nevertheless, current research suggests that gamification done according to sound principles yields benefits, but that the level of difficulty, soundness, and independence of thinking still needs to be kept high. There are many reasons why this could be so, and in the coming sections we outline the key insights and findings on the psychology behind gamification, on the pivotal role of fostering intrinsic motivation and a rich cognitive and social environment to increase educational outcomes, and on why gamification can work so well in an educational context.

When applied wisely, gamification can make life more fun, engaging, and effective. However, the potential benefits associated with gamification also raise potential dangers, and these should not be ignored. The psychological approach to studying the behavior of players is crucial in the field of gamification. It provides an understanding of player types or motivations, from which are derived the system's design and game balance unique to each player. This approach, however, is only a first step in the complete understanding of why users use and continue to use it. It has not been used systematically to study all game elements and how they interrelate. With various tasks developing within a game, research conducted so far found that both different levels of competence and influences of various motivations can be observed. (Zainuddin et al.2020)

4. THE RELATIONSHIP BETWEEN GAMIFICATION AND INNOVATION

The use of game elements is gradually becoming an important trend in today's organizations that want to innovate. Gamification can stimulate an innovation culture by involving employees in virtual tasks that mimic real problems and responsibilities. This suggests that, through game features such as narratives or rewards, employees may have an experience that is almost identical to working, which is beneficial for their organizations. During this process, they can practice and improve knowledge, skills, and abilities that add value to the organization and foster innovation, allowing the company to be in an advantageous position in the market and able to satisfy the customers' needs and desires. The subject of this research combines three concepts: Innovation Culture, Gamification, and Organizations. The increase in competitive intensity and the demand for greater dynamism and adaptation to changes by organizations and their social players makes it essential for employees to perform different and creative activities and be open to change and risk. Since generating innovative ideas is complex, unpredictable, time-consuming, and requires constant effort, and considering that organizations operate in less stimulating and change-resistant environments, applying game elements in everyday processes can make the culture of innovation flourish and enhance the flow of innovative ideas. (Abril & Gimenez-Fernandez, 2024)

4.1. How Gamification Enhances Innovation

Gamification is a game-changing strategy that promotes both the motivation of intrapreneurs and the substantive results of innovation. Gamification is a strategy for involving intrapreneurs in the process of achieving corporate objectives using the mechanics of games. This strategy, based on the principles instilled in gamification processes and systemic and cross-functional intention, is a dynamic force that promotes cooperation and motivation among players, with a proportional increase in the initiatives and innovative results obtained. Through work here, green processes and innovative results can be achieved. Through this chapter, professionals will be able to understand the potential that gamification represents in the innovation strategy, in the activation of intrapreneurs who are tired and disrupted by excess information as an instrument of greater internal innovation efficiency. Gamification offers innovation management opportunities, converting work into serious games and cool organizational environments. The multiplier effect of gamification in its applicable forms is discussed and analyzed in detail, as well as the benefits provided by some examples mentioned. The innovative model proposed in this chapter is called the hybrid SWOT model of gamification, capable of being compared with a common gamification control panel. It is noted that the processes related to this approach for organizations as games offer an effective market change. This study allowed an understanding of the characteristics of the potential that gamification represents in the innovative performance of organizations and in different competitive dynamics. (Patricio et al., 2020; Patricio et al., 2022)

4.2. Case Studies on Successful Implementation

Gamification has been successfully implemented in various organizations to foster innovation and enhance employee engagement. Below are specific case studies that illustrate how gamification strategies have led to significant improvements in innovation processes.

Example 1: Microsoft's Language Quality Game

Microsoft needed to improve the quality of software translations for its global user base. Traditional methods of localization were time-consuming and prone to errors. To address this, Microsoft developed the "Language Quality Game," a platform where employees and users could review and correct translation errors in Microsoft products. Participants earned points, badges, and appeared on leaderboards based on their contributions. This initiative resulted in thousands of translation errors being identified and corrected. It not only improved product quality but also engaged employees and users in a collaborative innovation process, fostering a culture of continuous improvement.

Example 2: SAP Community Network (SCN)

SAP aimed to enhance knowledge sharing and innovation within its global community of developers, customers, and partners. They integrated gamification into the SCN by awarding points, badges, and levels to members who contributed content, answered questions, or participated in discussions. High achievers gained recognition within the community. The gamified elements led to increased user engagement and a significant rise in content creation. This collaborative environment spurred innovation as members shared ideas, solved problems, and improved SAP's products and services.

Example 3: Deloitte Leadership Academy

Deloitte sought to increase engagement in its executive training programs to foster innovative leadership practices. The Deloitte Leadership Academy incorporated gamification by adding badges, leaderboards, and rewards for completing courses and participating in learning activities. The platform personalized learning paths and provided social features for collaboration. Engagement levels soared, with a 37% increase in the number of users returning weekly. Executives became more involved in their professional development, leading to the adoption of innovative strategies and improved leadership across the organization.

Example 4: IBM's Innov8 Simulation Game

IBM needed to educate clients and employees about complex business process management concepts to drive innovation in solutions. They created "Innov8," a series of immersive, 3D simulation games that allowed players to experience and solve real-world business challenges. The game encouraged creative problem-solving and collaboration. "Innov8" enhanced understanding of business processes and promoted innovative thinking. It was adopted by universities and businesses globally, contributing to a workforce better equipped with the skills necessary for innovation.

Example 5: Google's Internal Gamification for Innovation

Google wanted to encourage employees to contribute ideas and foster a culture of innovation. While not a traditional game, Google implemented the "Innovation Time Off" policy, allowing employees to spend 20% of their time on projects they were passionate about. This approach gamified work by introducing autonomy, mastery, and purpose. This policy led to the creation of groundbreaking products like Gmail, Google Maps, and AdSense. By giving employees the freedom to explore and innovate, Google harnessed gamification principles to drive significant innovation.

Example 6: Cisco's Employee Engagement through Gamification

Cisco aimed to improve employee expertise in cybersecurity and foster an innovative security culture. They introduced the "Cisco Security Ninja" program, where employees progressed through belt levels (white to black belt) by completing security training modules and contributing to security initiatives. Each level required mastering new skills and demonstrating innovation in security practices. The program increased participation in security training and encouraged employees to develop innovative solutions to cybersecurity challenges. It strengthened the organization's security posture and cultivated a proactive, innovative workforce.

Example 7: Siemens' Plantville Simulation Game

Siemens needed to educate and engage employees and customers in understanding industrial plant operations and promote innovative solutions. They developed "Plantville," a simulation game similar to "SimCity," where players managed a virtual plant. Players faced real-world challenges, requiring them to optimize processes, improve efficiency, and implement innovative technologies. The game enhanced understanding of Siemens' products and solutions, both internally and among customers. It promoted innovative thinking in plant management and showcased Siemens' commitment to innovation and education. (Viberg et al.2020; Patricio et al., 2022; Girdauskiene et al.2022; Breuer & Ivanov, 2020; Friedrich et al.2020; Spanellis et al., 2020)

5. DESIGNING EFFECTIVE GAMIFICATION STRATEGIES FOR INNOVATION

The extent to which organizations are successful in implementing gamification to foster innovation is contingent on the degree to which an innovative culture is embraced and the extent to which intrinsic motivations driving innovation within the workforce are much stronger in appeal than the extrinsic motivations that gamification provides. It is important to design and implement gamification strategies for innovation that drive more than mere extrinsic motivation. When gamification is only seen in this light and not supported or driven more by the intrinsic nature of the drive to innovate, then success will be limited. An innovative culture is far more powerful as an intrinsic motivation for employees to innovate, as it is strongly rooted in an individual's values and personal growth. The level of innovativeness is likely to grow further where intrinsic motivation is embraced alongside gamification that drives innovation at a more granular level.

The design of gamification strategies must not only address the issue of intrinsic and extrinsic motivation, but it should simultaneously do so at three levels: namely the individual, the group, and the organizational level, with creativity and innovation as the target behaviors. Once these levels are targeted, a 3D strategy is proposed. In this context, a 3D strategy is one that targets each of the three levels of intrinsically motivated, extrinsically motivated, and the organizational culture of motivation. The individual dimension should activate the intrinsic motivation of the workforce, initially inducing early adopters, followed by the early and late majority. The group dimension should then activate extrinsically motivated behavior to drive engagement and innovation. At the final stage, the organizational level, the intrinsic motivational force of the innovative culture is ignited. This will then facilitate the social and human collaboration that is critical in driving engagement and an organizational climate that fosters engagement and organizational innovation. This alignment of the three levels will ensure multiple opportunities to drive innovation at differing levels within the organizational workforce. The design of a suitable gamification strategy has to take into account the varying individuals and different stages of the innovation process, ultimately aiming at appropriate and sustainable innovation contributions. (Nguyen, 2020)

5.1. Key Components of Gamification Strategies

The experience of leading technology companies in the successful use of gamification components in their innovation programs requires special attention and careful consideration in corporations striving to implement such elements. The main components of gamification strategies encompass a wide range of techniques and approaches aimed at creating a more engaging and immersive experience for employees. These strategies include the introduction of rewards and recognition mechanisms into various business processes, creating a sense of achievement and progress that is often associated with the gaming context. Additionally, game mechanics are utilized to stimulate innovation and increase employee involvement in these tasks, fostering a culture of creativity and continuous improvement within the organization. By incorporating game-like elements into work-related activities, employees are encouraged to actively participate and contribute their unique perspectives and ideas.

Moreover, the creation of an atmosphere within the company that is conducive to innovation is of paramount importance. This entails establishing an environment that nurtures and supports innovative thinking, allowing employees to freely explore new ideas and experiment with different approaches. By fostering a workplace culture that values and encourages innovation, organizations can tap into the untapped potential of their workforce, uncovering new solutions and opportunities that can propel the company forward.

In order to foster growth and improvement among employees, it is essential to set specific goals for personal development. This can be achieved through various means, such as performance management or the identification and utilization of individual skills and talents. However, it is crucial to go beyond mere goal-setting and translate these objectives into game goals that are directly related to the development of professional skills. By aligning personal goals with game-like objectives, employees are motivated to proactively pursue their own development, gaining a sense of ownership and control over their growth process. This, in turn, fuels their intrinsic motivation and drive, leading to enhanced performance and productivity.

Notably, gamified business progress management systems provide a plethora of artifacts and tools that offer employees a comprehensive and tangible understanding of what it means to be "innovative". Through the use of interactive platforms and digital interfaces, employees are able to track their progress, receive real-time feedback, and gain insights into their strengths and areas for improvement. These systems not only facilitate performance management but also serve as a catalyst for continuous learning and development. By integrating gamified elements into business processes, companies can unlock the full potential of their employees, fostering a culture of innovation that drives sustainable growth and success.

In conclusion, the implementation of gamification components in innovation programs necessitates careful consideration and a tailored approach. By incorporating rewards and recognition mechanisms, utilizing game mechanics, and fostering an innovative atmosphere, companies can create a work environment that cultivates creativity, engagement, and continuous improvement. Moreover, by setting specific game goals that align with professional development objectives, organizations can stimulate proactivity and empower employees to take control of their growth journey. Lastly, gamified business progress management systems provide invaluable tools and resources that enable employees to enhance their performance and gain a comprehensive understanding of what it means to be innovative. By leveraging these strategies and approaches, companies can unlock the full potential of their workforce and drive long-term success. (Patrício et al.2021)

5.2. Best Practices in Gamification Design

Gamification is a powerful tool capable of addressing shortcomings that undermine the implementation and diffusion of innovation. Once innovation becomes a game—attracting, motivating, and engaging players who perform their best, often beyond their predisposed willingness—it can finally flourish. Although the popularity of gamification has recently soared, the theoretical and empirical academic knowledge is still in its infancy. Dominated by the application of traditional board or card games, with implemented mechanics, dynamics, and game design elements, enabling its intended use, adoption, and ensuring the desired change or development of the players' behavior, the true potential of gamification has barely been scratched.

However, when designing, developing, and integrating gamification, most efforts disregard the underlying scientifically multifaceted and multi-perspective supported knowledge. Multiple best practices can be found in publications and official portals to which actual developers and organizations, lacking the domain expertise needed for successful gamification design and implementation, may tend to ignore or pay little attention to. Therefore, we present an overview of the best practices for all phases of successful gamification design, embracing that marketing and economics-related knowledge provides a valuable precedence to the relatively new gamification domain. Furthermore, the most desirable game design parameters, when being different for the development of a game than the ones adjusting the dynamics of a system, are brought to the discussion with respect to system or process relevant rules. (Pospelova, 2020)

6. CHALLENGES AND LIMITATIONS OF GAMIFICATION IN INNOVATION

Although gamification is considered one of the innovative approaches to innovation in micro-level organizations, it has not been successfully applied due to several limitations and challenges. Indeed, our systematic review of the literature examines some of these challenges and limitations below in order to draw the attention of researchers to address and overcome such limitations.

It is difficult to empirically test the exact effect of gamification. Simulation and experimental methods could be useful in order to save time. However, when seeking social and organizational changes, there is a limit to the use of experimental methods that are criticized for not being able to perform realistic experiments, which makes application to real tasks difficult. Proceeding with behavioral experiments using lotteries or the like makes it difficult to relate the results to the organizational context. Many studies use a laboratory setting or ask people who are inexperienced in gamification games to participate. However, the participation motivation and effects of promoting human resources that the studies aim to investigate are severely limited. Despite the limitations, the importance of experimental empirical research and using laboratory settings is emphasized. (Trinidad et al., 2021)

6.1. Common Challenges Faced in Implementation

Over the last decade, organizations have adopted gamification strategies to increase engagement among employees, especially in areas of human resources and in learning and development. Although there is a growing body of research on gamification, findings from existing studies appear to be somewhat positive and defensive, while most studies focus on the effect on learning outcomes and results. So far, little research has focused on the reasons behind the success and failure of gamification, and even less research has studied the conditions associated with successful implementations in which little or no change can be seen in the recorded measurements. In gamification research, one key area that seems to be under-researched is around a broader set of effects on employee work, its effect on relationships, and its ability to encourage the organizational culture as a whole. A further area that appears to be under-researched is around challenges and implementation of gamification and its interconnectedness with the individual, the team, and the organizational context, as well as the role of leaders and organizations. This chapter applies a realist approach to a case study to better understand gamification through three separate reasoning cycles to identify common challenges faced in the implementation of a gamified solution, the potential impact of these challenges on the effectiveness of a gamified solution, and the measures and strategies that can be introduced to address these challenges in order to avoid the identified problems. (Gupta et al., 2022)

6.2. Addressing Ethical and Privacy Concerns

The sensitivity of a product's data can provoke users' defensive behaviors. Data privacy has always been a concern. However, blended with the shifting sense of identity, concerns about privacy can stifle the engagement experience. Having more users opt out of full engagement would result in a less effective solution. The platform addresses this very unsubtly at every touchpoint. To protect the privacy of the data, AI models run on each user's device to analyze and act on the information. This information is never sent to the server. The server even accepts any data formatting, and if a string of bad input data, which would generally be normal and human, is encountered, the server will accept it graciously and with a smile. The platform uses blockchain to associate anonymized user data with unique session IDs. This allows the user to remain anonymous to the platform, all other entities, and to all non-blockchain entities. However, a recognized pseudonym in the blockchain also increases the user's credibility by associating the user's usage data. People willfully opt in to receive the token-issuing association provided by the platform. Upon deployment, these associations will be further reinforced by cluster associations, profiles formed by members of different industries, and by gaming preferences. Information is shared broadly through the platform, being disseminated in this fashion to maintain its sense of community. A community adds authenticity to the proof of capability. (Alkadi et al., 2020)

7. MEASURING THE IMPACT OF GAMIFICATION ON INNOVATION

In the face of 80 percent of gamification initiatives failing, it is hard to measure the success of gamification. The success stories highlight gadgets and low-level engagement but not relationships or motivation and innovation processes in gaming. The absence of the position of gamification manager shows how gamification has not been embedded in organizations for a business outcome and has become simply another HR-sponsored, feel-good employee engagement routine. But as institutions steamroll us into the future, we will have an unintended avalanche of worker discontent and a shortage of new ideas to face the obvious challenges we are confronted with. Trends suggest a growing risk of collapse. When analyzing what factors are needed for us to embed innovation into the corporate culture to prepare for the future and what effects the journey may have, the role of gamification arises. The indications are that we have embraced word games for entrepreneurial development and brainstorming ideas for innovation during resting time and exploration in swaps. The question to consider is whether our gamified playtime can be extended to aid company innovation. We registered metrics that can be utilized to both create an environment where corporate-instituted gamification will benefit the firm and its employees and when the benefit will be realized. We further consider the type of play and event data needed to support play, and finally, the corporate managerial support of innovation resources that will encourage staff participation in gamified events and show that their leaders are innovative role models who understand and support employee work culture and processes. (Benitez et al., 2022)

7.1. Key Metrics for Evaluating Success

To correctly evaluate the ability of a gamification initiative to foster a culture of innovation, it is important as a first step to define which dimensions should be considered. Because the general purpose of gamification is to use game mechanisms to foster engagement in a defined context, for evaluating the success of a gamification project, we need to consider standard game constructs and then define appropriate key performance indicators. Game technology presents intrinsic qualities including the capability to motivate, persuasiveness, viral nature, and monitoring, which are inherited by gamification technology and could be exploited to engage users in the innovation process. Those attributes of gamification systems are usually summarized under the common name of 'gamification drivers'. The concept defines potential stimuli that can be engaged to prompt people's innovation or creativity abilities or to capture explicit innovation-related activities performed by the user in the scope of a predefined gamified context.

The capability to motivate measures how a system is able to attract the participation of a group of people in a predefined context. A wide set of factors that contribute to motivating engagement has been defined, including feedback, challenge, exploration, and control. Six are generally recognized as the basic needs that underpin an individual's intrinsic motivation and the capability of a task to be engaging. Satisfaction of these needs can lead to the individual's seeking out and thriving in challenging, novel, and optimal experiences, which in turn also contribute to the development and maintenance of personal well-being. Therefore, the presence of these factors in a gamification construct is crucial to assess the capability of the system to attract and maintain user attention and, in turn, to enable continuous participation and commitment. (Breuer et al.2023)

7.2. Tools and Methods for Data Collection

Companies use both automated and non-automated sensors in the workplace to collect data. While non-automated sensors require employee action to collect data, automated sensors record data whenever an employee is in the workplace. Through non-automated sensors, employees can provide qualitative, event-based data, either by pushing a button or by using voice recognition technology to log activities. However, logging is often voluntary, time-consuming, and requires specific, frontal commitment. Automated sensors, on the other hand, can detect things at a very exciting level. Examples include monitoring usage of kitchen appliances, access to workplace lockers, presence in the office, time spent at the desk, and browsing history.

A broad range of data on activities such as interpersonal, productivity, and work interruptions can be gathered through communication patterns. Such data have been used to measure the impact of workplace design on collaboration and have aided in the design of effective corporate programs to increase productive exchanges between employees. Sensors to track location, movement, and proximity of personnel can also be used to study social interactions. Data from such devices revealed that planners, particularly those in the top echelons of the company, had significantly more frequent and more prolonged interactions than did average workers, indicating the importance of social interaction and social density in promoting specific organizational and functional outcomes. In sum, there is a growing body of evidence that new workplace sensors offer tremendous potential for expanding the scope and rigor of organizational research. (Eisenberg, 2025)

8. FUTURE TRENDS AND EMERGING TECHNOLOGIES IN GAMIFICATION

The concept of gamification has been around for quite some time now, and during this period, it has undergone constant development in the construction, planning, and performance of tasks, covering both the professional and personal spheres. This chapter helped in understanding the concept itself and the benefits of using games as a motivational force in innovative companies. It is in light of emerging trends and technologies in gamified platforms that the future of the concept of gamification will be discussed in this chapter. It is noticeable how gamified environments are becoming increasingly common in companies, given the various motivational and rewarding technologies. Furthermore, the expansion and development of games have increased the range of possibilities for applying these technologies within companies, whose primary premise is to engage and stimulate innovative behavior in ideal employees. Such technologies allow employees to self-assess their task performance while directing them toward continuous improvement. It relies on constant feedback. In addition, such platforms also allow the identification of players' preferences, promoting more strategic decisions when establishing challenges or aligning objectives. As technology evolves and becomes easily accessible, there is no reason to doubt its applicability in terms of stimulating behaviors. Employees already understand intuitively and in personal use the rewards of immediate feedback, challenging goals, enjoyment, and fast-cycle assessments that changed platforms already provide. Other aspects of gamification include augmented reality and virtual reality. These technologies seem to be the crystallization of the ideal scenario for gamification. They allow individuals to experience and feel reality in an artificial form. Although their effective application range is still limited, their market is growing at a dizzying pace; companies continue to evolve and, indeed, invest in the creation of virtual simulations increasingly similar to reality. The potential of these technologies to revolutionize the way businesses operate is immense. With the use of augmented reality, employees can engage in hands-on training and simulations that mimic real-world scenarios, allowing for a more immersive and effective learning experience. Virtual reality, on the other hand, can transport individuals to entirely different environments, creating opportunities for team collaboration and problem-solving in a virtual space. These advancements in technology are paving the way for a new era of gamification, where companies can leverage the power of immersive experiences to drive employee engagement and productivity. Additionally, gamification can extend beyond the workplace and into various aspects of everyday life. From fitness apps that reward users for reaching their exercise goals to educational platforms that turn learning into a game, the potential applications of gamification are vast and ever-expanding. The key to successful gamification lies in thoughtful design and implementation. By understanding the motivations and preferences of users, companies can create compelling experiences that capture attention and drive desired behaviors. Whether it's through challenges, rewards, or friendly competition, gamification has the ability to tap into the innate human desire for achievement and mastery. As technology continues to advance and become more accessible, the future of gamification holds countless possibilities. It is an exciting time for businesses and individuals alike as they explore the full potential of gamified experiences to transform the way we work, learn, and interact. (Patrício et al.2021; Viberg et al.2020; Van et al.2020)

8.1. AI and Machine Learning in Gamification

Adopting AI and machine learning techniques can greatly complement the mechanics of gamification strategies. In fact, the integration of AI into gamification can revolutionize the way digitalization aspects are personalized and learned from user behavior to adjust goal setting and tangible objects or rewards. By leveraging the latest technological advancements, the gaming industry has the potential to universally underpin and drive the mechanics of gamification through AI and machine learning.

These tools have the unique capability to rapidly broaden the company context of implementing gamification interventions that are framed upon behavioral change.

To truly understand the transformative power of AI and machine learning in enhancing gamification, practitioners must delve into the potential of AI technologies to improve and personalize gamification functions. They are invaluable tools that enable the technology-enabled shaping of intended behavior. With AI and machine learning, it becomes possible to simulate, interact, or even hold a conversation with users. This level of interaction allows for a deep understanding of the principal causes behind behavior, enabling the design of tailored mechanics and fostering meaningful dialogue.

Exploring popular AI and machine learning approaches, such as reinforcement learning, deep learning, neural networks, and knowledge-based techniques, can provide valuable insights into modeling game players' behavior. By addressing potential challenges and obstacles, such as the integration of AI and machine learning for gamifying learning, we can debunk the theory that there is a lack of synergy between the respective fields of machine learning, AI, and gamification. On the contrary, there is a strong belief that a closer bond between these disciplines could create more empathy and interest among users.

In addition, it is important to disclose and address the technical challenges and limitations associated with developing AI-driven gamification. By anticipating and tackling these obstacles head-on, practitioners can pave the way for a future where AI and machine learning are seamlessly integrated into gamification efforts. Futuristic approaches that further link game theory with AI hold tremendous potential for revolutionizing the gaming industry and taking gamification to new heights. The possibilities are endless, and by embracing AI and machine learning, we can unlock a whole new world of gamification experiences. (Suresh and Dhakshina, 2024; Rane et al., 2023; Bezzina and Dingli, 2023)

8.2. Virtual Reality and Augmented Reality Integration

With respect to virtual reality (VR) and augmented reality (AR) integration, it has been receiving a great deal of research attention from several disciplines including science, technology, education, and medicine. With the growing number of VR applications and the increasing proliferation of AR, both have increasingly offered incredible opportunities to enhance education and training areas including workplace learning, cognitive skill acquisition, serious gaming, simulations, and creativity. This research addresses how to integrate VR and AR into a general gamified system, creating synergistic effects on user engagement and achievement. The research first introduces the concepts of VR and AR and systematically reviews ten related experiential studies conducted over the past 25 years. Then, it introduces the concept of entertainment technology (ET) to delineate an essential element to foster a user's intention for the ET system and describes the process of describing and comparing a novel ET (VR- and/or AR-integrated gamified type): on one hand, a gamified system encourages users to form the willingness to participate (entertained users in general), whereas, on the other hand, a non-gamified type ET application targets highly skilled users through high-effort applications; thus, both entertain and train users. Furthermore, incorporating VR and AR into gamified systems, respectively, can add effects of intrinsic motivation and four related theoretical constructs - namely, flow, presence, emotional involvement, and visual impact - into an efficient intention to foster the attributes of ET system use. Finally, the research provides substantial implications for producers and developers to promote the new wave of ET applications besides discussing recommendations and limitations of the research. (Lampropoulos et al.2022; Farooq et al.2022)

9. CONCLUSION

Gamification has emerged as a powerful strategy for fostering a culture of innovation within organizations. This paper has explored the multifaceted role of gamification, from its foundational concepts and psychological underpinnings to practical applications and future trends. By integrating game elements into non-game contexts, organizations can enhance motivation, engagement, and creativity among employees, leading to increased innovation and competitive advantage.

The key findings highlight that gamification enhances engagement by incorporating elements like points, badges, and leaderboards, which significantly boost employee participation in innovation processes. Understanding psychological drivers is crucial; recognizing the intrinsic and extrinsic motivations that influence employee behavior is essential for designing effective gamification strategies. Effective design is multidimensional, requiring careful consideration of individual, group, and organizational levels to align game mechanics with innovation goals. Challenges such as evaluation difficulties and ethical concerns must be addressed proactively, with organizations developing strategies to overcome these limitations. The integration of emerging technologies like AI, machine learning, virtual reality, and augmented reality holds great promise for the future of gamification in driving innovation.

The importance of gamification in promoting innovation cannot be overstated. In an era where businesses face rapid technological changes and increasing competition, fostering an innovative culture is vital for sustainability and growth. Gamification provides a unique approach to engaging employees, encouraging them to think creatively and collaborate effectively. It transforms routine tasks into engaging experiences, unlocking the full potential of the workforce.

From a practical standpoint, organizations should strategically implement gamification by designing strategies that align with their innovation objectives and consider the specific needs and motivations of their employees. Continuous evaluation is necessary to measure impact and make data-driven improvements. Ethical considerations are essential to maintain trust and ensure the long-term success of gamification efforts. Leveraging emerging technologies can enhance the effectiveness of gamification, providing immersive and personalized experiences that drive innovation.

Future research should focus on long-term impact studies to understand the sustained effects of gamification on innovation and organizational performance. Cross-cultural analysis can provide insights for global implementation, and exploring how gamification intersects with other organizational behavior theories may offer deeper understanding and more robust frameworks. Developing comprehensive guidelines to address ethical and privacy concerns associated with gamification technologies is also crucial.

In conclusion, gamification stands as a transformative approach that can significantly contribute to building and sustaining a culture of innovation. By thoughtfully integrating game design elements into organizational practices, companies can motivate their employees, stimulate creativity, and drive meaningful innovation. As technology continues to evolve, embracing gamification will be instrumental for organizations aiming to stay ahead in the dynamic landscape of the modern business world. (Bellosi et al., 2023; AlSaad and Durugbo, 2021; Sharma et al., 2024)

REFERENCES

Abril, C., & Gimenez-Fernandez, E. M. (2024). Using gamification to overcome innovation process challenges: A literature review and future agenda. Technovation. sciencedirect.comDOI: 10.1109/ACCESS.2022.3221473

Alkadi, O., Moustafa, N., & Turnbull, B. (2020). A review of intrusion detection and blockchain applications in the cloud: approaches, challenges and solutions. IEEE Access. ieee.orgDOI: 10.1109/ACCESS.2022.3221473

AlSaad, F. M., & Durugbo, C. M. (2021). Gamification-as-innovation: A review. [researchgate.net]. *International Journal on Management of Innovation & Technology*, 18(05), 2130002. DOI: 10.1142/S0219877021300020

Bellosi, F., Spadafora, M., & Rapaccini, M. (2023). Creating the Culture for Sustainable Innovation: A Gamified Approach. Sustainability. mdpi.comDOI: 10.1109/ACCESS.2022.3221473

Benitez, J., Ruiz, L., & Popovic, A. (2022). Impact of mobile technology-enabled HR gamification on employee performance: An empirical investigation. Information & Management. sciencedirect.comDOI: 10.1109/ACCESS.2022.3221473

Bezzina, S., & Dingli, A. (2023, July). Rethinking gamification through artificial intelligence. In International Conference on Human-Computer Interaction (pp. 252-263). Cham: Springer Nature Switzerland.

Breuer, H., Ivanov, K., & Abril, C. (2023). Management guidelines to address cultural challenges and facilitate values-based innovation through gamification. [uxberlin.com]. *International Journal of Entrepreneurship and Innovation Management*, 27(3-4), 208–236. DOI: 10.1504/IJEIM.2023.133383

Eisenberg, D. (2025). *The Future of Work in a Digital World*. Digital Transformation And Society.

Farooq, S. S., Rahman, H., Raza, S. A. N., Raees, M., & Jung, S. K. (2022). Designing gamified application: An effective integration of augmented reality to support learning. [ieee.org]. *IEEE Access : Practical Innovations, Open Solutions*, 10, 121385–121394. DOI: 10.1109/ACCESS.2022.3221473

Fasnacht, D., & Proba, D. (2024). Leveraging inter-organizational agility for innovation. Strategy & Leadership. researchgate.netDOI: 10.1109/ACCESS.2022.3221473

Friedrich, J., Becker, M., Kramer, F., Wirth, M., & Schneider, M. (2020). Incentive design and gamification for knowledge management. [e-tarjome.com]. *Journal of Business Research*, 106, 341–352. DOI: 10.1016/j.jbusres.2019.02.009

Girdauskiene, L., Ausrine Ciplyte, E., & Navickas, V. (2022). Gamification as an innovative instrument for employee engagement. Marketing i menedžment innovacij, (1), 10-17. zbw.eu Breuer, H. & Ivanov, K. (2020). Gamification to address cultural challenges and to facilitate values-based innovation. ISPIM Conference Proceedings. DOI: 10.21272/mmi.2022.1-01

Gupta, M., Behl, A., & Kumar, Y. L. N. (2022). "Prevention is better than cure": Challenges in engaging employees through gamification. *International Journal of Manpower*, 43(2), 380–394. DOI: 10.1108/IJM-03-2021-0172

Hanelt, A., Bohnsack, R., Marz, D., & Antunes Marante, C. (2021). A systematic review of the literature on digital transformation: Insights and implications for strategy and organizational change. [wiley.com]. *Journal of Management Studies*, 58(5), 1159–1197. DOI: 10.1111/joms.12639

Lampropoulos, G., Keramopoulos, E., Diamantaras, K., & Evangelidis, G. (2022). Augmented reality and gamification in education: A systematic literature review of research, applications, and empirical studies. applied sciences, 12(13), 6809. mdpi.comDOI: 10.1109/ACCESS.2022.3221473

Nguyen, T. M. (2020). Do extrinsic motivation and organisational culture additively strengthen intrinsic motivation in online knowledge sharing? An empirical study. *VINE Journal of Information and Knowledge Management Systems*, 50(1), 75–93. DOI: 10.1108/VJIKMS-02-2019-0019

Patricio, R., Moreira, A., Zurlo, F., & Melazzini, M. (2020). Co-creation of new solutions through gamification: A collaborative innovation practice. [ssrn.com]. *Creativity and Innovation Management*, 29(1), 146–160. DOI: 10.1111/caim.12356

Patrício, R., Moreira, A. C., & Zurlo, F. (2021). Enhancing design thinking approaches to innovation through gamification. [researchgate.net]. *European Journal of Innovation Management*, 24(5), 1569–1594. DOI: 10.1108/EJIM-06-2020-0239

Patricio, R., Moreira, A. C., & Zurlo, F. (2022). Gamification in innovation teams. International Journal of Innovation Studies. sciencedirect.comDOI: 10.1109/ACCESS.2022.3221473

Pospelova, T. (2020). Uncovering nudges in gamification and their application in organizational change. aalto.fiDOI: 10.1109/ACCESS.2022.3221473

Rane, N., Choudhary, S., & Rane, J. (2023). Education 4.0 and 5.0: Integrating artificial intelligence (AI) for personalized and adaptive learning. Available at *SSRN* 4638365. *ssrn.com* DOI: 10.2139/ssrn.4638365

Santos, A. C. G., Oliveira, W., Hamari, J., Rodrigues, L., Toda, A. M., Palomino, P. T., & Isotani, S. (2021). The relationship between user types and gamification designs. [springer.com]. *User Modeling and User-Adapted Interaction*, 31(5), 907–940. DOI: 10.1007/s11257-021-09300-z

Sharma, W., Lim, W. M., Kumar, S., Verma, A., & Kumra, R. (2024). Game on! A state-of-the-art overview of doing business with gamification. [sciencedirect.com]. *Technological Forecasting and Social Change*, 198, 122988. DOI: 10.1016/j.techfore.2023.122988

Spanellis, A., D rfler, V., & MacBryde, J. (2020). Investigating the potential for using gamification to empower knowledge workers. Expert Systems with Applications. strath.ac.uk

Suresh Babu, S., & Dhakshina Moorthy, A. (2024). Application of artificial intelligence in adaptation of gamification in education: A literature review. *Computer Applications in Engineering Education*, 32(1), e22683. DOI: 10.1002/cae.22683

Tongpaeng, Y., Nobnop, R., Wongwan, N., Homla, P., Intawong, K., & Puritat, K. (2024). Comparison of gamified and non-gamified mixed reality in enhancing museum visitor engagement, motivation, and learning outcome. *Journal of Heritage Tourism*, 19(6), 1–30. DOI: 10.1080/1743873X.2024.2351852

Trinidad, M., Calderón, A., & Ruiz, M. (2021). GoRace: a multi-context and narrative-based gamification suite to overcome gamification technological challenges. IEEE Access. ieee.orgDOI: 10.3389/fpsyg.2020.539363 PMID: 33584396

Van der Heijden, B. I. J. M., Burgers, M. J., Kaan, A. M., Lamberts, B. F., Migchelbrink, K., Van den Ouweland, R. C. P. M., & Meijer, T. (2020). Gamification in dutch businesses: An explorative case study. [sagepub.com]. *SAGE Open*, 10(4), 2158244020972371. DOI: 10.1177/2158244020972371

Vaska, S., Massaro, M., Bagarotto, E. M., & Dal Mas, F. (2021). The digital transformation of business model innovation: A structured literature review. [frontiersin.org]. *Frontiers in Psychology*, 11, 539363. DOI: 10.3389/fpsyg.2020.539363 PMID: 33584396

Viberg, O., Khalil, M., & Lioliopoulos, A. (2020). Facilitating ideation and knowledge sharing in workplaces: The design and use of gamification in virtual platforms. In Learning and Collaboration Technologies. Human and Technology Ecosystems: 7th International Conference, LCT 2020, Held as Part of the 22nd HCI International Conference, HCII 2020, Copenhagen, Denmark, July 19–24, 2020 [Springer International Publishing.]. *Proceedings*, 22(Part II), 353–369.

Zainuddin, Z., Chu, S. K. W., Shujahat, M., & Perera, C. J. (2020). The impact of gamification on learning and instruction: A systematic review of empirical evidence. *Educational Research Review*, 30, 100326. DOI: 10.1016/j.edurev.2020.100326

Compilation of References

Aadahl, M., & Bjerre-Nielsen, A. (2019). Leadership in remote teams: The case of a Danish healthcare organization. *Journal of Health Organization and Management*, 33(2), 125–140. DOI: 10.1108/JHOM-09-2018-0268

Abreu, M. M. V. (2020). O controle sanitário eo acesso a dispositivos médicos no Brasil: um estudo comparativo no cenário de convergência regulatória. fgv.br

Abril, C., & Gimenez-Fernandez, E. M. (2024). Using gamification to overcome innovation process challenges: A literature review and future agenda. Technovation. sciencedirect.comDOI: 10.1109/ACCESS.2022.3221473

Adebayo, Y. A., Ikevuje, A. H., Kwakye, J. M., & Esiri, A. E.Yetunde Adenike AdebayoAugusta Heavens IkevujeJephta Mensah KwakyeAndrew Emuobosa Esiri. (2024). Driving circular economy in project management: Effective stakeholder management for sustainable outcomes. *GSC Advanced Research and Reviews*, 20(3), 235–245. DOI: 10.30574/gscarr.2024.20.3.0351

Adeghe, E. P., Okolo, C. A., & Ojeyinka, O. T.Ehizogie Paul AdegheChioma Anthonia OkoloOlumuyiwa Tolulope Ojeyinka. (2024). A review of emerging trends in telemedicine: Healthcare delivery transformations. *International Journal of Life Science Research Archive*, 6(1), 137–147. DOI: 10.53771/ijlsra.2024.6.1.0040

Afonso, A. M., Cadwell, J. B., Staffa, S. J., Zurakowski, D., & Vinson, A. E. (2021). Burnout rate and risk factors among anesthesiologists in the United States. *Anesthesiology*, 134(5), 683–696. DOI: 10.1097/ALN.0000000000003722 PMID: 33667293

Agegnehu, W., Abdissa, D., & Alemayehu, D. (2022). Confirmatory and exploratory factor analysis for validating Allen and Meyer organizational commitment questionnaire for health professionals in Ethiopia—Amharic language. *Journal of Healthcare Leadership*, 14, 99–111. DOI: 10.2147/JHL.S364973 PMID: 35782682

Agner, L. (2023). Ergodesign e arquitetura da informação: trabalhando com o usuário. [HTML]

Aires, J. D. M. (2021). Avaliação de dinâmicas e orientações para a medição da inovação empresarial no turismo. [HTML]

Ajiga, D., Okeleke, P. A., Folorunsho, S. O., & Ezeigweneme, C. (2024). Methodologies for developing scalable software frameworks that support growing business needs. DOI: 10.1016/j.apenergy.2024.123789

Almasri, F. (2024). Exploring the impact of artificial intelligence in teaching and learning of science: A systematic review of empirical research. *Research in Science Education*, 54(5), 977–997. DOI: 10.1007/s11165-024-10176-3

Al-Mekhlafi, A. B. A., Isha, A. S. N., Chileshe, N., Abdulrab, M., Saeed, A. A. H., & Kineber, A. F. (2021). Modelling the relationship between the nature of work factors and driving performance mediating by role of fatigue. *International Journal of Environmental Research and Public Health*, 18(13), 6752. DOI: 10.3390/ijerph18136752 PMID: 34201674

Alotaibi, A., Habib, S. S., Al-Khlaiwi, T., Alodhayani, A., Rashed, Z. F., Al Mahdali, G., Alanazi, S., Al Hassan, S., Al-Anazi, S., Al Saif, R. A., & Alsaegh, N. A. (2024). Ambient conditions of the operating theatre and its correlation with fatigue and sleep quality of operating room workers: A cross-sectional survey. *Frontiers in Public Health*, 12, 1392950. DOI: 10.3389/fpubh.2024.1392950 PMID: 38813423

AlSaad, F. M., & Durugbo, C. M. (2021). Gamification-as-innovation: A review. [researchgate.net]. *International Journal on Management of Innovation & Technology*, 18(05), 2130002. DOI: 10.1142/S0219877021300020

Alves da Silva, A., de São Pedro Filho, F., Vasconcelos de Melo, J., Veludo Watanabe, C. Y., dos Santos, M. C., & Imam, A. (2015). Innovating the Organization through the Green Marketing Strategy. *International Journal of Research en Social Sciences*, 11(2), 165–178.

Alzahrani, A., & Alhalafawy, W. (2023). Gamified e-learning environments: Impact on student motivation and engagement. *Journal of Educational Technology & Society*, 26(1), 25–40. DOI: 10.1080/14364523.2023.0001

Amaral, C. M. (2021). Análise multicritério para apoio à seleção de fornecedores de dispositivos médicos. iscte-iul.pt

Amaral, M. B. & Rego, S. (2020). Doenças raras na agenda da inovação em saúde: avanços e desafios na fibrose cística. Cadernos de Saúde Pública. scielo.br

Ambrozio, A. M. H. P., & Dunham, F. B. (2024). Política industrial moderna: teoria e evidência empírica. bndes.gov.br

Anwar, A., Heller, K. O., Esper, S. A., & Ferreira, R. G. (2021). Nonoperating room anesthesia: Strategies to improve performance. *International Anesthesiology Clinics*, 59(4), 27–36. DOI: 10.1097/AIA.0000000000000339 PMID: 34456276

Arangüena, L., & Dorado, J. (2001). *Psicofisiologia: fundamentos metodológicos*. Ediciones Pirâmide.

Araujo, E. R., & Pereira, D. (2020). Entidades de mediação e constituição de parcerias institucionais locais: uma reflexão a partir do Famalicão made in, Portugal. DRd-Desenvolvimento Regional em debate, 10, 1123-1138. unc.br

Arora, V. M., & Kachalia, A. (2016). Leadership in healthcare: The importance of leadership for high-quality healthcare delivery. *Journal of the American Medical Association*, 316(10), 1063–1064. DOI: 10.1001/jama.2016.9472

Arshad, A. R., Rajashekar, M. R., & Srinivasan, . (2020). A Study on Mode of Injury, Types of Fractures and Associated Trauma in Unstable Pelvic Fractures. *Journal of Pharmaceutical Research International*, 32(12), 86–91. DOI: 10.9734/jpri/2020/v32i1230565

Asuquo, A.I., & Effiong, S.A., Tapang & Arzizeh, T. (2004). The effect of financial management practices on the Profitability of Small a Medium Enterprise in Nigeria. International Journal of Research in IT, Management and Engineering

Atanassov, A., Pilev, D., & Tomova, F. (2024). MULTIMODAL SYSTEM FOR FACIAL EMOTION RECOGNITION BASED ON DEEP LEARNING. *Journal of Chemical Technology and Metallurgy*, 59(3), 729–740. DOI: 10.59957/jctm.v59.i3.2024.29

Atkinson, A. A., & McCrindell, J. . (1997). Strategic performance measurement in government. *CMA Magazine*, •••, 20–23.

Averlid, G., & Høglund, J. S. (2020). The operating room as a learning arena: Nurse anaesthetist and student nurse anaesthetist perceptions. *Journal of Clinical Nursing*, 29(9-10), 1673–1683. DOI: 10.1111/jocn.15227 PMID: 32096572

Avritzer, L., Kerche, F., & Marona, M. (2021). Governo Bolsonaro: retrocesso democrático e degradação política. [HTML]

Babbie, E. (2010). *The Practice of Social Research* (12th ed.).

Baca, G. (2010). Evaluación de proyectos (69 ed.). Cidade do México: McGraw Hill Education.

Bach, S. (2021). Managing remote teams in healthcare: Strategies and challenges. *Health Services Management Research*, 34(1), 24–31. DOI: 10.1177/0951484820917712

Baig, M. S., Rocha, D. F. B., & Horwitz, D. S. (2021). *Injuries of the Pelvis*. Hoppenfeld's Treatment and Rehabilitation of Fractures.

Bak, P. (2012). Aspectos selecionados do planeamento financeiro em empresas mineiras. *AGH Journal of Mining and Geoengineering*, 36(3), 49–54.

Barañano, A. M. (2008). *Métodos e Técnicas de Investigação em Gestão*. Edições Sílabo.

Barcaui, A. B., Borba, D. B., Da Silva, I. M., & Neves, R. B. (2021). Gerenciamento de cronograma em projetos. [HTML]

Barrett, L. F., & Wager, T. D. (2006). The structure of emotion: Evidence from neuroimaging studies. *Current Directions in Psychological Science*, 15(2), 79–83. DOI: 10.1111/j.0963-7214.2006.00411.x

Basarah, J. C., Andry, A., & Tahjoo, A. (2022). Perceived accreditation benefits, participation and organizational commitment in hospital accreditation performance. *International Journal of Public Health Science*, 11(2), 527–536. DOI: 10.11591/ijphs.v11i2.20980

Bashar, S., Wang, D., & Rafiq, M. (2023). Adoption of green supply chain management in developing countries: Role of consumer cooperation, eco-design and green marketing. *Environmental Science and Pollution Research International*, 30(40), 92594–92610. DOI: 10.1007/s11356-023-28881-3 PMID: 37495804

Bauer, M. W., & Gaskell, G. (2017). *Qualitative research with text, image and sound: a practical manual*. Editora Vozes Limitada.

Belrhiti, Z., Bigdeli, M., Lakhal, A., Kaoutar, D., Zbiri, S., & Belabbes, S. (2024). Unravelling collaborative governance dynamics within healthcare networks: A scoping review. *Health Policy and Planning*, 39(4), 412–428. DOI: 10.1093/heapol/czae005 PMID: 38300250

Bento, K. D. (2020). Sustainability in shopping malls: The fusion between a green marketing tool and a competitive advantage strategy. *Revista Produção Online*, 20(3), 993–1016. DOI: 10.14488/1676-1901.v20i3.4049

Bezzina, S., & Dingli, A. (2023, July). Rethinking gamification through artificial intelligence. In International Conference on Human-Computer Interaction (pp. 252-263). Cham: Springer Nature Switzerland.

Birbaumer, N. (2006). Breaking the Silence: Brain–Computer Interfaces (BCI) for Communication and Motor Control. *Psychophysiology*, 43(6), 517–532. DOI: 10.1111/j.1469-8986.2006.00456.x PMID: 17076808

Bittencourt, P. F. & Rauen, A. T. (). Políticas de inovação: racionalidade, instrumentos e coordenação. RAPINI. researchgate.net

Blankertz, B., Müller, K. R., Curio, G., Vaughan, T. M., Schalk, G., Wolpaw, J. R., Schlögl, A., Neuper, C., Pfurtscheller, G., Hinterberger, T., Schröder, M., & Birbaumer, N. (2004). The BCI Competition 2003: Progress and Perspectives in Detection and Discrimination of EEG Single Trials. *IEEE Transactions on Biomedical Engineering*, 51(6), 1044–1051. DOI: 10.1109/TBME.2004.826692 PMID: 15188876

Bogar, P. Z., Virag, M., Bene, M., Hardi, P., Matuz, A., Schlegl, A. T., Toth, L., Molnar, F., Nagy, B., Rendeki, S., Berner-Juhos, K., Ferencz, A., Fischer, K., & Maroti, P. (2024). Validation of a novel, low-fidelity virtual reality simulator and an artificial intelligence assessment approach for peg transfer laparoscopic training. *Scientific Reports*, 14(1), 16702. DOI: 10.1038/s41598-024-67435-6 PMID: 39030307

Bogdan, R., & Biklen, S. (1994). Qualitative research in education: an introduction to theory and methods. Porto editora.

Bota, P. J., Wang, C., Fred, A. L. N., & Placido Da Silva, H. (2019). A Review, Current Challenges, and Future Possibilities on Emotion Recognition Using Machine Learning and Physiological Signals. *IEEE Access : Practical Innovations, Open Solutions*, 7, 140990–141020. DOI: 10.1109/ACCESS.2019.2944001

Boyle, G. J. (1984). Reliability and validity of Izard's differential emotions scale. *Personality and Individual Differences*, 5(6), 747–750. DOI: 10.1016/0191-8869(84)90124-7

Bradley, M. M., & Lang, P. J. (1994). Measuring emotion: The self-assessment manikin and the semantic differential. *Journal of Behavior Therapy and Experimental Psychiatry*, 25(1), 49–59. DOI: 10.1016/0005-7916(94)90063-9 PMID: 7962581

Braid, H. R. (2024). Development and Evaluation of a Surgical Simulator and Assessment Rubric for Standing Castration of the Horse. *Journal of Veterinary Medical Education*, e20230131. DOI: 10.3138/jvme-2023-0131 PMID: 39504222

Brandão, M. R. M., de Oliveira Alexandre, M. L., Anez, M. E. M., & Costa, B. K. (2011). Stakeholder influence on the adoption of green marketing strategies. *Pretexto Journal*, 12(4), 2.

Bremser, W. G., & Barsky, N. P. (2004). Utilizing the balanced scorecard for R&D performance measurement. *R & D Management*, 34(3), 229–238. DOI: 10.1111/j.1467-9310.2004.00335.x

Breuer, H., Ivanov, K., & Abril, C. (2023). Management guidelines to address cultural challenges and facilitate values-based innovation through gamification. [uxberlin.com]. *International Journal of Entrepreneurship and Innovation Management*, 27(3-4), 208–236. DOI: 10.1504/IJEIM.2023.133383

Brigham, E. F., & Ehrhardt, M. C. (2013). *Gestão Financeira: Teoria e Prática*. Cengage Learning.

Brigham, E. F., & Ehrhardt, M. C. (2019). *Gestão financeira: Teoria e prática* (159th ed.).

Brody, L. R., & Hall, J. A. (2008). Gender and Emotion in Context. In M. Lewis, J. M. Haviland-Jones, & L. F. Barrett (Eds.), *Handbook of Emotions* (3º ed., pp. 309-408). The Guilford Press.

Browne, J., Devlin, J., Rolstadas, A., & Andersen, B. (1997). Performance measurement: The ENAPS approach. *Int. J. Bus. Transform.*, 1, 73–84.

Bryman, A. (2012). *Social Research Methods* (4th ed.). Oxford University Press.

Cacioppo, J. T., Tassinary, L. G., & Berntson, G. (2017). *Handbook of Psychophysiology* (t. ed., Ed.). Cambridge University Press.

Cacioppo, J. T., & Gardner, W. L. (1999). Emotion. *Annual Review of Psychology*, 50(1), 191–214. DOI: 10.1146/annurev.psych.50.1.191 PMID: 10074678

Caetano, R. M. (). O uso da Inteligência Artificial na Saúde. MULTI DISCI PLINAR. ibra.edu.br

Canavarro, M. C. S. (1999). Inventário de Sintomas Psicopatológicos (BSI). In Simões, M. R., Gonçalves, M. M., & Almeida, L. S. (Eds.), *Testes e provas psicologias em Portugal* (Vol. 2, pp. 95–109). APPORT/SHO.

Canavarro, M. C. S. (2007). Inventário de Sintomas Psicopatológicos (BSI): Uma revisão crítica dos estudos realizados em Portugal. In Simões, M. R., Machado, C., Gonçalves, M. M., & Almeida, L. (Eds.), *Avaliação psicológica: Instrumentos validados para a população portuguesa* (Vol. III). Quarteto Editora.

Cançado, V. O. L. (2024). Avaliação de processos em laboratório de análises clínicas sob a ótica da segurança do paciente. unb.br

Carenzo, L., Cena, T., Carfagna, F., Rondi, V., Ingrassia, P. L., Cecconi, M., Violato, C., Della Corte, F., & Vaschetto, R. (2021). Assessing anaesthesiology and intensive care specialty physicians: An Italian language multisource feedback system. *PLoS One*, 16(4), e0250404. DOI: 10.1371/journal.pone.0250404 PMID: 33891626

Carlos, M. S. F. (2023). O papel do cluster da vinha e do vinho na internacionalização e inovação dos processos e produtos das empresas vitivinícolas portuguesas. utl.pt

Carmo, H., & Ferreira, M. (2008). Research Methodology–Guide for Self-Learning (2nd edition). *Lisbon: Universidade Aberta, 15*, 16.

Carmo, V. A. S., Pinheiro, R. R., Alvarenga, S. M., & Potrich, A. C. G. (2024). Ferramenta OKR aplicada ao agronegócio: Um estudo de caso. Seven Editora, 1350-1369. sevenpublicacoes.com.br

Carrasco, G., Pardo, J., & Utrilla, P. N. (2021). Gamification in healthcare: Challenges in adoption and integration. *Health Informatics Journal*, 27(4), 1–12. DOI: 10.1177/14604582211034567

Carstensen, L. L., Pasupathi, M., Mayr, U., & Nesselroade, J. R. (2000). Emotional experience in everyday life across the adult life span. *Journal of Personality and Social Psychology*, 79(4), 644–655. DOI: 10.1037/0022-3514.79.4.644 PMID: 11045744

Cascella, M., Cascella, A., Monaco, F., & Shariff, M. N. (2023). Envisioning gamification in anesthesia, pain management, and critical care: Basic principles, integration of artificial intelligence, and simulation strategies. *Journal of Anesthesia, Analgesia and Critical Care*, 3(1), 33. DOI: 10.1186/s44158-023-00118-2 PMID: 37697415

Chanel, G. (2009). *Emotion Assessment for Affective Computing Based on Brain and Peripheral Signals,* University of Geneve. https://theses.eurasip.org/theses/492/emotion-assessment-for-affective-computing-based/

Charsley, J., & Jarman, H. (2024). Assessment and management of pelvic fractures from high-energy trauma in adults. *Emergency Nurse*. PMID: 36880213

Chen, M. J., Ambardekar, A., Martinelli, S. M., Buhl, L. K., Walsh, D. P., Levy, L., & Mitchell, J. D. (2022). Defining and addressing anesthesiology needs in simulation-based medical education. *The Journal of Education in Perioperative Medicine : JEPM*, 24(2). PMID: 36051401

Chou, Y. K. (2016). *Actionable Gamification: Beyond Points, Badges, and Leaderboards*. Octalysis Media.

Christensen, L. B. (2007). *Experimental Methodology* (10th ed.). Pearson / Allyn & Bacon.

Christos Konstantinidis, M. D., Galanis, C., Sotiris Plakoutsis, M. D., Panagiotopoulos, V., Kotsias, C., Konidaris, K., & Dimitrios Giotis, M. D. (2024). Effectiveness of Pelvic Binders in Pre-Hospital Emergency Care: A Systematic Review of the Literature. *International Journal of Caring Sciences*, 17(1), 139–149.

Cleveland Clinic. (2020). **Telemedicine: A virtual visit for patients**. *Cleveland Clinic Newsroom*. https://newsroom.clevelandclinic.org/2020/03/31/telemedicine-a-virtual-visit-for-patients/

Coelho, J. B. L.Jr, Jurberg, C., Pinto, B. D. O. S., & de Barros, M. D. M. (2021). JOGO "DETROIT: BECOME HUMAN" COMO GUIA DE REFLEXÃO SOBRE A QUARTA REVOLUÇÃO INDUSTRIAL. [ufmt.br]. *Experiências em Ensino de Ciências*, 16(1), 105–120.

Cohen, S., Thiraios, D., & Kandilorou, M. (2008). Inter-relações dos parâmetros de desempenho numa perspetiva de balanced scorecard: Uma análise das empresas gregas. *Managerial Auditing Journal*, 23(5), 485–503. DOI: 10.1108/02686900810875307

Coleman, A., Croke, S., & Checkland, K. (2021). Improving care in care homes: What can Primary Care Networks learn from the Vanguards? *Journal of Integrated Care*, 29(1), 85–96. DOI: 10.1108/JICA-06-2020-0037

Cornelius, R. (2000). *Theoretical approaches to emotion* ISCA Tutorial and Research Workshop (ITRW) on Speech and Emotion, https://www.isca-archive.org/speechemotion_2000/cornelius00_speechemotion.html#

Correia, D. T. (2023). *Manual de psicopatologia - Psiquiatria & Psicologia Clínica - De Acordo com o DSM-5 e o CID-11* (3rd ed.). LIDEL.

Costa, R. M. P. (2024). O doente oncológico em programa de quimioterapia: Projeto de Desenvolvimento de Competências Clínicas Especializadas na Área de Enfermagem à Pessoa em …. rcaap.pt

COSTA. F. N. (2024). Questionamentos. Campinas, SP: Blog Cidadania & Cultura, 2024. 209p. 1. Papel dos Economistas. 2. História Econômica. 3. Organização Industrial. 4…. unicamp.br

Costa, A. P., Moreira, A., & Sá, P. (2021). Reflections on Research methodologies: data analysis (Vol. 3). *Aveiro: University of Aveiro.doi:* DOI: 10.34624/dws9-6j98

Costa, C., Rocha, G., & Acúrcio, M. (2004). *Research methodology*. Faculty of Sciences of the University of Lisbon.

Costa, E. A. M., & Costa, E. A. (2021). O dilema do reuso de dispositivos médicos de uso único: aspectos históricos e atuais. Vigilância Sanitária em Debate: Sociedade [redalyc.org]. *Ciência & Tecnologia*, 9(1), 91–98.

Coutinho, C. M. P. (2014). *Metodologia de Investigação em Ciências Sociais e Humanas* (2ª edição). Almedina.

Coutinho, C. P. (2014). *Research methodology in social and human sciences*. Leya.

Craig, J., & Moores, K. (2005). Balanced Scorecards para impulsionar o planeamento estratégico das empresas familiares. *Family Business Review*, XVIII(2), 105–122. DOI: 10.1111/j.1741-6248.2005.00035.x

Csikszentmihalyi, M., & Larson, R. (1987). Validity and reliability of the experience-sampling method. *The Journal of Nervous and Mental Disease*, 175(9), 526–536. DOI: 10.1097/00005053-198709000-00004 PMID: 3655778

Čudanov, M., Parlić, D., & Sofronijević, A. (2014). Proposed Framework for Gamifying Information Retrieval: Case of DART - European Research Theses Portal. *Proceedings of the Second International Conference on Technological Ecosystems for Enhancing Multiculturality*, 185–190. DOI: 10.1145/2669711.2669898

Cullen, P., Mackean, T., Walker, N., Coombes, J., Bennett-Brook, K., Clapham, K., Ivers, R., Hackett, M., Worner, F., & Longbottom, M. (2022). Integrating trauma and violence informed care in primary health care settings for first nations women experiencing violence: A systematic review. *Trauma, Violence & Abuse*, 23(4), 1204–1219. DOI: 10.1177/1524838020985571 PMID: 33573523

da Costa Júnior, J. F., Bezerra, D. D. M. C., dos Santos Cabral, E. L., Moreno, R. C. P., & Pires, A. K. S. (2021). A Matriz SWOT e suas subdimensões: Uma proposta de inovação conceitual. Research [rsdjournal.org]. *Social Development*, 10(2), e25710212580–e25710212580.

da Costa Teixeira, P., de Freitas, C. L. L., & de Brito, Z. M. (2024). A importância da gestão de custos para a lucratividade de micro e pequenas empresas: Um estudo de caso em Manacapuru-AM. [revistaacademicaonline.com]. *Revista Acadêmica Online*, 10(52), e235–e235. DOI: 10.36238/2359-5787.2024.v10n52.235

da Costa, M. I. F. (2023). tabilidade n. mcm.com.pt

da Cunha Machado, A. M. (2023). Contributos para a Estratégia de Internacionalização no Reino Unido: O Caso do Grupo ADA eo Mercado de Dispositivos Médicos. [HTML]

da Silva Lima, F., Vieira, G. B. B., Lazzari, F., Salvador, C. K., & Santos, C. H. S. (2024). Análise dos fatores críticos de sucesso na exportação: um estudo de empresas do setor metal-mecânico da Serra Gaúcha. Revista de Gestão e Secretariado, 15(8), e3973-e3973. revistagesec.org.br

da Silva, L. R. M. (2024). *Ciência*. Tecnologia e Sociedade. [HTML]

Dainotto, D. (2020). The Impact of a Pediatric Critical Incident Simulation on the Perceived Importance of and Need for a Critical Incident Stress Debriefing Protocol for Anesthesia. PMID: 36051401

Dai, Y., Wang, X., Zhang, P., Zhang, W., & Junfeng, C. (2018). Sparsity constrained differential evolution enabled feature-channel-sample hybrid selection for daily-life EEG emotion recognition. *Multimedia Tools and Applications*, 77(17), 21967–21994. Advance online publication. DOI: 10.1007/s11042-018-5618-0

Dallabrida, N. (2023). Brechas no Monólito Educacional: Classes Decundárias Experimentais e Inovação do Ensino Secundário nos Anos de 1950 e 1960. [HTML]

Dalmoro, M., Venturini, J. C., & Pereira, B. A. D. (2009). Green marketing: Social and environmental responsibility integrated into the marketing environment. *RBGN: Brazilian Journal of Business Management*, 11(30), 38–52. DOI: 10.7819/rbgn.v11i30.232

Davi, S. G. (2021). Impactos com a implantação da certificação da norma ABNT NBR ISO 9001: 2015 em um laboratório de um órgão público. ufmg.br

David, A. (2023). Navigating Critical Care: Anesthesia and Surgical Considerations in Emergency Situations. PMID: 36051401

Davis, M., & Kohn, L. T. (2019). Leadership strategies in remote healthcare environments: A review of the literature. *International Journal of Healthcare Management*, 12(3), 205–211. DOI: 10.1080/20479700.2019.1630481

DE ANDRADE. P. I. (). IMPORTÂNCIA E BENEFÍCIOS DO PLANEJAMENTO E DO SETOR TRIBUTÁRIO PARA A TOMADA DE DECISÃO NAS ORGANIZAÇÕES EMPRESARIAIS. repositorio.pgsscogna.com.br. pgsscogna.com.br

de Araújo, L. F., & de Almeida Barros, A. C. (2021). PROPOSTA DE DESENVOLVIMENTO DE UM PLANEJAMENTO ESTRATÉGICO PARA UMA CLÍNICA DE OTORRINOLARINGOLOGIA EM MACEIÓ–AL. Ideias e Inovação-Lato Sensu, 6(2), 122-122. set.edu.br

De Carli, J. P. (2024). O PAPEL DA ODONTOLOGIA E DA PSICOLOGIA NA SAÚDE DA PESSOA IDOSA INSTITUCIONALIZADA. editoracientifica.com.br

de Castro Gil, J. P. (2023). Taxa de Sucesso da Ancoragem Ortodôntica com Recurso a Mini-Implantes Interradiculares no Maxilar Superior-Revisão Sistemática. [HTML]

de Faria, S. R. (2022). Análise da contribuição do lean na redução do impacto ambiental em obras de urbanização. unicamp.br

de Jesus Costa, I. J. (2024). Avaliação dos resultados do planejamento estratégico no Grupo Santa Casa de Belo Horizonte no ciclo 2016 a 2020. ufmg.br de Lima Maia, I. C. V., Peixoto, M. D. G. B., Schwermann, L. P., da Silva, D. L. L., & Maia, D. C. G. (2020). Construções coletivas na formação médica sobre planejamento em saúde. [unirioja.es]. *Temas em Educação e Saúde*, 16(2), 720–734. DOI: 10.26673/tes.v16i2.13823

de Menezes, F. G. (2021). Acesso ao Mercado: Conhecendo os caminhos de acesso no mercado de saúde. [HTML]

de Moraes, L. R., de Araújo Neto, L. T., de Azevedo Garcia, L. H., Mendonça, M. A. B., dos Santos, R. R., & Neto, O. C. (2024). BENEFÍCIOS, DESAFIOS E LEGISLAÇÕES PARA UTILIZAÇÃO DE DRONES NA PRODUÇÃO AGRÍCOLA: UMA REVISÃO DA LITERATURA. Revista Multidisciplinar do Nordeste Mineiro, 3(3). unipacto.com.br

de Nefrologia, S. P. (2024). Abstracts of 37th Congress of the Portuguese Society of Nephrology. Portuguese Kidney Journal.

de Oliveira, J. P. R. (). GESTÃO TRIBUTÁRIA E BENEFÍCIOS FISCAIS APLICADOS A EMPRESAS DA CONSTRUÇÃO CIVIL. bib.pucminas.br. pucminas.br

de Oliveira, C. P., & Sousa, B. M. (2020). Green consumer behavior and its implications for brand marketing strategy. In *Green Marketing as a positive driver for corporate sustainability* (pp. 69-95). IGI Global. Sustainable Management Practices: Green Marketing as A Source for Organizational Competitive Advantage. *Journal of Social and Environmental Management*, 18(4).

de Sousa, L. G., de Oliveira, L. V., de Oliveira, L. V., Rampanelli, G., Felix, D. R., Borba, L. D. O. F., & de Andrade, M. P. D. O. (2024). ABORDAGENS AVANÇADAS NO TRATAMENTO DE DOENÇAS CRÔNICAS. *Brazilian Journal of Implantology and Health Sciences*, 6(9), 1194–1201. emnuvens.com.br. DOI: 10.36557/2674-8169.2024v6n9p1194-1201

de Souza, D. C. (2023). A IMPORTÂNCIA DA CONTROLADORIA CONTÁBIL EM OPERADORAS DE PLANOS DE SAÚDE: UMA ANÁLISE ABRANGENTE. Revista GeTeC. fucamp.edu.br

de Souza, F. R. (2023). Economia circular na indústria eletroeletrônica: o caso da empresa ABC. Revista Produção Online. producaoonline.org.br

de Souza, L. F. R., Vogel, P. T., Venâncio, L. G., & Lopes, L. L. S. R. (2024). Foca nas novas opções de tratamento para reduzir a progressão da doença e melhorar a qualidade de vida dos pacientes. sevenpublicacoes.com.br

de Vianna Tiné, J. P. (2024). Impacto da Tecnologia e Suas Transformações na Área da Saúde. Unirepositório. unirepositorio.education

Deleuze, G. (2004). *A imagem-movimento: Cinema 1* (Godinho, R., Trans.). Assírio & Alvim.

Deloof, M. (2003). Does Working Capital Management Affect Profitability of Belgian Firms? *Journal of Business Finance & Accounting*, 30(3), 573–587. DOI: 10.1111/1468-5957.00008

Denzin, N. K., & Lincoln, Y. S. (2006). Qualitative research design: Theories and approaches. *The Art of Medication*.

Deterding, S., Dixon, D., Khaled, R., & Nacke, L. (2011). From Game Design Elements to Gamefulness: Defining Gamification. *Proceedings of the 2011 Annual Conference Extended Abstracts on Human Factors in Computing Systems* - CHI EA '11. https://doi.org/DOI: 10.1145/1979742.1979575

Deuchler, S., Scholtz, J., Ackermann, H., Seitz, B., & Koch, F. (2022). Implementation of microsurgery simulation in an ophthalmology clerkship in Germany: A prospective, exploratory study. *BMC Medical Education*, 22(1), 599. DOI: 10.1186/s12909-022-03634-x PMID: 35922857

Diallo, M. S., Tan, J. M., Heitmiller, E. S., & Vetter, T. R. (2022). Achieving greater health equity: An opportunity for anesthesiology. *Anesthesia and Analgesia*, 134(6), 1175–1184. DOI: 10.1213/ANE.0000000000005937 PMID: 35110516

Dias da Silva, C., & Moreira Peixoto, J. F. (2023). APITERAPIA: FINS TERAPÊUTICOS ATRAVÉS DA APITOXINA E OUTROS PRODUTOS DA ABELHA APIS MELLIFERAS. Revista Foco (Interdisciplinary Studies Journal), 16(9). [HTML]

do Aguiar, C. S. (2024). O USO DA TECNOLOGIA EM APOIO AO SISTEMA DE SAÚDE NACIONAL. Unirepositório. unirepositorio.education

dos Santos, M. M., Alencar, R. A., Schneider, F. F., Fernandes, G. X. D. A., Melo, A. B., Dias, L. A., . . . Farias, J. D. A. (2024). A eficácia das intervenções de saúde pública: avaliação de programas e políticas. Periódicos Brasil. Pesquisa Científica, 3(2), 94-110. emnuvens.com.br

DOS SANTOS. T. J. (). A APLICABILIDADE DAS FERRAMENTAS DO PLANEJAMENTO ESTRATÉGICO PARA AS MICRO E PEQUENAS ORGANIZAÇÕES. repositorio.pgsscogna.com.br. pgsscogna.com.br

dos Santos, N. M., & da Luz, E. R. (2024). Social responsibility and sustainability under the influence of social marketing: A case study of a hospital. *Brazilian Journal of Business*, 6(3), e72215. DOI: 10.34140/bjbv6n3-017

Drago, H. F. (2023). Capacidades dinâmicas produtivas, comportamento estratégico e desempenho organizacional: um estudo nas microcervejarias artesanais. ufsm.br

Dury, C., & El-Shishini, H. (2005). Division Performance Measurement: An Edwards, D., & Thomas, J. C. (2005). Developing a Municipal Performance- Measurement System: Reflections on the Atlanta Dashboard. *Public Administration Review*, 65(3), 369–376. DOI: 10.1111/j.1540-6210.2005.00461.x

Edmondson, A. C. (2018). *The Fearless Organization: Creating Psychological Safety in the Workplace for Learning, Innovation, and Growth*. John Wiley & Sons.

Edmondson, A. C., & Harvey, J. F. (2018). Cross-boundary teaming for innovation: Integrating research on teams and knowledge in organizations. *Human Resource Management Review*, 28(4), 347–360. DOI: 10.1016/j.hrmr.2017.03.002

Eisenberg, D. (2025). *The Future of Work in a Digital World*. Digital Transformation And Society.

Ekman, P. (1999). Basic Emotions. In *Handbook of Cognition and Emotion* (pp. 45-60). https://doi.org/DOI: 10.1002/0470013494.ch3

Ekman, P. (1972). Universals and cultural differences in facial expressions of emotion. *Nebraska Symposium on Motivation*, Lincoln.

Ekman, P. (2008). An argument for basic emotions. *Cognition and Emotion*, 6(3-4), 169–200. DOI: 10.1080/02699939208411068

Ekman, P., & Cordaro, D. (2011). What is Meant by Calling Emotions Basic. *Emotion Review*, 3(4), 364–370. DOI: 10.1177/1754073911410740

Ekman, P., & Friesen, W. V. (1971). Constants across cultures in the face and emotion. *Journal of Personality and Social Psychology*, 17(2), 124–129. DOI: 10.1037/h0030377 PMID: 5542557

Ekman, P., Friesen, W. V., O'Sullivan, M., Chan, A., Diacoyanni-Tarlatzis, I., Heider, K., Krause, R., LeCompte, W. A., Pitcairn, T., Ricci-Bitti, P. E., Scherer, K., Tomita, M., & Tzavaras, A. (1987). Universals and cultural differences in the judgments of facial expressions of emotion. *Journal of Personality and Social Psychology*, 53(4), 712–717. DOI: 10.1037/0022-3514.53.4.712 PMID: 3681648

El Sibaii, M., Granja, J., & Azenha, M. (2024, May). Transformação digital na indústria da construção: Capacitando a gestão de dados através de uma plataforma de modelos de dados de produtos (PDT). In 5º Congresso Português de Building Information Modelling Volume 2 (p. 87). UMinho Editora. uminho.pt

Elgeziry, A., Mumtaz, N., Thodika, A. V., & Mallal, K. A. (2022). Non-technical Skills for Anesthesia Technician. In *Improving Anesthesia Technical Staff's Skills* (pp. 1–10). Springer International Publishing. DOI: 10.1007/978-3-030-88849-7_1

Epstein, D., Lavin, P. M., Withall, J., & Wong, D. (2024). Empowering Nurses to Increase Certification Rates in a Postanesthesia Care Unit: A Collaborative Team Approach. *Journal of Perianesthesia Nursing*. Advance online publication. DOI: 10.1016/j.jopan.2024.05.004 PMID: 39115477

Eriksson-Liebon, M., Roos, S., & Hellström, I. (2021). Patients' expectations and experiences of being involved in their own care in the emergency department: A qualitative interview study. *Journal of Clinical Nursing*, 30(13-14), 1942–1952. DOI: 10.1111/jocn.15746 PMID: 33829575

ESTRATÉGICO, D. D. E. U. M. P. (2022). DIGITALIZAÇÃO DE UM CENTRO DE INVESTIGAÇÃO CLÍNICA: DESENHO DE UM PLANO ESTRATÉGICO TRABALHO DE PROJETO. unl.pt

Evangelista, J. R. (2021). Gerenciamento de risco de equipamentos eletromédicos para segurança eletromagnética em estabelecimentos assistencias de saúde. unicamp.br

Fadilah, R. A., Sukmaningtyas, W., & Burhan, A. (2023). *The The Correlation between Motivation and Anesthetists' Working Performance in Banyumas Regency: English*. Java Nursing Journal.

Falcão, M. S. I. (2021). Modelo regulamentar integrado no sector do medicamento e produtos de saúde: o caso português (passado, presente e futuro). ul.pt

Fangueiro, C. S. P. (2021). [Numa Adega. uminho.pt]. *Otimização da Implementação da Norma ISO*, 22000, 2018.

Faridullah, S. (2024). Indian IT Firms: A systematic review of existing literature with reference to prominent employee engagement theory and models. Educational Administration: Theory and Practice.

Fenech, M. (2024). The business development role of Maltese listed entity CFOs. DOI: 10.3390/su16135800

Fincher, E. L. (2023). Increasing Anesthesia Provider Knowledge on Noise and Cognitive Overload in the Operating Room.

Firth-Cozens, J. & King, J. (2023). Are psychological factors linked to performance?. Understanding doctors' performance.

Fischer, A. H., Rodriguez Mosquera, P. M., van Vianen, A. E., & Manstead, A. S. (2004). Gender and culture differences in emotion. *Emotion (Washington, D.C.)*, 4(1), 87–94. DOI: 10.1037/1528-3542.4.1.87 PMID: 15053728

Fitzgerald, L., & McDermott, A. (2017). *Challenging Perspectives on Organizational Change in Health Care* (1st ed.). Routledge., DOI: 10.4324/9781315690735

Folstein, M. F., Folstein, S. E., & McHugh, P. R. (1975). "Mini-mental state". A practical method for grading the cognitive state of patients for the clinician. *Journal of Psychiatric Research*, 12(3), 189–198. DOI: 10.1016/0022-3956(75)90026-6 PMID: 1202204

Fonseca, J. R. S. (2008, July). Quantitative methods in sociology: difficulties of a research methodology. In *VI Portuguese Congress of Sociology–Social Worlds: Knowledge and Practices. Universidade Nova de Lisboa: Faculty of Social Sciences and Humanities* (p. 8).

Fordson, P., Xing, X., Guo, K., & Xu, X. (2022). Emotion Recognition With Knowledge Graph Based on Electrodermal Activity. *Frontiers in Neuroscience*, 16, 911767. DOI: 10.3389/fnins.2022.911767 PMID: 35757534

Friedrich, J., Becker, M., Kramer, F., Wirth, M., & Schneider, M. (2020). Incentive design and gamification for knowledge management. [e-tarjome.com]. *Journal of Business Research*, 106, 341–352. DOI: 10.1016/j.jbusres.2019.02.009

Friend, T. & Zaleski, L. (2022). The Development of an Assessment Plan for Wellness and Risk for Substance Use in Nurse Anesthesia Students.

Gaba, D. M. (). … of simulation in health care share a common Vision of a future revolution in health care organization, with simulation as a key enabling technique. Simulation is …. simulatorcentrum.se.

Gafsou, B., Becq, M. C., Michelet, D., Julien-Marsollier, F., Brasher, C., & Dahmani, S. (2021). Determinants of work-related quality of life in French anesthesiologists. *Anesthesia and Analgesia*, 133(4), 863–872. DOI: 10.1213/ANE.0000000000005397 PMID: 33543868

Gansel, B. (2005). *Toward a framework of financial planning in new venture creation. Documento de investigação, Otto-von-Guericke-Universität Magdeburg*. Alemanha.

Garcia, D. B., Pereira, F. H., & Ribeiro, E. R. (2023). Evaluation of Third-Year Anesthesiology Residents Knowledge on Patient Safety: Descriptive Study. [IJAP]. *International Journal of Anesthesiology and Practice*, 1(1).

Garcia-Marcinkiewicz, A. G., & Titler, S. S. (2022). Lactation in anesthesiology. *Anesthesiology Clinics*, 40(2), 235–243. DOI: 10.1016/j.anclin.2022.01.014 PMID: 35659397

Ghellere, J. C., de Oliveira, P. H. P., de Aguiar, E. C., de Oliveira Pereira, H. J., Marin, B. T., Fernandes, A. C. S., & Ferreira, A. F. L. (2023). Técnicas Minimamente Invasivas em Cirurgia Geral: Benefícios, Limitações e Futuras Perspectivas. *Brazilian Journal of Implantology and Health Sciences*, 5(5), 3025–3041. emnuvens.com.br. DOI: 10.36557/2674-8169.2023v5n5p3025-3041

Girdauskiene, L., Ausrine Ciplyte, E., & Navickas, V. (2022). Gamification as an innovative instrument for employee engagement. Marketing i menedžment innovacij, (1), 10-17. zbw.eu Breuer, H. & Ivanov, K. (2020). Gamification to address cultural challenges and to facilitate values-based innovation. ISPIM Conference Proceedings. DOI: 10.21272/mmi.2022.1-01

Gold, A. H., Malhotra, A., & Segars, A. H. (2001). Knowledge Management: An Organizational Capabilities Perspective. *Journal of Management Information Systems*, 18(1), 185–214. https://www.jstor.org/stable/40398521. DOI: 10.1080/07421222.2001.11045669

Gomes, M. A. (2024). Certificação de um Sistema de Gestão da Qualidade NP EN ISO 9001: 2015 numa Empresa de Injeção de Plástico. ipleiria.pt

Gootenberg, D. B., Kurtzman, N., O'Mara, T., Jennifer, Y. G., Chiu, D., Shapiro, N. I., & Dagan, A. (2021). Developing a pulse oximetry home monitoring protocol for patients suspected with COVID-19 after emergency department discharge. *BMJ Health & Care Informatics*, 28(1), e100330. DOI: 10.1136/bmjhci-2021-100330 PMID: 34301725

Gosselin, M. (2005). An empirical study of performance measurement in manufacturing organizations. *International Journal of Productivity and Performance Management*, 54(5/6), 419–437. DOI: 10.1108/17410400510604566

Gottumukkala, V., Vetter, T. R., & Gan, T. J. (2023). Perioperative medicine: What the future can hold for anesthesiology. *Anesthesia and Analgesia*, 136(4), 628–635. DOI: 10.1213/ANE.0000000000006412 PMID: 36928147

Graglia, M. V. & Huelsen, P. (2023). Inovação e competitividade. [HTML]

Guedes, M. M. (2024). ...: Um Contributo da Enfermagem Perioperatória-Desenvolvimento de competências clínicas especializadas na área de Enfermagem Médico-Cirúrgica, na área da .... rcaap.pt

Guerra, D. K. H., da Rocha Legoff, W. G., Menezes, P. H. S. D. S., Dias, M. V. S., Alves, L. P., Sacchi, J., ... & Simplicio, W. K. G. (2024). ESTRATÉGIAS NO DIAGNÓSTICO E CONDUTA DO MELANOMA: UMA ABORDAGEM DERMATOLÓGICA. Revista CPAQV-Centro de Pesquisas Avançadas em Qualidade de Vida, 16(2). cpaqv.org

Guerreiro, M., Botelho, M. A., Leitão, O., Castro-Caldas, A., & Garcia, C. (1994). *Adaptação à população portuguesa na tradução do Mini Mental State Examination*. Reunião da Primavera da Sociedade Portuguesa de Neurologia.

Guerreiro, V. (2011). *Desenvolvimento moral: relações entre consistência do raciocínio moral, a atribuição de emoções e ação moral*. ISPA.

Gunawan, J. (2023). Exploring the future of nursing: Insights from the ChatGPT model. *Belitung Nursing Journal*, 9(1), 1–5. DOI: 10.33546/bnj.2551 PMID: 37469634

Gupta, A. K., & Govindarajan, V. (2000). Knowledge flows within multinational corporations. *Strategic Management Journal*, 21(4), 473–496. https://doi.org/https://doi.org/10.1002/(SICI)1097-0266(200004)21:4<473:AID-SMJ84>3.0.CO;2-I. DOI: 10.1002/(SICI)1097-0266(200004)21:4<473::AID-SMJ84>3.0.CO;2-I

Gupta, M., Behl, A., & Kumar, Y. L. N. (2022). "Prevention is better than cure": Challenges in engaging employees through gamification. *International Journal of Manpower*, 43(2), 380–394. DOI: 10.1108/IJM-03-2021-0172

Haavik, T. K., & Våpenstad, C. (2020). The role of simulators in interdisciplinary medical work. Multimodal Technologies and Interaction. Abaalkhayl, M. (2024). IMPACT OF SIMULATED ANESTHESIA CRISIS MANAGEMENT TRAINING ON INTRAOPERATIVE COMPLICATIONS. *Gland Surgery*.

Hafeez K., Zhang YB., Malak N. (2002) Determining key capacidades de uma empresa utilizando o processo de hierarquia analítica.

Hafermalz, E. (2021). Out of the Panopticon and into Exile: Visibility and control in distributed new culture organizations. *Organization Studies*, 42(5), 697–717. DOI: 10.1177/0170840620909962

Hamari, J., Hassan, L., & Dias, A. (2018). Gamification, quantified-self or social networking? Matching users' goals with motivational technology. *User Modeling and User-Adapted Interaction*, 28(1), 35–74. DOI: 10.1007/s11257-018-9200-2

Hamari, J., Koivisto, J., & Sarsa, H. (2014). Does gamification work? - A literature review of empirical studies on gamification. *Proceedings of the Annual Hawaii International Conference on System Sciences*. DOI: 10.1109/HICSS.2014.377

Hammer, M., & Champy, J. (1994). *Reengineering the Corporation – A Manifesto for Business*. Nicholas Breale.

Hamza, I., & Tóvölgyi, S. (2022). Empirical Analysis of the Influence of Gamification on Employees' Behavior. *Dynamic Relationships Management Journal*, 11(2). Advance online publication. DOI: 10.17708/DRMJ.2022.v11n02a05

Hanelt, A., Bohnsack, R., Marz, D., & Antunes Marante, C. (2021). A systematic review of the literature on digital transformation: Insights and implications for strategy and organizational change. [wiley.com]. *Journal of Management Studies*, 58(5), 1159–1197. DOI: 10.1111/joms.12639

Harif, M., Osman, H., & Ho, C. (2010). Efficient financial management practices: An in-depth study among the CEOs of Small and Medium Enterprises (SMEs). *International Review of Busines Research Papers*, 4(6), 13–35.

Harrell, K., Horwood, C., & Burlew, C. C. (2023). Current Management of Hemodynamically Unstable Patients with Pelvic Fracture. *Current Surgery Reports*, 11(4), 92–100. DOI: 10.1007/s40137-023-00348-x

Harris, D. M., & Franceschini, D. (2022). The Unpredictable Future of High-Fidelity Patient Simulation in Biomedical Science Education: The Price Must Be Right. In *Technologies in Biomedical and Life Sciences Education: Approaches and Evidence of Efficacy for Learning* (pp. 493–517). Springer International Publishing. DOI: 10.1007/978-3-030-95633-2_16

Harrison, W. (2022). *Optimizing Patient Care: Synergy between Anesthesia, Surgery, and Radiology*. Cosmic Journal of Biology.

Hawkins, A. D., Strobel, R. J., Mehaffey, J. H., Hawkins, R. B., Rotar, E. P., Young, A. M., Yarboro, L. T., Yount, K., Ailawadi, G., Joseph, M., Quader, M., & Teman, N. R. (2024, June). Operating room versus intensive care unit extubation within 6 hours after on-pump cardiac surgery: Early results and hospital costs. [). WB Saunders.]. *Seminars in Thoracic and Cardiovascular Surgery*, 36(2), 195–208. DOI: 10.1053/j.semtcvs.2022.09.013 PMID: 36460133

Hayward, P. (2009). *Terror tracks: music, sound and horror cinema*. Equinox.

Health Organization, W. (2020). Avaliação externa conjunta das principais capacidades do RSI da República de Cabo Verde: relatório de missão, 4-8 novembro 2019. google.com

Heckl, D., & Moormann, J. (2010). Process performance management. In *Handbook on Business Process Management* (Vol. 2, pp. 115–135). Springer. DOI: 10.1007/978-3-642-01982-1_6

Hedrik, V. (2008) Performance Evaluation of Foreign Subsidiaries: A Critical Analysis.

Hessen, J. (2001). *Filosofia dos valores*. Almedina.

Hofmann, R., Curran, S., & Dickens, S. (2021). … non-technical skills in simulation-based medical education: Findings from an integrated scoping review of research and content analysis of curricular learning…. *Studies in Educational Evaluation*, 71, 101093. DOI: 10.1016/j.stueduc.2021.101093

Hong, T., Case, V., Farcas, A. M., Whitfield, D., Muller, G., Schlesinger, S. A., Haamid, A. S., Middleton, M. T., Breyre, A., Buaprasert, P., Whitten-Chung, K., Lichtenbelt, K. J. C., Joiner, A. P., Pereira, C., & Brown, J. (2024). Caring for Transgender and Gender Diverse Prehospital Patients: A NAEMSP Position Statement and Resource Document. *Prehospital Emergency Care*, •••, 1–13. DOI: 10.1080/10903127.2024.2411723 PMID: 39422378

Hood, C., & Peters, G. (2004). O Envelhecimento Médio da Nova Gestão Pública: Into the Age of Paradox? *Journal of Public Administration: Research and Theory*, 14(3), 267–282. DOI: 10.1093/jopart/muh019

Hopwood, A. G. (1972). An empirical study of the role of accounting data in performance evaluation. investigação empírica em contabilidade: Estudos selecionados. *Journal of Accounting Research*, 10, 156–182. DOI: 10.2307/2489870

Howe, T. J., Claireaux, H., Fox, H., Morgan, G., McMenemy, L., Masouros, S. D., & Ramasamy, A. (2023). Mechanical assessment of proprietary and improvised pelvic binders for use in the prehospital environment. *BMJ Military Health*, e002398. DOI: 10.1136/military-2023-002398 PMID: 37541678

Huang, Y., Chen, Y., & Wang, L. (2020). Cultural adaptation in the implementation of gamification in healthcare: A review of challenges and practices. *Journal of Global Health*, 10(2), 020432. DOI: 10.7189/jogh.10.020432 PMID: 33403104

Hu, H., Cohen, G., Sharma, B., Yin, H., & McConnell, R. (2022). Sustainability in health care. *Annual Review of Environment and Resources*, 47(1), 173–196. DOI: 10.1146/annurev-environ-112320-095157

Hunicke, R., Leblanc, M., & Zubek, R. (2004). MDA: A Formal Approach to Game Design and Game Research. *Proceedings of the AAAI Workshop on Challenges in Game AI*, 4(1). https://www.researchgate.net/publication/228884866

Hu, Q., Dollard, M. F., & Taris, T. W. (2022). Organizational context matters: Psychosocial safety climate as a precursor to team and individual motivational functioning. *Safety Science*, 145, 105524. DOI: 10.1016/j.ssci.2021.105524

Hwang, U., Dresden, S. M., Vargas-Torres, C., Kang, R., Garrido, M. M., Loo, G., Sze, J., Cruz, D., Richardson, L. D., Adams, J., Aldeen, A., Baumlin, K. M., Courtney, D. M., Gravenor, S., Grudzen, C. R., Nimo, G., Zhu, C. W., Abraham, G., Amoko, C., & Sumberg, D. (2021). Association of a geriatric emergency department innovation program with cost outcomes among Medicare beneficiaries. *JAMA Network Open*, 4(3), e2037334–e2037334. DOI: 10.1001/jamanetworkopen.2020.37334 PMID: 33646311

Iurilli, M., Dentice, S., Di Nitto, M., Coclite, D., Napoletano, A., Bruno, V., & Papa, G. (2024). Availability and quality assessment of Clinical Practice Guidelines on Orthoplastic surgery treatment of open fractures of the lower limb using AGREE II tool: A systematic review. *Journal of Plastic, Reconstructive & Aesthetic Surgery; JPRAS*. PMID: 39700849

Izard, C. E. (1977). *Human Emotions*. Plenum Press. DOI: 10.1007/978-1-4899-2209-0

Izard, C. E. (1991). *The psychology of emotions*. Springer Science & Business Media. DOI: 10.1007/978-1-4899-0615-1

Izard, C. E. (2009). Emotion theory and research: Highlights, unanswered questions, and emerging issues. *Annual Review of Psychology*, 60(1), 1–25. DOI: 10.1146/annurev.psych.60.110707.163539 PMID: 18729725

Izard, C. E., Dougherty, F. E., Bloxom, B. M., & Kotsch, W. E. (1974). *The differential emotions scale: A method of surveying the subjective experience of discrete emotions*. Vanderbilt University Press.

Jaafer, M. A., & Mohammad, F. S. (2012). The Relationship between capital structure and profitability. *International Journal of Business and Social Science*, 3(16).

Jianlan, R., Mei, Y., Chunyan, Y., Rendie, X., Yiping, B., & Li, L. (2024). Exploring anesthesiology nurse'presenteeism in China: Cross-sectional study. *BMC Public Health*, 24(1), 2008. DOI: 10.1186/s12889-024-19476-9 PMID: 39060992

Jia, Y., Xu, B., Karanam, Y., & Voida, S. (2016). Personality, targeted gamification: A survey study on personality traits and motivational affordances. *Conference on Human Factors in Computing Systems - Proceedings*, 2001–2013. DOI: 10.1145/2858036.2858515

Jonathan, H. (2020). *Organizational commitment scale validation in tanzanian context*. Res Humanit Soc Sci.

Joseph, A. L., Borycki, E. M., & Kushniruk, A. W. (2021). Alert fatigue and errors caused by technology: a scoping review and introduction to the flow of cognitive processing model. Knowledge management & e-learning, (4), 500.

Juba, O. O. (2024). Impact of workplace safety, health, and wellness programs on employee engagement and productivity. International Journal of Health. *Medicine and Nursing Practice*, 6(4), 12–27.

Júlio, A. M. P. (2023). Relatório de Estágio: Um Olhar Sobre os Benefícios Fiscais com Foco No SIFIDE II. [HTML]

JUNER, R. & RODRIGUES, S. (2022). SBIdC-MPH: SISTEMA BASEADO EM INTERNET DAS COISAS PARA O MONITORAMENTO DE PACIENTES COM HIPERTENSÃO. ufscar.br

Kabariti, C. M. C., Cardoso, M. N., & Costa, L. C. (2024). ENVELHECIMENTO E SAUDE, A URGENCIA DOS CUIDADOS PALIATIVOS. Revista Cedigma, 1(1), 53-70. cedigma.com.br

Kang, S., Park, C. Y., Kim, A., Cha, N., & Lee, U. (2022). *Understanding Emotion Changes in Mobile Experience Sampling*. https://doi.org/DOI: 10.1145/3491102.3501944

Kao, K. Y., Hsu, H. H., Lee, H. T., Cheng, Y. C., Dax, I., & Hsieh, M. W. (2022). Career mentoring and job content plateaus: The roles of perceived organizational support and emotional exhaustion. *Journal of Career Development*, 49(2), 457–470. DOI: 10.1177/0894845320946399

Kaplan, R. S., & Atkinson, A. A. (198). Advanced Management Accounting (terceira ed.), 3 Prentice-Hall, EUA.

Kaplan, R. S., & Norton, D. P. (1992). The balanced scorecard: Measures that drive performance. *Harvard Business Review*, •••, 71–79. PMID: 10119714

Kaplan, R. S., & Norton, D. P. (1993). Using the balanced scorecard as a strategic management system. *Harvard Business Review*, 71(5), 134–148.

Karekla, M., Pollalis, Y., & Angelopoulos, M. (2021). Key drivers of digital transformation in greek businesses: Strategy vs. technology. *Central European Management Journal*, 29(2), 33–62. DOI: 10.7206/cemj.2658-0845.45

Kastner, F., Escamilla, E. Z., Langenberg, S., & Ng, M. S. (2025). Adoption of Life Cycle Thinking: Impact-driven comparative assessment of Japanese construction corporations' trends in practices. *Building and Environment*, 267, 112131. DOI: 10.1016/j.buildenv.2024.112131

Kelly, F. E., Frerk, C., Bailey, C. R., Cook, T. M., Ferguson, K., Flin, R., Fong, K., Groom, P., John, C., Lang, A. R., Meek, T., Miller, K. L., Richmond, L., Sevdalis, N., & Stacey, M. R. (2023). Implementing human factors in anaesthesia: guidance for clinicians, departments and hospitals: guidelines from the Difficult Airway Society and the Association of Anaesthetists. *Anaesthesia*, 78(4), 458–478. DOI: 10.1111/anae.15941 PMID: 36630725

Keung, P., & Kawalek, P. (1997). Goal-based Business Process Models: Creation and Business Process. *Management Journal*, 3(1), 17–38.

Kim, B., & Jo, S. (2019). *An Affective Situation Labeling System from Psychological Behaviors in Emotion Recognition*. https://doi.org//arXiv.1911.01158DOI: 10.48550

Kim, B. (2015). Chapter 2: Gamification: Examples, Definitions, and Related Concepts. *Library Technology Reports*, 51, 10.

Kim, B. H., Jo, S., & Choi, S. (2020). A-Situ: A computational framework for affective labeling from psychological behaviors in real-life situations. *Scientific Reports*, 10(1), 15916. DOI: 10.1038/s41598-020-72829-3 PMID: 32985534

Klein, G. F. (2024). Tecnologia no processo de antecipação de recebíveis: O caso da Securitizadora Digital SA. ufsc.br

Klein, C. J., Dalstrom, M. D., Weinzimmer, L. G., Cooling, M., Pierce, L., & Lizer, S. (2020). Strategies of advanced practice providers to reduce stress at work. *Workplace Health & Safety*, 68(9), 432–442. DOI: 10.1177/2165079920924060 PMID: 32491978

Koufteros, X. A., Vonderembse, M. A., & Doll, W. J. (1998). Developing measures of time-based manufacturing. *Journal of Operations Management*, 16(1), 21–41. DOI: 10.1016/S0272-6963(97)00027-2

Kowatsch, T., Otto, L., Harperink, S., Civit, C., & Denecke, K. (2021). Gamified e-learning as a facilitator for medical training: Implications for health professionals. *Medical Education Online*, 26(1), 1895035. DOI: 10.1080/10872981.2021.1895035

Ladeiro, J. G. (2020). Critérios para um Centro de Investigação Clínica de Referência. uc.pt

Lange, R., & Houran, J. (1998). Delusions of the paranormal: A haunting question of perception. *The Journal of Nervous and Mental Disease*, 186(10), 637–645. DOI: 10.1097/00005053-199810000-00008 PMID: 9788641

Lang, P. J., Bradley, M. M., & Cuthbert, B. N. (1997a). *International Affective Picture System (IAPS): Technical Manual and Affective Ratings*. Center for the Study of Emotion and Attention.

Lang, P. J., Bradley, M. M., & Cuthbert, B. N. (1997b). Motivated attention: Affect, activation, and action. In *Attention and orienting: Sensory and motivational processes* (pp. 97–135). Lawrence Erlbaum Associates Publishers.

Lanka, E., Lanka, S., Rostron, A., & Singh, P. (2020). Why we need qualitative research in management studies. *Journal of Contemporary Administration*, 25(2), e200297.

Larán, J. A., & Rossi, C. A. V. (2006). Surpresa e a formação da satisfação do consumidor. *RAE Eletrônica*, 5(1). Advance online publication. DOI: 10.1590/S1676-56482006000100002

Larradet, F., Niewiadomski, R., Barresi, G., Caldwell, D. G., & Mattos, L. S. (2020). Toward Emotion Recognition From Physiological Signals in the Wild: Approaching the Methodological Issues in Real-Life Data Collection. *Frontiers in Psychology*, 11, 1111. DOI: 10.3389/fpsyg.2020.01111 PMID: 32760305

Lau, C. H., & Sholihin, M. (2005). Financial and non-financial performance measures: Como é que elas afectam a satisfação no trabalho? *The British Accounting Review*, 37, 389–413. DOI: 10.1016/j.bar.2005.06.002

Lee, K., Ko, G. H., Lee, C. H., & Geong, Y. S. (2023). Detection Performance Analysis Based on EEG Signals for Visual BCI. *IEEE Access : Practical Innovations, Open Solutions*, 11, 2516–2526. DOI: 10.1109/ACCESS.2023.9887523

Lengler, F. (2023). Avaliação de metodologias forenses de análise de cronograma aplicadas à um caso de construção industrial. ufrgs.br

Leong, G. K., Snyder, D. L., & Ward, P. T. (1990). Research in the process and content of manufacturing strategy. *Omega*, 18(2), 109–122. DOI: 10.1016/0305-0483(90)90058-H

Leoni, M. (2024). A Ciência dos Gatilhos Mentais: Desvendando a Mente. [HTML]

Lewis, P. M. J. (2007). *Gendering emotions in organizations*. Palgrave Macmillan. DOI: 10.1007/978-1-137-07297-9

Libby, T., & Lindsay, R. M. (2010). Para além da orçamentação ou a orçamentação reconsiderada? A survey of North American budgeting practice. [London: Grin Verlag GmbH.]. *Management Accounting Research*, 21(1), 56–75. DOI: 10.1016/j.mar.2009.10.003

Lima, E. J. A., da Silva, J. V. V., Tenorio, C. M. P., de Lima, C. G., de Melo, D. C., de Lima, R. E., & Pinheiro, T. D. S. A. (2023). Relação entre doenças crônicas não transmissíveis e o tempo de internação de idosos em Unidade de Terapia Intensiva. *Brazilian Journal of Implantology and Health Sciences*, 5(4), 2620–2632. emnuvens.com.br. DOI: 10.36557/2674-8169.2023v5n4p2620-2632

Lisann-Goldman, L., Cowart, C., Lin, H. M., Orlando, B., & Mahoney, B. (2022). Well-being in anesthesiology graduate medical education: Reconciling the ideal with reality. *Anesthesiology Clinics*, 40(2), 383–397. DOI: 10.1016/j.anclin.2022.01.011 PMID: 35659409

Liu, D., Santhanam, R., & Webster, J. (2017). Toward Meaningful Engagement: A Framework for Design and Research of Gamified Information Systems. *Management Information Systems Quarterly*, 41(4), 1011–1034. DOI: 10.25300/MISQ/2017/41.4.01

Li, X. Y., Wang, J., Zhang, R. X., Chen, L., He, C. K., Wang, C. Y., Ke, J., Wang, Y., Zhang, Z., & Song, X. M. (2020). Psychological status among anesthesiologists and operating room nurses during the outbreak period of COVID-19 in Wuhan, China. *Frontiers in Psychiatry*, 11, 574143. DOI: 10.3389/fpsyt.2020.574143 PMID: 33343417

Lodgaard, E., & Schulte, K. Ø. (2019). Knowledge Sharing in Product Development Teams. In Wang, K., Wang, Y., Strandhagen, J., & Yu, T. (Eds.), *Advanced Manufacturing and Automation VIII. IWAMA 2018. Lecture Notes in Electrical Engineering* (Vol. 484). Springer., DOI: 10.1007/978-981-13-2375-1_54

López, M. A. (2016). The Role of Emotions in the Consumer: Theoretical Review and Analysis of Components. *World Academy of Science, Engineering and Technology, International Journal of Social, Behavioral, Educational, Economic. Business and Industrial Engineering*, 10(3), 890–894.

Maan, J. (2013). Social Business Transformation Through Gamification. [IJMIT]. *International Journal of Managing Information Technology*, 5(3), 9–16. DOI: 10.5121/ijmit.2013.5302

Mabunda, L. C. (2021). Avaliação da regulamentação dos dispositivos médicos em Moçambique e seu enquadramento no contexto global. ul.pt

MacDonald, R. D., & Soel, M. S. M. (2023). Articles That May Change Your Practice: Pelvic Binders Revisited. *Air Medical Journal*, 42(2), 88–90. DOI: 10.1016/j.amj.2023.01.003 PMID: 36958878

Machado, A. M. C. (2023). Contributos para a estratégia de internacionalização no Reino Unido: o caso do Grupo ADA eo mercado de dispositivos médicos. uminho.pt

Machado, L. P. (2024). Proposta de um Plano Estratégico de Marketing para um Sistema Inteligente de Apoio ao Diagnóstico do Cancro da Mama: O caso de Estudo do Projeto …. [HTML]

Machado, L. P. (2024). Proposta de um Plano Estratégico de Marketing para um Sistema Inteligente de Apoio ao Diagnóstico do Cancro da Mama: O caso de Estudo do Projeto …. [HTML].

Madsen, J. E., Flugsrud, G. B., Hammer, N., & Puchwein, P. (2024). Emergency treatment of pelvic ring injuries: State of the art. *Archives of Orthopaedic and Trauma Surgery*, 144(10), 1–15. DOI: 10.1007/s00402-024-05447-7 PMID: 38970673

Magretta, J., & Stone, N. (2002). What Management is: How it Works and Why it's Everyone's Business. Free Press, New York, NYManagement Accountants Mason: South-Western College Pub.

Marczewski, A. (2013). *Gamification: A simple introduction & a bit more*. CreateSpace Independent Publishing Platform.

Margolis, R. D., & Ku, C. M. (2021). *The "Difficult Learner" in anesthesiology: challenges, pitfalls, and recommendations*. Pediatric Anesthesia.

Markets, M. (2023). Gamification market trends, analysis, and growth prospects in 2023. Market Research Reports. Available at: https://www.marketsandmarkets .com/gamification2023

Markus, H. R., & Kitayama, S. (1991). Culture and the self: Implications for cognition, emotion, and motivation. *Psychological Review*, 98(2), 224–253. DOI: 10.1037/0033-295X.98.2.224

Maroco, J. (2007). *Análise estatística: com utilização do SPSS (3ª Edição)*. Edições Sílabo.

Marôco, J. (2021). *Análise Estatística com o SPSS Statistics*. ReportNumber.

Marsh, A. A., Elfenbein, H. A., & Ambady, N. (2003). Nonverbal "accents": Cultural differences in facial expressions of emotion. *Psychological Science*, 14(4), 373–376. DOI: 10.1111/1467-9280.24461 PMID: 12807413

Marshall, M. N., Hiscock, J., & Sibbald, B. (2002). Attitudes to the public release of comparative information on the quality of general practice care: Qualitative study. *BMJ (Clinical Research Ed.)*, 325(7375), 1278. DOI: 10.1136/bmj.325.7375.1278 PMID: 12458248

Martínez-Peláez, R., Ochoa-Brust, A., Rivera, S., Félix, V. G., Ostos, R., Brito, H., Félix, R. A., & Mena, L. J. (2023). Role of digital transformation for achieving sustainability: Mediated role of stakeholders, key capabilities, and technology. *Sustainability (Basel)*, 15(14), 11221. DOI: 10.3390/su151411221

Martins, J. Z. (2024). O uso da metodologia BIM no gerenciamento e coordenação de projetos. unb.br

Martins, M. I. (2022). Relatórios de Estágio e Monografia intitulada Epilepsia Canina: Contributo dos Dispositivos Médicos. uc.pt

Massonini Ngoma, R. G. T., Abraham Mahanga Tsoni, C. G., Meng, X., & Bashiru Danwana, S. (2023). The impact of the mining equipment, technological trends, and natural resource demand on climate change in Congo. *Sustainability (Basel)*, 15(2), 1691. DOI: 10.3390/su15021691

Mathis, M. R., Schonberger, R. B., Whitlock, E. L., Vogt, K. M., Lagorio, J. E., Jones, K. A., & Kheterpal, S. (2022). Opportunities beyond the anesthesiology department: Broader impact through broader thinking. *Anesthesia and Analgesia*, 134(2), 242–252. PMID: 33684091

Mavroeidi, A. G., Kitsiou, A., Kalloniatis, C., & Gritzalis, S. (2019). Gamification vs. privacy: Identifying and analysing the major concerns. *Future Internet*, 11(3), 67. Advance online publication. DOI: 10.3390/fi11030067

Mayo Clinic. (2020). **Virtual care: Patient-centered remote healthcare services**. *Mayo Clinic Social Media Network*. https://socialmedia.mayoclinic.org/2020/05/12/virtual-care-patient-centered-remote-healthcare-services/

Mazzarol, T., (2005, setembro). Caraterísticas de planeamento e crescimento dos proprietários- gestores de pequenas empresas. Barcelona: 359 Conferência sobre Empreendedorismo, Inovação e Pequenas Empresas (EISB).

McCormack, B., & McCance, T. (2021). The Person-Centred Nursing Framework. In Dewing, J., McCormack, B., & McCance, T. (Eds.), *Person-centred Nursing Research: Methodology, Methods and Outcomes*. Springer., DOI: 10.1007/978-3-030-27868-7_2

Mcevoy, M. D., & Abernathy, J. J. (2023). *Perioperative Safety Culture, An Issue of Anesthesiology Clinics*. E-Book.

Mearns, K., Whitaker, S. M., & Flin, R. (2003). Safety climate, safety management practice and safety performance in offshore environments. [Measurement.]. *Safety Science*, 41(8), 641–680. DOI: 10.1016/S0925-7535(02)00011-5

Medina, A. S. A., Bonilla, M. I. A., Giraldo, I. D. R., Palacios, J. F. M., Gutiérrez, D. A. C., & Liscano, Y. (2024). Electroencephalography-Based Brain-Computer Interfaces in Rehabilitation: A Bibliometric Analysis (2013–2023). *Sensors (Basel)*, 24(22), 7125. DOI: 10.3390/s24227125 PMID: 39598903

Melo, J. C. (2024). Alinhamento entre o planejamento estratégico eo orçamento: um estudo de caso em uma instituição de ensino superior. ufrn.br

Mendes, E., Timóteo, J., & Cabral, A. S. (2014). Aspetos médico-legais em psiquiatria. In C. B. Saraiva & J. Cerejeira (Eds.), *Psiquiatria fundamental* (Vol., pp. 507-520). LIDEL – Edições Técnicas, Lda.

Mendes, J. C. V. (2024). Exposição a Dispositivos Eletrónicos em Idades Precoces–Seu Impacto no Desenvolvimento e Regulação Emocional de Crianças em Idade Pré-Escolar. uminho.pt

Mendes, M. M. (2024). Planejamento estratégico para o desenvolvimento da implementação de franquias de micro e pequenas empresas. unipampa.edu.br

Meng, X., & Minoque, M. (2011). Performance Measurement Models in Facility Management: A Comparative Study. *Facilities*, 29(11/12), 472–484. Advance online publication. DOI: 10.1108/02632771111157141

Mennen, A. H., Lommerse, M., Hemke, R., Willems, H. C., Maas, M., Bloemers, F. W., Ponsen, K. J., & Van Embden, D. (2024). Does regional implementation of a clinical pathway for older adult patients with pelvic fragility fractures after low-energy trauma improve patient outcomes (PELVIC): A multicentre, stepped-wedge, randomised controlled trial. *BMJ Open*, 14(8), e083809. DOI: 10.1136/bmjopen-2023-083809 PMID: 39142675

Meyer, M., & Schaeffer, J. (2019). Challenges in remote healthcare delivery: Perspectives from healthcare leaders. *Health Affairs*, 38(8), 1346–1354. DOI: 10.1377/hlthaff.2019.00412

Meyer, T., Selb, M., Kiekens, C., Grubišić, F., Arienti, C., Stucki, G., & Negrini, S. (2020). Toward better reporting standards of patients' characteristics in rehabilitation trials: Applying a new conceptual framework to current standards. *American Journal of Physical Medicine & Rehabilitation*, 99(3), 216–223. DOI: 10.1097/PHM.0000000000001375 PMID: 31860587

Mickan, S. M., & Rodger, S. A. (2005). Effective health care teams: A model of six characteristics developed from shared perceptions. *Journal of Interprofessional Care*, 19(4), 358–370. DOI: 10.1080/13561820500165142 PMID: 16076597

Millan, J. R., Renkens, F., Mourino, J., & Gerstner, W. (2004). Noninvasive Brain-Actuated Control of a Mobile Robot by Human EEG. *IEEE Transactions on Biomedical Engineering*, 51(6), 1026–1033. DOI: 10.1109/TBME.2004.827086 PMID: 15188874

Modell, S. (2009). Institutional research on performance measurement and management in the public sector accounting literature: A review and assessment. Financial Accountability & Management, 25(3), 277-303. DOI: . 00477.xDOI: 10.1111/j.1468- 0408.2009

Mohadeseh, R., Mohaddeseh, M., Azam, M., & Mahboobeh, K. (2021). Correlation of Moral Courage and Organizational Commitment in Operating Room Nurses. *Siriraj Medical Journal*, 73(3), 183–190. DOI: 10.33192/Smj.2021.24

Mohajan, H. (2017). The Impact of Knowledge Management Models for the Development of Organizations. *Journal of Environmental Treatment Techniques*, 5(1), 12–33. https://mpra.ub.uni-muenchen.de/83089/1/MPRA_paper_83089.pdf

Mokarami, H., Gharibi, V., Kalteh, H. O., Faraji Kujerdi, M., & Kazemi, R. (2020). Multiple environmental and psychosocial work risk factors and sleep disturbances. *International Archives of Occupational and Environmental Health*, 93(5), 623–633. DOI: 10.1007/s00420-020-01515-8 PMID: 31955238

Monteiro, T. A., Giuliani, A. C., Pizzinatto, A. K., & de Toledo Pitombo, T. C. D. (2014). Consumer ecological awareness and green marketing: a case study on sustainable marketing practices in Brazil/ ecological awareness of the consumer and green marketing: a case study of sustainable marketing practices in brazil. [Santo Agostinho University Center]. *FSA Journal*, 11(2), 84–97.

Mora, A., Riera, D., Gonzalez, C., & Arnedo-Moreno, J. (2015, October 9). A Literature Review of Gamification Design Frameworks. VS-Games 2015 - *7th International Conference on Games and Virtual Worlds for Serious Applications*. https://doi.org/DOI: 10.1109/VS-GAMES.2015.7295760

Moreira, K. T. D. (2024). Responsabilidade civil em cirurgias robóticas: desafios e perspectivas no contexto brasileiro.. unisc.br

Moreira, C. V. (2015). Green marketing as a sustainable competitive advantage for an organization. *Revista Foco*, 8(2), 133–144. DOI: 10.28950/1981-223x_revistafocoadm/2015.v8i2.183

Morgan, S. E., Mosser, A., Ahn, S., Harrison, T. R., Wang, J., Huang, Q., Reynolds, A., Mao, B., & Bixby, J. L. (2021). Developing and evaluating a team development intervention to support interdisciplinary teams. *Journal of Clinical and Translational Science*, 5(1), e166. DOI: 10.1017/cts.2021.831 PMID: 34733543

Moss, E., Seifert, P. C., & O'Sullivan, A. (2016). Registered Nurses as Interprofessional Collaborative Partners: Creating Value-Based Outcomes. *Online Journal of Issues in Nursing*, 21(3), 4. DOI: 10.3912/OJIN.Vol21No03Man04 PMID: 27857055

Motta, S. L. S., & Oliveira, B. (2007). Ecological marketing as a competitive advantage. *REGE Management Journal*, 14(2), 49–59.

Mount Sinai Health System. (2021). *The Mount Sinai Health System's telehealth initiative: Expanding access to care*. Mount Sinai Health System News.

Moy, A. J., Hobensack, M., Marshall, K., Vawdrey, D. K., Kim, E. Y., Cato, K. D., & Rossetti, S. C. (2023). Understanding the perceived role of electronic health records and workflow fragmentation on clinician documentation burden in emergency departments. *Journal of the American Medical Informatics Association : JAMIA*, 30(5), 797–808. DOI: 10.1093/jamia/ocad038 PMID: 36905604

Mulualen, M. (2011). The impacts of working capital management of firms' profitability. Msc thesis Addis Ababa University. Addis ababa- Ethiopia

Murteira, B. J. F. (2004). *Análise exploratória de dados: estatística descritiva*. McGraw-Hill.

Neely, A., Gregory, M., & Platts, K. (2005). Performance measurement system design: A literature review and research agenda. *International Journal of Operations & Production Management*, 25(12), 1228–1263.

Nguyen, , P. N. D., Nguyen, L. L. K., & LE, D. N. T. (2021). The impact of extrinsic work factors on job satisfaction and organizational commitment at higher education institutions in Vietnam. *The Journal of Asian Finance, Economics and Business*, 8(8), 259–270.

Nguyen, T. M. (2020). Do extrinsic motivation and organisational culture additively strengthen intrinsic motivation in online knowledge sharing? An empirical study. *VINE Journal of Information and Knowledge Management Systems*, 50(1), 75–93. DOI: 10.1108/VJIKMS-02-2019-0019

Nielsen, J. (2019). *Designing user-friendly digital interactions: The gamification perspective*. Morgan & Claypool Publishers.

Nigg, C. R., Fuchs, R., Gerber, M., Jekauc, D., Koch, T., Krell-Roesch, J., Lippke, S., Mnich, C., Novak, B., Ju, Q., Sattler, M. C., Schmidt, S. C. E., van Poppel, M., Reimers, A. K., Wagner, P., Woods, C., & Woll, A. (2020). Assessing physical activity through questionnaires–A consensus of best practices and future directions. *Psychology of Sport and Exercise*, 50, 101715. DOI: 10.1016/j.psychsport.2020.101715

Nilashi, M., Keng Boon, O., Tan, G., Lin, B., & Abumalloh, R. (2023). Critical data challenges in measuring the performance of sustainable development goals: Solutions and the role of big-data analytics. *Harvard Data Science Review*, 5(3), 3–4. DOI: 10.1162/99608f92.545db2cf

Nolan, R.Jr, & Foran, R. (1983). Strategic financial planning. *Journal - American Water Works Association*, 75(9), 436–440. DOI: 10.1002/j.1551-8833.1983.tb05190.x

Nuryakin, N., & Maryati, T. (2022). Do green innovation and green competitive advantage mediate the effect of green marketing orientation on SMEs' green marketing performance? *Cogent Business & Management*, 9(1), 2065948. Advance online publication. DOI: 10.1080/23311975.2022.2065948

Nuttin, J. (2014). *Future time perspective and motivation: Theory and research method*. Psychology Press. DOI: 10.4324/9781315802244

Nwosu, N. T. (2024). *Reducing operational costs in healthcare through advanced BI tools and data integration*. World Journal of Advanced Research and Reviews.

Oliveira, D., Campelo, F., Poblete, J., Herszkowicz, L., Ribas, R., & Rodrigues, R. (2021). Planejamento estratégico da Viação Paraty: uma proposta com ênfase na inovação e eficiência operacional. itl.org.br

Oliveira, MLD (2019). Sustainable consumption behavior in thrift stores: an analysis of the influence of sociocultural factors on the purchase decision process.

Oliveira, A. G. (2009). *Bioestatística, epidemiologia e investigação: teoria e aplicações*. LIDEL.

Oliveira, B. S. D. S. B., Neto, C. F., Damasceno, D. L. N. G., da Costa, E. R., de Paiva Brasil, L. G., Velho Filho, O. P., & Lima, S. C. (2024). ANÁLISE E EVOLUÇÃO DA TELEMEDICINA NO BRASIL NOS ANOS 2019-2023 E SUA ATUAL IMPORTÂNCIA. [revistacontemporanea.com]. *Revista Contemporânea*, 4(10), e6123–e6123. DOI: 10.56083/RCV4N10-088

Ordunez, P., & Campbell, N. R., GP, G. A., Angell, S. Y., Lombardi, C., Brettler, J. W., ... & Sharman, J. E. (2022). HEARTS in the Americas: innovations for improving hypertension and cardiovascular disease risk management in primary careHEARTS nas Américas: inovações para melhorar a gestão do risco de hipertensão e de doenças cardiovasculares na atenção primária. Revista Panamericana de Salud Publica= Pan [HTML]. *American Journal of Public Health*, 46, e197–e197. PMID: 36284552

Ortega, A., (2008). Planeamento financeiro estratégico. Cidade do México: McGraw Hill Interamericana.

Otley, D. (2003) "Measuring Performance, the Accounting Perspective in Business Performance

Otta, E., & Fiquer, J. (2004). Subjective well-being and emotional regulation. *Psicologia em Revista*, 10(15), 144–149. https://periodicos.pucminas.br/index.php/psicologiaemrevista/article/view/204

Pacevičiūtė, A., & Razbadauskaitė-Venskė, I. (2023). The role of green marketing in creating a sustainable competitive advantage. *Regional training and development studies: journal of social sciences .*, (2), 89-98.

Pacheco, R. P. V. Q. (2023). Desafios na implementação e manutenção de um sistema de gestão integrado* numa organização multisite* âmbitos: qualidade, ambiente, segurança e saúde no .... ipl.pt

Padilla-Lozano, C. P., & Collazzo, P. (2022). Corporate social responsibility, green innovation, and competitiveness–causality in manufacturing. *Competitiveness Review*, 32(7), 21–39. DOI: 10.1108/CR-12-2020-0160

Paige, J. T., Garbee, D. D., Bonanno, L. S., & Kerdolff, K. E. (2021). Qualitative analysis of effective teamwork in the operating room (OR). *Journal of Surgical Education*, 78(3), 967–979. DOI: 10.1016/j.jsurg.2020.09.019 PMID: 33160940

Panditrao, M. M., & Panditrao, M. M. (2024). "Burnout syndrome" in anesthesiologists and remedial measures-A narrative review. *Journal ofAnaesthesiology, Clinical Pharmacology*, 40(2), 206–216. DOI: 10.4103/joacp.joacp_322_22 PMID: 38919431

Panksepp, J. (2003). At the interface of the affective, behavioral, and cognitive neurosciences: Decoding the emotional feelings of the brain. *Brain and Cognition*, 52(1), 4–14. DOI: 10.1016/S0278-2626(03)00003-4 PMID: 12812799

Panksepp, J. (2004). *Affective Neuroscience: The Foundations of Human and Animal Emotions*. Oxford University Press.

Papalia, D. E., Martorell, G., & Feldman, R. D. (2021). *Desenvolvimento Humano* (14.ª ed.). McGraw Hill.

Parker, W. J., Johnston, L. R., Atwood, R., Walker, P., & Bradley, M. J. (2024). Initial Management of Pelvic Fractures. *Current Trauma Reports*, •••, 1–7.

Parlindungan, H. H., Masatip, A., & Manurung, H. (2021). Tourism investment and financial digital. European Journal of Science. *Innovation and Technology*, 1(4), 30–44.

Parmenter, D. (2009). *Key Performance Indicators: Developing, Implementing, and Using Winning KPIs*. Wiley.

Parmenterg, D. (2007). *Key Performance Indicators: developing, implementing, and using winning KPIs*. Wiley.

Parnikh, H., Torabizadeh, C., Najafi Kalyani, M., & Soltanian, M. (2022). A Study of the Relationship between Professional Communication and Professional Commitment in Operating Room Nurses. *Nursing Research and Practice*, 2022(1), 5871846. DOI: 10.1155/2022/5871846 PMID: 35847234

Patrício, R., Moreira, A. C., & Zurlo, F. (2021). Enhancing design thinking approaches to innovation through gamification. [researchgate.net]. *European Journal of Innovation Management*, 24(5), 1569–1594. DOI: 10.1108/EJIM-06-2020-0239

Patricio, R., Moreira, A. C., & Zurlo, F. (2022). Gamification in innovation teams. *International Journal of Innovation Studies*, 6(3), 156–168. DOI: 10.1016/j.ijis.2022.05.003

Patricio, R., Moreira, A., Zurlo, F., & Melazzini, M. (2020). Co-creation of new solutions through gamification: A collaborative innovation practice. [ssrn.com]. *Creativity and Innovation Management*, 29(1), 146–160. DOI: 10.1111/caim.12356

Pechim, M. D. F. (2024). O PAPEL ESTRATÉGICO DO DEPARTAMENTO CONTÁBIL: PRÁTICAS, DESAFIOS E INOVAÇÕES. RECIMA21-Revista Científica Multidisciplinar-ISSN 2675-6218, 5(5), e555290-e555290. recima21.com.br

Pereira Pinheiro, C. M., Schreiber, D., Cherutti, M., & Schmidt, S. (2020). Processo criativo em moda: redes de colaboração entre microempreendedores individuais gaúchos. Diálogo com a Economia Criativa, 5(14). [HTML]

Pereira, C. A. (2023). Impacto das redes sociais na medicina dentária na vertente social e económica em Portugal. rcaap.pt

Pereira, T. P. C. (2024). Explorando os limites da responsabilidade civil: o impacto do desenvolvimento tecnológico dos procedimentos cirúrgicos robóticos.. 52.186.153.119

Pereira, R., & Gomes, L. (2022). Exploring gamified learning in higher education: Student perspectives and outcomes. *Journal of Interactive Learning Research*, 33(3), 213–229. DOI: 10.1007/s11423-022-10045-x

Perez, J. F. L. U. (2020). Modos de convergência regulamentar entre medicamentos e dispositivos médicos no quadro da União Europeia. ul.pt

Pfister, R. A., & Eppler, M. J. (2012). The benefits of sketching for knowledge management. *Journal of Knowledge Management*, 16(2), 372–382. DOI: 10.1108/13673271211218924

Pfurtscheller, G., Neuper, C., Guger, C., Harkam, W., Ramoser, H., Schlogl, A., Obermaier, B., & Pregenzer, M. (2000). Current Trends in Graz Brain–Computer Interface (BCI) Research. *IEEE Transactions on Rehabilitation Engineering*, 8(2), 216–219. DOI: 10.1109/86.847821 PMID: 10896192

Pham, H.T. (2010). The effect of efficient financial management practices on Profitability of Small and Medium

Philips, P., & Louvieris, P. (2005). Sistemas de medição do desempenho em pequenas, médias e grandes empresas de turismo, hotelaria e lazer. *Journal of Travel Research*, 44, 201–211. DOI: 10.1177/0047287505278992

Picard, R. W. (2000). *Affective computing*. The MIT Press. DOI: 10.7551/mitpress/1140.003.0008

Pinyavat, T., & Mulaikal, T. A. (2020). Fostering physician well-being in anesthesiology. *International Anesthesiology Clinics*, 58(4), 36–40. DOI: 10.1097/AIA.0000000000000300 PMID: 32841965

Pio Abreu, J. L. (2015). *Introdução à psicopatologia compreensiva*. Fundação Calouste Gulbenkian.

Pio Abreu, J. L., & Vaz Patto, M. L. (1981). A Utilização de uma Escala de Rastreio em Epidemiologia Clínica. *Psiquiatria Clínica*, 2, 119–133.

Plsek, P. E., & Greenhalgh, T. (2001). Complexity science: The challenge of complexity in health care. *BMJ (Clinical Research Ed.)*, 323(7313), 625–628. DOI: 10.1136/bmj.323.7313.625 PMID: 11557716

Pollak, J., & Adams, P. (2011). *PAM: A Photographic Affect Meter for frequent, in situ measurement of affect*. https://doi.org/DOI: 10.1145/1978942.1979047

Pols J. (2017). Good relations with technology: Empirical ethics and aesthetics in care. *Nursing philosophy: an international journal for healthcare professionals, 18*(1), . https://doi.org/DOI: 10.1111/nup.12154

Pontin, A. L., Angélica, C., Miragem, B., & Santorsula, C. B. (2020). Compliance na área da saúde. [HTML]

Porto, I. G. C. (2024). Processo de regulamentação de dispositivos médicos no brasil: da anvisa até o consumidor final. ufscar.br

Probst, T., Pryss, R., Langguth, B., & Schlee, W. (2016). Emotion dynamics and tinnitus: Daily life data from the "TrackYourTinnitus" application. *Scientific Reports*, 6(1), 31166. DOI: 10.1038/srep31166 PMID: 27488227

Purwanti, I., Abadi, M. D., Suyanto, U. Y., & Ahmad, S. T. I. E. K. (2019). Green marketing: Strategy for achieving sustainable competitive advantage in industry 4.0. *Management Bisnis*, 9(2), 176–193.

Queirós, C. C. (2022). Análise do custo-efetividade da PET/CT com 68Ga-PSMA nos doentes de carcinoma da próstata em recidiva bioquímica após prostatectomia radical. ipl.pt

Radons, D. L., Battistella, L. F., & Grohmann, M. Z. (2012). Competitive advantage of companies: What is the influence of green innovation? *Brazilian Journal of Scientific Administration*, 3(3), 97–111.

Ralph, P., & Monu, K. (2015). Toward a Unified Theory of Digital Games. *The Computer Games Journal*, 4(1–2), 81–100. DOI: 10.1007/s40869-015-0007-7

Rane, N., Choudhary, S., & Rane, J. (2023). Education 4.0 and 5.0: Integrating artificial intelligence (AI) for personalized and adaptive learning. Available at *SSRN* 4638365. *ssrn*.com DOI: 10.2139/ssrn.4638365

Rathore, S. (2008). *International Accounting*. PHI Learning Private Limited.

Rattan, A., Joshi, M. K., Mishra, B., Kumar, S., Sagar, S., & Gupta, A. (2021). Profile of injuries in children: Report from a level I trauma center. *Indian Pediatrics*, 58(6), 553–555. DOI: 10.1007/s13312-021-2239-x PMID: 32893835

Rauch, M. (2013). Best practices for using enterprise gamification to engage employees and customers. *In Lecture Notes in Human Computer Science* (pp. 276–283). https://doi.org/DOI: 10.1007/978-3-642-39262-7_31

Reato, F., Bresil, A., D'Angelo, C., Gorli, M., Ivziku, D., Lommi, M., & Carcano, G. (2024, September). Toward the Definition of a Repertoire of Technical Professional Specialist Competencies for Operating Room Nurses: An Ethnographic Study. In Healthcare (Vol. 12, No. 17, p. 1774). MDPI.

Reis, E. (2006). *Estatística multivariada aplicada* (2.ª ed.). Edições Sílabo.

Reis, M. A. B. M. N., & Horta, M. P. (2015). O papel das emoções na relação confiança-exatidão do testemunho. *Psicologia USP*, 26(2), 231–239. DOI: 10.1590/0103-656420140003

Riar, M., Morschheuser, B., Zarnekow, R., & Hamari, J. (2022). Gamification of cooperation: A framework, literature review and future research agenda. *International Journal of Information Management,* Volume 67, 102549, ISSN 0268-4012, DOI: 10.1016/j.ijinfomgt.2022.102549

Ribeiro, V. T. R. (2024). Avaliação e implementação de arquitetura distribuída para disponibilização de serviços de telemedicina em computação em borda. ufcg.edu.br

Ribeiro, A., & Monteiro, L. (2015). Induction affective scenarios virtual reality: Assessment of the sensation of presence. *Psicologia Clínica*, 27(1), 139–160. DOI: 10.1590/0103-56652015000100008

Robson, K., Plangger, K., Kietzmann, J. H., McCarthy, I., & Pitt, L. (2015). Is it all a game? Understanding the principles of gamification. *Business Horizons*, 58(4), 411–420. https://doi.org/https://doi.org/10.1016/j.bushor.2015.03.006. DOI: 10.1016/j.bushor.2015.03.006

Rodrigues, F. L. B. (2024). Proposta de planejamento estratégico para uma revista científica da área da administração. ufsc.br

Rolstadås, A. (1998). Enterprise performance measurement. *International Journal of Operations & Production Management*, 18(9/10), 989–999. DOI: 10.1108/01443579810225577

Rositch, A. F., Unger-Saldaña, K., DeBoer, R. J., Ng'ang'a, A., & Weiner, B. J. (2020). The role of dissemination and implementation science in global breast cancer control programs: Frameworks, methods, and examples. *Cancer*, 126(S10), 2394–2404. DOI: 10.1002/cncr.32877 PMID: 32348574

Röttger, S., & Krey, H. (2021). Experimental study on the effects of a single simulator-based bridge resource management unit on attitudes, behaviour and performance. *Journal of Navigation*, 74(5), 1127–1141. DOI: 10.1017/S0373463321000436

Roveda, A. (2024). Mapeamento de depósitos de patentes referentes a tecnologias utilizadas na detecção do Transtorno do Espectro do Autismo (TEA) no mundo. ufsc.br

Ruhi, U. (2015). Level Up Your Strategy: Towards a Descriptive Framework for Meaningful Enterprise Gamification. *Technology Innovation Management Review*, 5(8), 5–16. DOI: 10.22215/timreview/918

Russell, J. A. (1980). A Circumplex Model of Affect. *Journal of Personality and Social Psychology*, 39(6), 1161–1178. DOI: 10.1037/h0077714

Russell, J. A., & Barrett, L. F. (1999). Core affect, prototypical emotional episodes, and other things called emotion: Dissecting the elephant. *Journal of Personality and Social Psychology*, 76(5), 805–819. DOI: 10.1037/0022-3514.76.5.805 PMID: 10353204

Sá, J., Lins, N., Fonseca, R., & Santos, R. (2017). Green marketing-an analysis of Shell 's "make the future" campaign . *Veredas FAVIP: Electronic Journal of Science and Culture, 10* (1).

Sadler-Smith, E., Spicer, D. P., & Chaston, I. (2001). Learning orientations and growth in smaller organizations. *Long Range Planning*, 34(2), 139–158. DOI: 10.1016/S0024-6301(01)00020-6

Sailer, M., Hense, J. U., Mayr, S. K., & Mandl, H. (2017). How gamification motivates: An experimental study of the effects of specific game design elements on psychological need satisfaction. *Computers in Human Behavior*, 69, 371–380. DOI: 10.1016/j.chb.2016.12.033

Sales, J. L. (2023). Estudo bibliométrico sobre o Sistema de Gestão Integrada (SGI) no Brasil. ufc.br

Santos Toscas, F. (2021). Abordagens do monitoramento do horizonte tecnológico e prospecção tecnológica em dispositivos médicos. JBES: Brazilian Journal of Health Economics/Jornal Brasileiro de Economia da Saúde, 13(3). [HTML]

Santos Toscas, F., & Alves Teixeira, L. A. (2022). Mapeamento dos bancos de dados em dispositivos médicos: revisão narrativa e o cenário brasileiro para avaliação com dados de mundo real (RWD). JBES: Brazilian Journal of Health Economics/Jornal Brasileiro de Economia da Saúde, 14. [HTML]

Santos Toscas, F., de Morais Oliveira, V. C., & Silveira Silva, A. (2022). O papel da sociedade civil na inovação e incorporação de dispositivos médicos no Brasil. JBES: Brazilian Journal of Health Economics/Jornal Brasileiro de Economia da Saúde, 14. [HTML] Machado, A. M. C. (2023). Contributos para a estratégia de internacionalização no Reino Unido: o caso do Grupo ADA eo mercado de dispositivos médicos. uminho.pt

Santos, A. L. G. (2023). Proposta de planejamento estratégico em uma microempresa: estudo de caso em um comércio especializado no serviço de sinalização de trânsito. ufc.br

Santos, B. S. O. (2023). Gestão de risco em engenharia clínica: revisão sistemática. ufrn.br

Santos, A. C. G., Oliveira, W., Hamari, J., Rodrigues, L., Toda, A. M., Palomino, P. T., & Isotani, S. (2021). The relationship between user types and gamification designs. [springer.com]. *User Modeling and User-Adapted Interaction*, 31(5), 907–940. DOI: 10.1007/s11257-021-09300-z

Savakus, J. C., Skacel, T., Jindia, M., Al-Madani, Y., Spoletini, L., Ross, R. C., & Stinner, D. J. (2024). Biomechanical validation of the field-expedient pelvic splint. *BMJ Military Health*, military-2024-002815. DOI: 10.1136/military-2024-002815 PMID: 39521613

Savioz, P., & Blum, M. (2002). Strategic forecast tool for SMEs: How the opportunity landscape interacts with business strategy to anticipate technological trends. *Technovation*, 22(2), 91–100. DOI: 10.1016/S0166-4972(01)00082-7

Sawang, S. (2011). Key Performance Indicators for Innovation Implementation: Perception vs. Actual Usage. *Asia Pacific Management Review*, 16(1), 23–29.

Schechowiz, R. (2021). Contributions of chief financial officers working as interim managers to organisation success in small and medium-sized companies. DOI: 10.1155/2022/8669348

Scherer, K. R. (2003). Vocal communication of emotion: A review of research paradigms. *Speech Communication*, 40(1-2), 227–256. DOI: 10.1016/S0167-6393(02)00084-5

Scherer, K. R., Schorr, A., & Johnstone, T. (2001). *Appraisal Processes in Emotion*. Oxford University Press., DOI: 10.1093/oso/9780195130072.001.0001

Schindler, C. R., Sturm, R., Hörauf, J. A., Marzi, I., & Störmann, P. (2023). The sequence of the treatment of combined fractures of the pelvis, spine, and extremities in polytraumatized patients. *EFORT Open Reviews*, 8(5), 372–381. DOI: 10.1530/EOR-23-0046 PMID: 37158361

Schmutz, J. B., Meier, L. L., & Manser, T. (2019). How effective is teamwork really? The relationship between teamwork and performance in healthcare teams: A systematic review and meta-analysis. *BMJ Open*, 9(9), e028280. DOI: 10.1136/bmjopen-2018-028280 PMID: 31515415

Segurado, M. A. P. (1980). *Biomatemática: matemática aplicada para estudantes de biologia, farmácia e medicina* (Vol. 1). Plátano Editora.

Serrano, G. P. (1994). *Investigation qualitative: straight and questioning* . Madrid: The wall .

Severi, L. D. M. (2024). Conectividade e saúde: uma revisão crítica da literatura sobre a inserção da IoT no contexto médico. ufscar.br

Shah, M. K., Gandrakota, N., Cimiotti, J. P., Ghose, N., Moore, M., & Ali, M. K. (2021). Prevalence of and Factors Associated With Nurse Burnout in the US. *JAMA Network Open*, 4(2), e2036469. DOI: 10.1001/jamanetworkopen.2020.36469 PMID: 33538823

Shah, N. K., & Emerick, T. D. (2021). Lean Six Sigma methodology and the future of quality improvement education in anesthesiology. *Anesthesia and Analgesia*. Advance online publication. DOI: 10.1213/ANE.0000000000005636 PMID: 34142980

Sharma, W., Lim, W. M., Kumar, S., Verma, A., & Kumra, R. (2024). Game on! A state-of-the-art overview of doing business with gamification. [sciencedirect.com]. *Technological Forecasting and Social Change*, 198, 122988. DOI: 10.1016/j.techfore.2023.122988

Shaukat, F., & Ming, J. (2022). Impact of green marketing orientation on business performance: Case of Pakistani pharmaceutical industry. *Frontiers in Psychology*, 13, 940278. DOI: 10.3389/fpsyg.2022.940278 PMID: 36237687

Shetti, A. N. (2024). Battling Burnout: A Comprehensive Exploration of The Impact on Anaesthesiologists and Strategies for Resilience. *Jour Med Dent Fron*, 1, 5–15.

Shu, L., Xie, J., Yang, M., Li, Z., Li, Z., Liao, D., Xu, X., & Yang, X. (2018). A Review of Emotion Recognition Using Physiological Signals. *Sensors (Basel)*, 18(7), 2074. DOI: 10.3390/s18072074 PMID: 29958457

Siddiqui, S., Bartels, K., Schaefer, M. S., Novack, L., Sreedharan, R., Ben-Jacob, T. K., Khanna, A. K., Nunnally, M. E., Souter, M., Simmons, S. T., & Williams, G. (2021). Critical care medicine practice: A pilot survey of US anesthesia critical care medicine–trained physicians. *Anesthesia and Analgesia*, 132(3), 761–769. DOI: 10.1213/ANE.0000000000005030 PMID: 32665465

Silva, A. C. (2022). Equipamento rapha® para a cura do pé diabético: uma abordagem translacional em saúde. unb.br

Silva, F. A. C. (2023). O financiamento às atividades inovativas na indústria nas regiões brasileiras. ufc.br

Silva, M. L. S. (2021). Análise do protocolo RPL em redes LLNs no ambiente de internet das coisas, healthcare. ufu.br

Silva, S. C. S. (2021). Impacto das Novas ISO 14001: 2015 e ISO 9001: 2015 Nos Sistemas Integrados: Análise de Um Percurso de Transição. [HTML]

Silva, T. G. (2022). Desenvolvimento de um bloco operatório: projeto, construção, equipamentos médicos e vídeo-integração. rcaap.pt

Silva, P. C. D., Teixeira, R. L. P., & de Araújo Brito, M. L. (2022). The role of green marketing in advertising campaigns of cosmetics companies: an analytical and linguistic approach to the metaphorization of green: green marketing in cosmetics companies advertising campaigns: an analytical and linguistic approach to the metaphorization of Green. *Journal of Social and Environmental Management*, 16(2), e02996–e02996.

Simons, R. (2000). Performance Measurement and Control Systems for Implementing Slovene Multinational Companies ". [Strategy. New Jersey: Prentice- Hall.]. *Management*, 9(1), 53–73.

Şimşek, P., Tayfur, İ., Gunduz, A., & Bayramoglu, B. (2025). Effectiveness of a training program for emergency nurses on pelvic binder application and patient care: A single-group pretest–posttest study. *International Emergency Nursing*, 78, 101528. DOI: 10.1016/j.ienj.2024.101528 PMID: 39612718

Smith, E., & Mackie, D. (2008). Intergroup Emotions. In M. Lewis, J. M. Haviland-Jones, & L. F. Barrett (Eds.), *Handbook of Emotions* (3ª ed., pp. 428-439). The Guildford Press. https://doi.org/DOI: 10.4324/9780203361993

Sobh, R., & Perry, C. (2006). Research design and data analysis in realism research. *European Journal of Marketing*, 40(11/12), 1194–1209. DOI: 10.1108/03090560610702777

Sousa, I. A. M. (2023). Inovação na Administração de Terapêutica Endovenosa: Aperfeiçoamento da Seringa DUO. uc.pt

Sousa, T., Lopes, L., & Esteves, S. (2023). Sustainability and marketing: marketing strategies applied to green marketing and consumer perceptions. *IV International Meeting on Portuguese Language and Lusophone Relations*, 246-254. Steiner[1], VL, & Calgaro, C. Sustainability indicators and corporate social responsibility: a tool for assessing organizational sustainability indicators and corporate social responsibility: a tool for organizational assessment.

Sousa, D. G., Carvalho, R. B., & Castro, J. M. (2020). Análise da contribuição de mapeamento tecnológico (Roadmapping) para a gestão estratégica da inovação: Estudo de caso de uma multinacional do setor automotivo. Revista Inovação [uninove. br]. *Projetos e Tecnologias*, 8(1), 13–24. DOI: 10.5585/iptec.v8i1.17400

Spanellis, A., D rfler, V., & MacBryde, J. (2020). Investigating the potential for using gamification to empower knowledge workers. Expert Systems with Applications. strath.ac.uk

Streckenbach, S., Lai, Y., Bas, H., Crowley, J., Salzsieder, H., Mela, T., & Dalia, A. A. (2021). Starting an Anesthesia-based perioperative device management service: A practical guide to training anesthesiologists. *Journal of Cardiothoracic and Vascular Anesthesia*, 35(4), 1006–1017. DOI: 10.1053/j.jvca.2020.11.044 PMID: 33341343

Suarez, V., Lesneski C., Denison D. (2011). Defender a utilização de indicadores financeiros nas agências locais de saúde pública. Jornal Americano de Saúde Pública, Vol 101, No.3, pp.419.-425

Sugianto, S., Hasriani, H., & Noor, R. M. (2024). Inovações na medição e gestão de riscos para decisões estratégicas de financiamento. *Advances in Management & Financial Reporting*, 2(2), 59–71. DOI: 10.60079/amfr.v2i2.263

Suresh Babu, S., & Dhakshina Moorthy, A. (2024). Application of artificial intelligence in adaptation of gamification in education: A literature review. *Computer Applications in Engineering Education*, 32(1), e22683. DOI: 10.1002/cae.22683

Su, Y., & Zeng, Y. (2023). Simulation based training versus non-simulation based training in anesthesiology: A meta-analysis of randomized controlled trials. *Heliyon*, 9(8), e18249. DOI: 10.1016/j.heliyon.2023.e18249 PMID: 37576292

Tan, M., Naegle, J. A., Boscardin, C. K., Chang, D. P., Chang, J. M., Sullivan, K. R., & Sinskey, J. L. (2023). Drivers of Well-Being and Burnout in Anesthesiology Residents. *The Journal of Education in Perioperative Medicine : JEPM*, 25(4). PMID: 38162705

Teixeira, L. D. M. (2024). Barreiras e potencialidades para educação médica permanente e continuada em saúde mental na atenção primária: uma revisão de escopo. unb.br

Teladoc Health. (2020). **Leadership during crisis: Adapting to remote healthcare delivery**. *Teladoc Health Blog*. https://www.teladochealth.com/leadership-during -crisis/

Thomasian, N. M., & Adashi, E. Y. (2021). Cybersecurity in the internet of medical things. *Health Policy and Technology*, 10(3), 100549. DOI: 10.1016/j.hlpt.2021.100549

Thomas, J.III, & Evanson, R. V. (1987). An Empirical investigation of association between financial ratio use and small business success. *Journal of Business Finance & Accounting*, 14(4), 555–571. DOI: 10.1111/j.1468-5957.1987.tb00112.x

TI, S., Santos, B. J., & Bock, E. G. P. (2023). O preço da vida: entendendo os custos de um dispositivo de assistência ventricular no Brasil. researchgate.net

Tongpaeng, Y., Nobnop, R., Wongwan, N., Homla, P., Intawong, K., & Puritat, K. (2024). Comparison of gamified and non-gamified mixed reality in enhancing museum visitor engagement, motivation, and learning outcome. *Journal of Heritage Tourism*, 19(6), 1–30. DOI: 10.1080/1743873X.2024.2351852

Toscas, F., Oliveira, V., & Silva, A. (2022). O papel da sociedade civil na inovação e incorporação de dispositivos médicos no Brasil. Jornal Brasileiro de Economia da Saúde. jbes.com.br

Toscas, F. S., de Morais Oliveira, V. C., & Silva, A. S. (2022). The role of civil society in the innovation and incorporation of medical devices in Brazil/O papel da sociedade civil na inovacao e incorporacao de dispositivos medicos no Brasil. [HTML]. *Jornal Brasileiro de Economia da Saúde*, 14(2), 146–155. DOI: 10.21115/JBES.v14.Suppl2.p146-54

Tourna, E., & Germanos, G. (2000). *The role of accounting information on business strategy. United Nations Industrial Development Organization. (2009).* Investment Opportunities for Development Mekelle.

Tran, V. (2020). Positive Affect Negative Affect Scale (PANAS). In Gellman, M. D. (Ed.), *Encyclopedia of Behavioral Medicine* (pp. 1708–1709). Springer International Publishing., DOI: 10.1007/978-3-030-39903-0_978

Trinidad, M., Calderón, A., & Ruiz, M. (2021). GoRace: a multi-context and narrative-based gamification suite to overcome gamification technological challenges. IEEE Access. ieee.orgDOI: 10.3389/fpsyg.2020.539363 PMID: 33584396

Trist, E. L., & Bamforth, K. W. (1951). Some Social and Psychological Consequences of the Longwall Method of Coal-Getting: An Examination of the Psychological Situation and Defences of a Work Group in Relation to the Social Structure and Technological Content of the Work System. *Human Relations*, 4(1), 3–38. DOI: 10.1177/001872675100400101

Tuan, L. H. A. (2023). The entrepreneurial pathway of Vietnamese super-rich. The sources of their successful business performance. *International Journal of Entrepreneurship and Small Business*, 10, 1–17.

Tylee, M. J., Rubenfeld, G. D., Wijeysundera, D., Sklar, M. C., Hussain, S., & Adhikari, N. K. (2020). Anesthesiologist to patient communication: A systematic review. *JAMA Network Open*, 3(11), e2023503–e2023503. DOI: 10.1001/jamanetworkopen.2020.23503 PMID: 33180130

Tzamaras, H. M., Brown, D., Gonzalez-Vargas, J., Moore, J., & Miller, S. R. (2024). Evaluating the effects of comprehensive simulation on central venous catheterization training: A comparative observational study. *BMC Medical Education*, 24(1), 745. DOI: 10.1186/s12909-024-05661-2 PMID: 38987803

Utterback, J. M., & Abernathy, W. J. (1975). A dynamic model of process and product innovation. *Omega*, 3(6), 639–656. DOI: 10.1016/0305-0483(75)90068-7

Van der Heijden, B. I. J. M., Burgers, M. J., Kaan, A. M., Lamberts, B. F., Migchelbrink, K., Van den Ouweland, R. C. P. M., & Meijer, T. (2020). Gamification in dutch businesses: An explorative case study. [sagepub.com]. *SAGE Open*, 10(4), 2158244020972371. DOI: 10.1177/2158244020972371

Värbu, K., Muhammad, N., & Muhammad, Y. (2022). Past, Present, and Future of EEG-Based BCI Applications. *Sensors (Basel)*, 22(9), 3331. DOI: 10.3390/s22093331 PMID: 35591021

Vazquez, F. J. B. (2024). Política de resposta a incidentes cibernéticos e estratégias de aderência à legislação brasileira. Dataset Reports. royaldataset.com

Veiga Neto, AR, de Paula Costa, F., Pereira da Silva, AW, Abbas El- Aouar, W., & de Lima Dantas, BL (2019). Environmental Marketing as a Business Strategy: Determining Factors According to Brazilian Advertisers. *Electronic Journal of Strategy & Business, 12* (1).

Velyako, V., & Musa, S. (2024). The relationship between digital organizational culture, digital capability, digital innovation, organizational resilience, and competitive advantage. *Journal of the Knowledge Economy*.

Venkatraman, N., & Ramanujam, V. (1986). Measurement of business performance in strategy research: A comparison of approaches. *Academy of Management Review*, 11(4), 801–814. DOI: 10.2307/258398

Verkuyl, M., Lapum, J. L., Hughes, M., Romaniuk, D., & Garcia, S. (2021). Emergency response training using gamification: Impact on collaboration among nurses. *Nurse Education Today*, 100, 104835. DOI: 10.1016/j.nedt.2021.104835

Viberg, O., Khalil, M., & Lioliopoulos, A. (2020). Facilitating ideation and knowledge sharing in workplaces: The design and use of gamification in virtual platforms. In Learning and Collaboration Technologies. Human and Technology Ecosystems: 7th International Conference, LCT 2020, Held as Part of the 22nd HCI International Conference, HCII 2020, Copenhagen, Denmark, July 19–24, 2020 [Springer International Publishing.]. *Proceedings*, 22(Part II), 353–369.

Viegas, A. M. P. F. A. (2021). A cooperação global na regulação do medicamento e os desafios para o acesso à inovação. ul.pt Perez, J. F. L. U. (2020). Modos de convergência regulamentar entre medicamentos e dispositivos médicos no quadro da União Europeia. ul.pt Oliveira, D. J. S. & Ckagnazaroff, I. B. (2024). A colaboração como um dos princípios de governo aberto. Revista Gestão & Conexões. unirioja.es

VIEIRA, M. (2024). Integrando a Agenda 2030 e os Objetivos de Desenvolvimento Sustentável-ODS na Disciplina de Projetos Sociais/IFCE. RCMOS-Revista Científica Multidisciplinar O Saber, 1(1). submissoesrevistacientificaosaber.com

Viswa, C. A., Bleys, J., Leydon, E., Shah, B., & Zurkiya, D. (2024). *Generative AI in the pharmaceutical industry: Moving from hype to reality*. McKinsey & Company.

Völz, V. K., Pereira, A. S., Walker, E., & Porciúncula, G. S. (2023). Avaliação de maturidade da Indústria 4.0 em uma empresa fabricante de produtos eletromédicos. [furg.br]. *VETOR-Revista de Ciências Exatas e Engenharias*, 33(1), 80–96. DOI: 10.14295/vetor.v33i1.14662

Vucomanovic, M., Radujkovic, M., & Nahod, M. (2010). Leading, Lagging and Performance Measures in the Construction Industry. International Journal of Organization. *Technology and Management in Construction*, 2(1), 103–111.

Wager, T. D., Phan, K. L., Liberzon, I., & Taylor, S. F. (2003). Valence, gender, and lateralization of functional brain anatomy in emotion: A meta-analysis of findings from neuroimaging. *NeuroImage*, 19(3), 513–531. DOI: 10.1016/S1053-8119(03)00078-8 PMID: 12880784

Wahyuni, D. (2012). The research design maze: Understanding paradigms, cases, methods, and methodologies. *Journal of applied management accounting research, 10* (1), 69-80.

Wang, Y., Luo, J., Guo, Y., Du, Q., Cheng, Q., & Wang, H. (2021). Changes in EEG Brain Connectivity Caused by Short-Term BCI Neurofeedback-Rehabilitation Training: A Case Study. *Frontiers in Human Neuroscience*, 15, 627100. DOI: 10.3389/fnhum.2021.627100 PMID: 34366808

Wärnberg, H. & Oliv, A. (2022). Designing Effective Post-Simulator Training Session Feedback Reports.

Warren, C., & Reeve, J. (2006). *Financial and Managerial Accounting* (9th ed.).

Watkins, C., Gill, S., Loudon, G., Hall, J., Carwardine, M., Ngua, C. W., & Jackson, J. (2022). The challenges of parachute design: The development of a low cost, fit for purpose trauma pack for use in Namibia. *Journal of Desert Research*, 20(1), 1–34. DOI: 10.1504/JDR.2022.125874

Watkins, S. C., & Hensley, N. B. (2023). Team Dynamics in the Operating Room: How Is Team Performance Optimized? *Anesthesiology Clinics*, 41(4), 775–787. DOI: 10.1016/j.anclin.2023.05.004 PMID: 37838383

Watson, D., Clark, L., & Tellegen, A. (1988). Development and Validation of Brief Measures of Positive and Negative Affect: The PANAS Scales. *Journal of Personality and Social Psychology*, 54(6), 1063–1070. DOI: 10.1037/0022-3514.54.6.1063 PMID: 3397865

Weer, C. H., & Greenhaus, J. H. (2020). … of employees' organizational career growth opportunities: The role of extra-role performance, work engagement, and perceived organizational commitment. *Journal of Career Development*, 47(3), 280–295. DOI: 10.1177/0894845317714892

Weichbroth, P., & Łysik, Ł. (2020). Mobile security: Threats and best practices. *Mobile Information Systems*, 2020, 1–15. DOI: 10.1155/2020/8828078

Wendling, A. P., Paiva, M., & Provezano, A. (2020). APLICAÇÃO DA ANÁLISE SWOT COMO FERRAMENTA DO PLANEJAMENTO ESTRATÉGICO: UM ESTUDO DE CASO EM UMA EMPRESA DE LÁCTEOS LOCALIZADA NA ZONA DA MATA MINEIRA. Gestão da Produção: Organização e Planejamento. academia.edu

Werbach, K., & Hunter, D. (2012). For the Win: How Game Thinking Can Revolutionize Your Business. *In Wharton Digital Press*. Wharton Digital Press. DOI: 10.1017/CBO9781107415324.004

Weretecki, P., Greve, G., Bates, K., & Henseler, J. (2021). Information management can't be all fun and games, can it? How gamified experiences foster information exchange in multi-actor service ecosystems. *International Journal of Information Management*, 61, 102391. DOI: 10.1016/j.ijinfomgt.2021.102391

West, M., Armit, K., Loewenthal, L., Eckert, R., West, T., & Lee, A. (2015). *Leadership and leadership development in health care: The evidence base.*

Whaley, J. K. (2022). IMPLEMENTATION OF UNIT COUNCIL IN THE ANESTHESIA DEPARTMENT.

White, G. P. (1996). A survey and taxonomy of strategy-related performance measures for manufacturing. *International Journal of Operations & Production Management*, 16(3), 42–61. DOI: 10.1108/01443579610110486

Wirani, R., Sutanto, R., & Nugroho, D. (2022). The role of gamification in enhancing student engagement in online learning: A systematic review. *Education and Information Technologies*, 27(4), 567–589. DOI: 10.1007/s10639-021-10756-3

Wolf-Fordham, S. (2020). Integrating government silos: Local emergency management and public health department collaboration for emergency planning and response. *American Review of Public Administration*, 50(6-7), 560–567. DOI: 10.1177/0275074020943706

Wolpaw, J. R., Heetderks, W. J., McFarland, D. J., Peckham, P. H., Schalk, G., Donchin, E., Quatrano, L. A., Robinson, C. J., & Vaughan, T. M. (2000). Brain–Computer Interface Technology: A Review of the First International Meeting. *IEEE Transactions on Rehabilitation Engineering*, 8(2), 164–173. DOI: 10.1109/TRE.2000.847807 PMID: 10896178

Wong, C., & Laschinger, H. K. (2019). The influence of authentic leadership on nurses' outcomes in a remote healthcare setting. *Journal of Nursing Management*, 27(6), 1095–1102. DOI: 10.1111/jonm.12786

Wood, B., & Sacks, G. (2023). The influence of share buybacks on ill-health and health inequity: An exploratory analysis using a socio-ecological determinants of health lens. *Globalization and Health*, 19(1), 3. DOI: 10.1186/s12992-023-00905-0 PMID: 36631805

Xavier, R. N., & Chiconatto, P. (2014). The Direction of Green Marketing in Organizations: Concept, Opportunities and Limitations. *Scientific-Electronic Capital Journal (RCC)- ISSN 2177-4153, 12* (1), 133-147.

Xi, N., & Hamari, J. (2020). Does gamification affect brand engagement and equity? A study in the context of branded apps. *Journal of Business Research*, 109, 449–460. DOI: 10.1016/j.jbusres.2019.11.058

Xu, W., Yang, L., Niu, Z., Wang, S., Wang, Y., Zhu, Z., & Cui, P. (2024). Thermodynamic and economic analysis of a novel DME-power polygeneration system based on the integration of biomass gasification and alkaline electrolysis of water for hydrogen production. *Energy*, •••, 134185.

Yerkes, R., & Dodson, J. (1908). The relation of strength of stimulus to rapidity of habit-formation. *The Journal of Comparative Neurology and Psychology*, 18(5), 459–482. http://psychclassics.yorku.ca/Yerkes/Law/. DOI: 10.1002/cne.920180503

Yu, L.-C., Lee, L.-H., Hao, S., Wang, J., He, Y., Hu, J., Lai, K., & Zhang, X. (2016). *Building Chinese Affective Resources in Valence-Arousal Dimensions.*

Zahid, M. A., Ali, P., Saddique, F., Khan, B., Rehman, M. A., & Kumar, A. (2023). Resilience unveiled: Empowering Pakistani anesthetists in challenging low-resource environment. *Anaesthesia, Pain & Intensive Care*, 27(5), 592–598. DOI: 10.35975/apic.v27i5.2299

Zainuddin, N., Jaafar, M., & Harris, J. (2022). Gamified remote monitoring for chronic illness: Engaging patients and healthcare teams. *International Journal of Medical Informatics*, 162, 104749. DOI: 10.1016/j.ijmedinf.2022.104749

Zainuddin, Z., Chu, S. K. W., Shujahat, M., & Perera, C. J. (2020). The impact of gamification on learning and instruction: A systematic review of empirical evidence. *Educational Research Review*, 30, 100326. DOI: 10.1016/j.edurev.2020.100326

Zaman, M. (2004) "The Role of Financial and Nonfinancial Evaluation Measures in

Zhang, C., & Pandit, J. J. (2023). Getting operating theatre metrics right to underpin quality improvement: Understanding limitations of NHS Model Hospital calculations. *British Journal of Anaesthesia*, 131(1), 130–134. DOI: 10.1016/j.bja.2023.03.032 PMID: 37169629

Zheng, H., Wu, J., Song, R., Guo, L., & Xu, Z. (2024). Predicting financial enterprise stocks and economic data trends using machine learning time series analysis. *Applied and Computational Engineering*, 87(1), 26–32. DOI: 10.54254/2755-2721/87/20241562

Zheng, X., Chen, M., Zhuang, Y., Xu, J., Zhao, L., Qian, Y., Shen, W. M., & Chu, Y. (2024). Hemostatic Interventions and All-Cause Mortality in Hemodynamically Unstable Pelvic Fractures: A Systematic Review and Meta-Analysis. *Emergency Medicine International*, 2024(1), 6397444. DOI: 10.1155/2024/6397444 PMID: 39224863

Zhu, Q., & Sarkis, J. (2016). Green marketing and consumerism as social change in China: Reviewing the literature. *International Journal of Production Economics*, 181, 289–302. DOI: 10.1016/j.ijpe.2016.06.006

Ziervogel, G., Enqvist, J., Metelerkamp, L., & van Breda, J. (2022). Supporting transformative climate adaptation: Community-level capacity building and knowledge co-creation in South Africa. *Climate Policy*, 22(5), 607–622. DOI: 10.1080/14693062.2020.1863180

Zuin, D. A. (2022). Os Efeitos da 4a Revolução Industrial nas Relações de Trabalho: entre o livre-arbítrio ea exploração. [HTML]

About the Contributors

Ricardo Marcão, and MedTech consulting strategies by integrating gamification to enhance engagement and adherence, while also improving project management efficiency across global operations. In 2021, Ricardo revolutionized risk management approaches by introducing a new strategic control framework, which resulted in a 20% increase in direct project margins and strengthened overall business sustainability. Between 2022 and 2023, Ricardo led global CRM projects for some of the largest pharmaceutical companies worldwide, working with a New York City-based global Pharma leader to enhance customer relationship management (CRM) strategies. His expertise in enterprise CRM implementation, process optimization, and digital transformation played a crucial role in streamlining commercial operations and improving market engagement across multiple international markets. Beyond his corporate impact, Ricardo is a seasoned academic and editor, shaping the discourse on strategic management, innovation, and performance evaluation in business and healthcare. As the coordinator of several advanced programs at ISLA Santarém, including MBAs and post-graduate programs in Project Management, Quality Management, and Diplomacy and Financial-Economic Management, Ricardo plays a pivotal role in shaping future business leaders through a strategic lens that integrates healthcare, technology, and global governance. A distinguished international speaker, Ricardo actively contributes to transatlantic relations between the US and Europe, focusing on strategy, leadership, and competitive intelligence. His memberships in SCIP Portugal, APMP in NYC, PMI Portugal, and PMI South Florida reflect his ongoing commitment to excellence in strategic intelligence, business consultancy, and project management.

Stéphanie Monteiro is a Senior Quality Engineer at Nemotec, specializing in medical devices. She holds an MSc in Biomedical Technology and is a PhD researcher in Biomedical Engineering, focusing on medical devices and simulator development. Stéphanie has extensive expertise in quality management, medical devices, medical prototypes, and the pharmaceutical industry. She is a Certified Six Sigma Black Belt™ and has significant experience as a CSV Engineer and QA Technical Specialist, focusing on quality systems and continuous improvement. Additionally, she is affiliated with the Institute for Systems and Robotics (ISR-Lisboa), where she contributes as a Medical Devices Researcher, advancing innovation in healthcare technology.

***

Lara Mendes Bacalhau holds a PhD in Management with specialization in Marketing and Strategy, and Master's degree in Data Analysis and Decision Support Systems on University of Porto. Her academic journey includes also two Bachelor's degrees: Mathematics from the University of Coimbra and another in Business Management from the Coimbra Business School (CBS|ISCAC)of the Politechnic University of Coimbra. Since 2003, she has been a lecturer at CBS|ISCAC, teaching courses in Marketing, Business Management, Accounting, and Taxation. Currently, she coordinates the Bachelor's program in Marketing and International Business and belong of the Master's direction. She actively contributes to Marketing and Business Management research. She is full researcher in CEOS.PP, a peer reviewer, and co-authors scientific publications, and participates, also, in national and international research projects.

Hugo Miguel Carvalho is a university professor, CEO of Neuro IT, member of the board of FISICARE, Business Angel, teacher, researcher and clinician. PhD in Applied Neurosciences in Emotions for Brain Mapping and Neurophysiological Signal Collection from the University of Beira Interior- Portugal. She is a specialist in Communication Sciences and in Marketing and Advertising, both by public exams, from ISCIA Aveiro and has a Master's degree in Design and Neurosciences with a specialization in Cognitive Rehabilitation from the University of Aveiro. He is part of the clinical team, being director of the Mental Health Unit at FISCARE, in Aveiro-Portugal, he is a researcher at CIDETH, ISCIA and Lipis- Pontifical Catholic University of Rio de Janeiro- Brazil. He is General Manager and Research Director of Neuro IT, Administration Advisor of Fisicare and Business Angel. He is a professor at ISCIA, University of Beira Interior (UBI), ISCAP, Isla Gaia, CESPU, IEES, European University and AEAAV. He is the founder of the project "Negócios à (sobre)mesa", "Pigo", "Abac- Aveiro Business Angels Club", "Geisertech", he is also a national ambassador of "Ignite Portugal". Co-author of the book Business Management with People on Board, author of the book Corporator: How to avoid the main management mistakes and coordinator, co-author of the book Networking

One Hundred (100)Scenes Vol I and II and the book Strategia: Analysis of the Strategic Environment of Companies.

Patrícia David is an experienced Quality Assurance and Control professional specializing in the pharmaceutical industry, medicinal cannabis, medical devices, and medical prototypes. She is recognized as one of the key experts in Portugal for these fields, with extensive expertise in GxP, GMP, and GACP compliance, quality management systems (QMS), and project management. Patrícia has successfully led various quality assurance initiatives, including internal audits, supplier evaluations, and regulatory compliance projects, both nationally and internationally. She is skilled in continuous improvement using Lean Six Sigma tools and holds a Green Belt certification. Patrícia is dedicated to maintaining high-quality standards, managing teams effectively, and ensuring compliance in complex regulatory environments, making her a significant figure in the pharma and life sciences sectors.

Filipa Martinho is an assistant professor at ISLA Santarém. Master in health psychology (ISPA, Portugal)and degree in Applied Psychology (ISPA, Portugal). Postgraduate in Management (ISLA, Portugal). Integrated researcher at CEPESE/UP (Center for Population, Economy, and Society Studies). Author of scientific articles and book chapters. Research areas: management, psychology, and human resources management.

Cindy Monteiro is a nurse specialized in Intensive Care, with professional experience at Hospital Santa Maria and Hospital das Forças Armadas. With extensive experience in the care of critically ill patients, she has also worked in the Emergency Department at Hospital de Cascais, developing essential skills in emergency and trauma situations. She holds a Master's degree in Medical-Surgical Nursing, with a specialization in Nursing Care for Critically Ill Patients. In addition to her practical experience, Cindy Monteiro is a certified instructor in Basic Life Support and Automated External Defibrillation by INEM and holds further certifications in Advanced Life Support (ALS), ITLS (International Trauma Life Support), and MRMI (Medical Response in Major Incidents). Her career is defined by a commitment to excellence in patient care and training other healthcare professionals, with a focus on preparing for emergency situations and intensive care.

Stéphanie Monteiro is a Senior Quality Engineer at Nemotec, specializing in medical devices. She holds an MSc in Biomedical Technology and is a PhD researcher in Biomedical Engineering, focusing on medical devices and simulator development. Stéphanie has extensive expertise in quality management, medical devices, medical prototypes, and the pharmaceutical industry. She is a Certified Six Sigma Black Belt™ and has significant experience as a CSV Engineer and QA

Technical Specialist, focusing on quality systems and continuous improvement. Additionally, she is affiliated with the Institute for Systems and Robotics (ISR-Lisboa), where she contributes as a Medical Devices Researcher, advancing innovation in healthcare technology.

Vasco Santos holds a PhD in Business Sciences with specialization in Marketing (Fernando Pessoa University, Portugal), a PhD in Tourism (Seville University, Spain), a Post-Doc in Innovation Management applied to Sustainable Luxury Tourism (Aveiro University, Portugal), an Habilitation in Management (European University, Portugal), an MSc in Marketing and Tourism Promotion, and a BA in Hospitality Management (Higher School of Tourism and Maritime Technology, Polytechnic of Leiria). Lecturer at the Polytechnic University of Tomar. Lecturer at the Higher Institute of Management and Administrationof Santarém. Full researcher in GOVCOPP (Competitiveness, Innovation and Sustainability Research Group), University of Aveiro. Effective and founding member of PNT - National Tourism Platform. Author of several scientific papers and book chapters. Research areas: tourism, marketing, employer branding and management.

Bharti Singh is a BBA student at Christ University, specializing in Human Resources and Organizational Behavior. With a keen interest in leadership and remote healthcare systems, she has engaged in various internships and projects focused on crowdfunding, employee engagement, and organizational management. Bharti's practical experience includes her role as an HR intern at Mensa Brands, where she contributed to employee onboarding and engagement strategies. She is also passionate about addressing gender disparities in the workplace and exploring innovative approaches to enhance team performance in digital health environments. As a budding researcher, Bharti aims to leverage her academic background and practical insights to contribute to the evolving landscape of remote healthcare leadership.

Bruno Barbosa Sousa is Professor Coordenador of Marketing at Polytechnic Institute of Cávado and Ave (IPCA), Portugal and PhD in Marketing and Strategy in Universidade do Minho, Portugal. Head of Masters Program - Tourism Management and Marketing Tourism (IPCA); CiTUR – Center for Tourism Research, Development and Innovation and UNIAG research member. He has published in the Journal of Enterprising Communities, Tourism Management Perspectives, Current Issues in Tourism, Journal of Organizational Change Management, World Review of Entrepreneurship, Management and Sust. Development, among others.

Maria José Sousa has a PhD in Management with Habilitation in Management and Public Management. She was Pro-Rector for the Development of Distance

Learning and is a professor and a research fellow at ISCTE/Instituto Universitário de Lisboa, Portugal. She has assumed a postdoc position from 2016-2018, researching that field, with several publications in journals with high impact factor and has worked as an expert in a project of the European Commission for the creation of a new category regarding digital skills to be integrated with the European Innovation Scoreboard (EIS). Her research interests currently are public policies of Innovation and Education. She is a bestselling author in Research Methods, ICT and People Management and has co-authored over 180 articles and book chapters in high-level journals (such as the Journal of Business Research, Management Decision, European Planning Studies, Information Systems Frontiers, Systems Research, and Behavioral Science, Computational and Mathematical Organization Theory, Future Generation Computer Systems, and others), and she is the guest-editor of several Special Issues from reputed publishing houses as Springer and Elsevier. She was/ is the coordinator of several European projects of innovation (funded by programs as Erasmus +, Horizon Europe, and ICMPD)and is also External Expert of COST Association - European Cooperation in Science and Technology.

Index

I

M

N

O

P

R

S

T

V

W

www.ingramcontent.com/pod-product-compliance
Lightning Source LLC
LaVergne TN
LVHW080904300926
849162LV00003B/550
* 9 7 9 8 3 6 9 3 8 5 9 8 2 *